Gontran Sennwald

# The Wrist

## Anatomical and Pathophysiological Approach to Diagnosis and Treatment

Forewords by
J.-J. Comtet and G. Segmüller

Adapted for the English edition by
R.G. McCormack

With 343 Figures
Illustrations and Diagrams by the Author

Springer-Verlag
Berlin Heidelberg NewYork
London Paris Tokyo

Dr. Gontran Sennwald

Kantonsspital
Klinik für Orthopädische Chirurgie
CH-9007 St. Gallen

Adapted for the English edition by:

Robert G. McCormack, M.D.

310–1076 West 14th Ave.
Vancouver
British Columbia
Canada V6H-1P3

Translated from the French by:

David Le Vay

Dewhurst Lodge
Wadhurst
Sussex TN5 6QB
Great Britain

Original French edition
L'entité radius-carpe


ISBN-13: 978-3-642-71624-9 e-ISBN-13: 978-3-642-71622-5
DOI: 10.1007/978-3-642-71622-5

Library of Congress Cataloging-in-Publication Data. Sennwald, Gontran, 1943- The wrist. Translation of: L'entité radius-carpe. Includes bibliographies and index. 1. Wrist. 2. Wrist – Diseases. 3. Wrist – Surgery. I. Title. [DNLM: 1. Wrist. 2. Wrist Injuries. WE 830 S478L] RD559.S4713 1987 617'.574 86-33911



Reproduction of figures: Gustav Dreher GmbH, Stuttgart.

Typesetting, printing, and bookbinding: Universitätsdruckerei H. Stürtz AG, Würzburg.
2124/3130-543210

*Love and friendship form the foundations of this book. Thanks to the constant and active support of my wife, I have been able to complete it; thanks to the well-founded and stimulating advice of Dr. Segmüller, the ideas contained in it have come to full fruition; its precision I owe to my friend Wolfram Fischer, mathematician and information technologist.*

*My profound thanks*

# Foreword

In the space of only a few years, reconstructive surgery of the skeleton of the hand has become a focus of attention. The reason for this has been the advent of principles and techniques of stable internal fixation, the unparalleled advantages of which are particularly evident in the treatment of the complex, multi-structural lesions so typical of injuries of the hand, and also in procedures such as replantation or revascularisation.

What a striking contrast on the other hand is to be seen in the slow and painful progress made in our understanding of the biomechanics of the radiocarpal joint! This is most eloquently illustrated by the embryonic state of prosthetic surgery of the wrist, compared with the sophisticated advances made in hip and knee surgery. Yet it is undeniable that painful conditions involving dysfunctions of the wrist are increasing in number and affect young people in particular; this should spur us on to seek more effective therapeutic solutions.

The very complexity of the carpus has been a subject of theoretical interest. Still, it was not until 1943 that our knowledge of the wrist acquired a clinical dimension: Gilford, Bolton and Lambrinudi formulated the notion of a joint consisting of a chain of intercalated small bones. They determined the axes of each bone and were thus able to define instability of the carpus in terms of deviations from these axes. Ever since, clinicians and anatomists have been increasingly successful in their efforts to gain a better understanding of the principles of mobility as well as of stability of the carpus.

These endeavours constitute the basis of this stimulating monograph by G. Sennwald, who has amply succeeded in setting forth a unified concept of the anatomy, function and pathology of the carpus. Dr. Sennwald both presents a critical analysis of the body of literature published on this subject around the world and at the same time, examines with equal thoroughness a large group of patients treated in the unit for hand surgery at the Kantonsspital, St. Gall, Switzerland. From this body of data, he formulates a theory of the global function of the radiocarpal joint, which also constitutes a rationale for proposals of patient care. Not only does this volume represent a benchmark for the progress made in surgery of the hand; it also underscores the paramount position this field of surgery has come to occupy in modern reconstructive surgery. There can be no doubt that this book will earn the respect it deserves from clinicians and future researchers alike.

G. SEGMÜLLER

# Foreword

This is a book that is original and personal in content and style. It provides a mine of information and ideas to consider: a description of the carpal ligaments clarified by a functional classification, a new concept of carpal stability, ingenious hypotheses on pathogenesis of certain traumatic disorders, and analyses of results of tested operative techniques.

Tedious, purely morphological description of the different carpal ligaments is replaced by classification into restraining, stabilizing and guiding ligaments. The presence of restraining ligaments is related to the existence of the distal carpal row monolith. Failure of the stabilizing ligaments accounts for displacements, and even dislocations. Failure of the guiding ligaments is responsible for malalignment.

The author's concept of carpal stability rejects the notion of a "central column", which is hardly admissible in the virtual absence of an effective luno-capitate ligament. How could it be otherwise, when at its very centre there is a point of such weakness that every perilunate dislocation disrupts this column!

At last, the lunate has been accorded its proper place as the keystone of the carpal edifice. Firmly buttressed against the radius, it supports its two lateral partners. And, as the scaphoid is too loosely attached to the distal monolith to coordinate the mobility of the two carpal rows, with all respect to Gilford, this coordinating function can only be ascribed to the distal V ligament.

We are then presented with the consequences of hyperextension injuries: the ligamentous tears (or the alternative fractures) originate at one side of the lunate and progress around the bone in direction one or the other. The author explains how to read the radiographs in order to identify the signs of these tears or fracture: disjunction, arthrographic leakage, or final disalignment or dislocation, until ultimately the lunate loses its radial attachments.

Fractures of the distal ends of the two forearm bones and fractures of the carpus are not merely bony lesions. The author shows how they fall within the setting of a lesion of the radiocarpal entity, where the ligamentous injuries worsen the prognosis. This applies especially to pseudarthroses of the scaphoid, when they are associated with instability requiring ligamentoplasties and pins to secure fixation of the site and correction of disalignment. Nevertheless, taking all categories together, these pseudarthroses unite in 85% of cases.

The author is clearly not in favour of the use of Silastic, whether for pseudarthroses of the scaphoid or for Kienböck's disease. It is true that, despite encapsulation, the implant never acquires ligamentous attachments, and can be maintained in position only by some form of intracarpal arthrodesis. In this field, although the outright condemnation of scapho-lunate arthrodesis is possibly debatable, the review of the different methods of fusion between the carpal bones provides an excellent basis for discussion.

In the chapters on surgical technique, the author gives an account of his own experience with precision and sincerity, and this section is one to be readily resorted to before undertaking a particular operation. However, younger surgeons should resist the temptation to bypass the first part of the book, however arduous it may seem, for quality of surgical procedure and the proper choice of indications are to be achieved by global understanding of the radio-carpal entity.

At the end of the work the author, in his direct, personal and sometimes nonconformist style, addresses himself directly to his readers. Perhaps I may be allowed to reply on their behalf. Persuaded by your concepts, we shall adopt your proposals for standardization of the clinical and radiological approach to radio-carpal lesions. "Treatment will continue to develop, thanks to the elaboration of a common language as the basis for progress and research". We congratulate and thank Dr. Sennwald for this youthful and stimulating book.

J.-J. Comtet

# Preface

Is it really necessary to add yet another book to the already very long catalogue of medical literature? Aware of the responsibilities that this implies, and thoroughly absorbed in my hospital activities, I needed strong motivation to write this monograph on the carpus. By means of this modest work it is my earnest hope to bring to colleagues who, though interested, but possibly overworked or out of touch, a digest of my experience, my reading and my own research and studies on a fascinating but difficult subject; to make it more accessible to them.

I also hope to stimulate research workers to abolish all my question-marks by devoting themselves to new studies, with their inventive and scientific spirit, and evermore-refined modern techniques. I hope to assist surgeons anxious to make a precise diagnosis, and to thereby choose the appropriate treatment methods; and I hope to contribute to the eradication of certain popular but erroneous ideas that are harmful to the rehabilitation of patients.

To satisfy these ambitions, I have attempted to extract the gist of what the best authors and researchers have supplied us with so far, and also of what I have learned from clinical and operative experience, the dissecting-room and the analytical study of results obtained. In reviewing the classical anatomy I have striven to simplify the facts without loss of accuracy, with the overriding aim of being essentially practical and therefore useful. This has sometimes led me to entirely new concepts. The statistical study complies with the modern scientific spirit, but also with the desire to comfort all those who talk about "medical flair", well realizing that this boils down to a fine brew of anatomical knowledge, technical competence and clinical experience.

If our approach to the carpus, in that it is different and novel, manages to stimulate the mind and arouse contradiction, then my task will not have been in vain; progress may come through confrontation which leads to revision of one's opinions and, sometimes, to an opening of new pathways.

It is in this spirit that I set out here a new concept of the stability of the carpus; a global radiological approach to the injured wrist; a broadening of the spectrum of treatment of pseudarthrosis of the scaphoid, necessitated by ligamentous instability; and a new classification of, and new ideas concerning, fracture of the distal radius, so common and yet so misunderstood, especially as regards its clinical and anatomical consequences, those of the associated radio-carpal ligamentous lesions in particular.

I acknowledge the assistence of Dr. David Le Vay in the primary translation and the Springer Verlag for their cooperation for the success of the English edition. Again I thank Robert McCormack, M.D., F.R.C.S., Vancouver (Canada), who added his skill to make this English edition possible.

Thus, whether the reader be a trainee or an experienced surgeon, or perhaps a research worker, I believe that he or she will find something to ponder. It is with optimism that I entrust the reader with the fruits of my reflections.

G. SENNWALD

# Contents

CHAPTER IV

**Fractures of the Distal Radius**



CHAPTER V

**Operative Techniques and Indications**

# Introduction

Ever since man acquired an upright position he has had the privilege of falling. And falling is common! It begins early in infancy, when the child with its first steps, awkwardly tries to imitate the adult. However, neither the adolescent, the adult, nor the aged are spared. In the great majority of cases the fall is broken by the hand, with the wrist extended. Thanks to the muscles and reflexes which make it possible to spread the damaging energy throughout the upper limb, the wrist sustains the shock without mishap on most occasions. If this is not the case, the resulting injury is unpredictable; it varies not only in relation to the trauma itself, but also depends on age and sex. Thus, the epiphyseal fracture of the radius and ulna, by definition, affects only the child. The scaphoid fracture appears in adolescence, when it is on even terms with the epiphyseal fracture, but it also affects young men. Women once seemed to be spared, but doubtless this will be less and less the case as they take their place in sport!

Weber and Chao (1978) demonstrated that only the scaphoid fractures occurred beyond 95° of dorsiflexion of the wrist. According to this, we would expect an increase of this type of fracture with the progressive weakening of age. But it is the fracture of the distal radius which becomes most frequent after age 30. Furthermore, though the distal radial fractures affect both sexes equally between age 30 and 50, it becomes more common in women, as if they reserve the privilege of falling, or as if all men leave this world prematurely. The demarcation between these different conditions exists but is certainly not always so clear-cut; the exceptions prove the rule. It will be interesting to try to understand the reasons for this unexpected distribution of injuries.

As for our knowledge about the ligamentous lesions, this is very limited. The parcelling-out of the carpus into different disorders that are apparently independent of each other, the complexity of the anatomy and pathomechanics of the wrist and the absence of standardized radiographs have all, up to the present time, prevented understanding of the relationships that exist between the various lesions observed. Frykmann (1967) and Mayfield (1980) both analysed the consequences of hyperextension; the mechanism of injury may be identical, but not the results of or the conclusions from their experiments. Even today, there are still too few surgeons who realize that scapho-lunate dissociation is the ligamentous equivalent of scaphoid fracture. Triquetro-lunate dissociation is another uncommonly recognized injury. How many patients have been charged with malingering because the surgeon was unaware of this hyperextension injury? In the subsequent chapters we will present a comprehensive approach to these diverse lesions.

These problems and their radiological assessment may appear to be new but Castaing (1964) reminds us that the lateral movements of the ulna have been known since 1828. However, he gives only a very rough sketch of how to measure the radio-ulnar angles and index. In fact, it is possible to measure two frontal angles according to the landmarks chosen (Fig. II.5a, b), and it is important to decide which one to consider when treating a fracture of the distal radius. We shall study this in the chapter on the possibilities and limits of conservative management of this kind of fracture. It should also be realized, what Castaing seemed to ignore, that the radio-ulnar index differs significantly depending on whether it is measured in pronation or in supination (Epner et al. 1982; Palmer et al. 1982). These findings are not well known and suggest that we should review our concepts, particularly concerning routine radiological examination.

With the explosion in medical costs becoming a major issue, is it really proper to discuss new supplementary methods of examination and sophisticated treatments for what seem to be commonplace problems? While these lesions are extremely common, they are expensive in social terms. According to the Swiss National Insurance Office, the duration of incapacity of work and the degree of permanent disability resulting from carpal injuries are higher than other lesions of the hand (Morger 1985). A hand-surgery service such as our own is confronted daily with the consequences of hyperextension injuries. An awareness of the magnitude of these problems demands an endeavour to improve our knowledge of their pathophysiology, anatomy and mechanics; that is the price of progress.

It will be apparent to the reader that the wrist is a controversial and complicated area of study. We hope, therefore, that this work will contribute, no doubt modestly, to a better definition of the clinical and radiological approach to this complex joint. To put them into perspective, we have systematically incorporated the opinions of different authors into our discussions. The references will be found at the end of each chapter, and not at the end of the book, and they are limited to the absolute minimum required for the discussion.

## References


Castaing J (1964) Les fractures récentes de l'extrémité inférieure du radius. Rev Chir Orthop 50:581–696

Epner RA, Bowers WH, Guilford WB (1982) Ulnar variance – the effect of wrist positioning and Roentgen filming technique. J Hand Surg 7:298–305

Frykmann G (1967) Fracture of the distal radius including sequelae shoulder-hand-finger syndrome, disturbance in the distal radio-ulnar joint

and impairment of nerve function. Acta Orthop Scand 108 [suppl]: 5–143
Mayfield JK, Johnson RP, Kilcoyne RK (1980) Carpal dislocations: pathomechanics and progressive perilunar instability. J Hand Surg 5: 226–241
Morger W (1985) Le point de vue des assureurs, premières expériences avec la nouvelle LAA. 72nd annual meeting of the Société Suisse de Chirurgie, together with the Société Suisse de Médecine des Accidents et des Maladies Professionnelles and the Société Suisse de Chirurgie de la Main. Interlaken, 15.6.85
Palmer AK, Glisson RR, Werner FW (1982) Ulnar variance determination. J Hand Surg 7: 376–379
Weber ER, Chao EY (1978) An experimental approach to the mechanism of scaphoid waist fracture. J Hand Surg 3: 142

# History

## The Carpus

According to Daremberg's translation (1854), Gallien thought that the different bones which make up the carpus must be mobile between themselves. On the other hand, Allieu (1984) reminds us that this notion was refuted by Charles Bell in 1833 without clinical confirmation. He likened the carpus to a single bone, which can well be understood when one studies examples of congenital synostoses (see figure below). This patient was able to live without apparent difficulty for over 50 years; there is virtually no arthrosis between the radius and this single carpus. Such a malformation, congenital and bilateral, appears to support Gallien's opponent. Henke, in 1859, seems to have been the first to demonstrate, in the cadaver, the differential mobility of the carpal bones between themselves.

The advent of radiology was decisive and allowed Bryce (1897) to confirm in vivo this intracarpal mobility in relation to the position of the hand. His work, extremely precise and detailed, is of great value and deserves to be better known. We call attention here to some of his observations which seem not only judicious but still valid today.

- "The centre of the shadow of the styloid process of the ulna is, in the supine position, 12 mm removed from the central point of the transverse axis of the wrist, while in pronation the distance is increased to 25 mm."

The importance of this preliminary observation lies in the fact that, to explain the movement of translation, it is necessary to

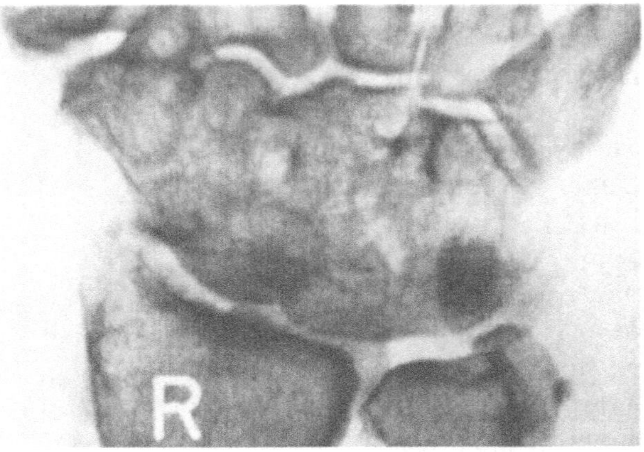


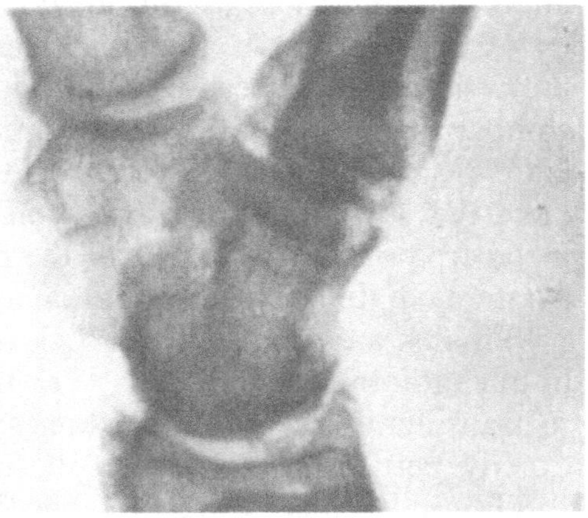

50-year-old man, synostosis, no pain

involve the entire forearm and the elbow! Furthermore, translation is impossible without distinct rotation of the humerus, and therefore of the shoulder. This simple observation makes it clear that the hand forms an integral part of the entire upper extremity. He stated subsequently, when comparing radiological films with anatomical dissections, that the first row of the carpus functions independently of the second, confirming the work of Henke: "I think it must be admitted that the rays are released from one another in a manner not represented in traditional figures".

However, he went further in his analysis, and affirmed that in radial and ulnar deviation the scaphoid undergoes not only rotational movement, but also translation. Thus, in radial deviation, the scaphoid becomes more vertical, and glides in a palmar direction, while the reverse is the case in ulnar deviation, i.e. the scaphoid becomes more horizontal (its axis becoming parallel to that of the radius), while undergoing dorsal translation. He stated that the lunate follows the movements of the scaphoid, though only in part, and that the triquetrum exhibits dorsal or palmar gliding opposite to that of the scaphoid. Without explaining it completely, he realized that the scapho-lunate ligament permits differentiated movements of these two bones. It was for Kauer later (1980) to better understand both the movement and the anatomy.

The studies of Bryce stimulated other anatomists and in 1898 Virchow published corresponding studies and his conclusions were similar to those of Bryce. In 1901, Fick, in his paper *On the Movements of the Wrist-Joint,* laid down the foundations of modern radiology. The terms in the introduction to this work, now 84 years old, remain remarkably contemporary. I quote: "In view of the uncommonly frequent transillumination of the hand with X-rays by physicians and anatomists one may really expect the mechanism of movement of the wrist-joints to be completely clarified thereby. Nothing less than this..." and he goes on to quote other authors and divergent opinions.

In addition, he affirmed a fact that is sometimes obvious, but too often forgotten: "The 'mid-position' of any joint is in fact, in mechanical and practical respects, actually the most important and most useful position". Like every rule, this has its exceptions, but it remains essential in orthopaedics, since the rest position is easy to reproduce, and therefore useful in comparisons. It is rare for an injured person to be unable to place his limb in this neutral position. Fick states that in the hand this so-called normal position is with the axis of the third metacarpal in line with that of the radius, and that the position is intermediate between pronation and supination.

Finally, a quotation from Fick that is also too often ignored in our radiological analyses: "For many problems it is essential to transilluminate individual bones in the three main positions exactly perpendicular to the photographic plate". Thanks to this he analysed accurately the positions and shapes of the bones of the carpus in the different positions of the hand. From this viewpoint his work remains valid, even if the films he analysed were taken in supination (contradicting his assertions about the importance of standardization of X-ray positioning!).

Destot, in 1923, published a remarkable radiological text describing the movement of the scaphoid particularly well. He spoke of a "handbell" movement; for that period, and for those who once knew these handbells, this image is very expressive. Mouchet and Belot, in 1934, published the first case of a post-traumatic snapping wrist. This concerned a doctor's wife who sustained a contusion of the wrist in a car accident. This particular snap occurred with dorsiflexion and on grasping, with the subluxed wrist reducing spontaneously and easily in palmar flexion. Radiologically, the subluxation took place between the first and second rows of the carpus.

In 1943, Gilford, Bolton and Lambrinudi analysed the special position of the scaphoid, bridging the first and second rows of carpal bones. This led them to suppose that it has a dual function: to buffer and to constrain the movements of the first row in relation to the second. Fisk (1970) used this work as a basis to explain the collapse of the carpus secondary to fracture of the scaphoid. Linscheid et al., in 1972, concurred with this viewpoint, while attaching importance to the two following structures:

1. The *scapho-lunate couple*, bound by a powerful ligament synchronizing their movements
2. The *scapho-trapezo-trapezoid articulation*, a distal stabilizer of the scaphoid

In this view, the scaphoid has a role analogous to that proposed by Gilford. However, Linscheid's explanation is difficult to understand, probably because it contains only part of the truth, and does not take into account the other constraints, notably of the palmar ligaments joining the lunate to the two bones of the forearm.

In the same article, Linscheid defined the concept of traumatic instability of the carpus and the radiological factors permitting its diagnosis. He stated that instability, associated with a fracture or pseudarthrosis of the scaphoid, has a worse prognosis. He also referred to instability associated with fracture of the radius, but seems to have ascribed this more to mechanical disturbances than to a concomitant ligamentous lesion.

It was not until the work of Mayfield et al. (1980) that it was better understood that the radius and the carpus are an anatomical and functional unit that cannot be dissociated and apportioned into numerous disparate elements. A comprehensive approach is necessary. Weber (1980) supports this concept and proposed a classification of the scaphoid fractures in relation to the associated ligamentous lesions and the displacement of the fragments. This supplants the classification of Trojan and Mourgues (1959) based on structural appearance alone.

Youm et al., in 1978, showed that the carpus has two centres of rotation, depending on whether one considers the frontal or the sagittal plane. This mechanical fact helps one better understand why, nowadays, total prostheses of the wrist are not well accepted, whereas the hip prosthesis has acquired world-wide acceptance. They demonstrated a constant relationship between the length of the third metacarpal and the depth of the wrist. Such a relationship also exists between the prolongation of the axis of the ulna and the centre of rotation of the capitate. All these data contribute to the analysis of the radiological films, and help to define "normality".

## The Concept of Stability

As long as the carpus seemed to be an anatomical monolith, it was superfluous to seek to understand its function. After the work of Bryce and Fick demonstrating the functional independence of the proximal and distal rows of the carpus, it became necessary to explain the interrelationships between the different bones.

Navarro, in 1919 (he published his studies in 1937), seems to have been the first to establish a theory seeking to explain both function and carpal interrelationship. According to him, the hamate, capitate and lunate are the "vertebral column" of the carpus, thanks to the powerful ligamentous system that unites them. Thanks to their mobility, the triquetrum, on the one hand, and the scaphoid, trapezoid and trapezium on the other are centres of rotation permitting adduction and abduction of the wrist. It may be interesting to emphasize that Bryce, back in 1897, contested this point of view; according to him, the trapezoid and the trapezium could not be bound closely to the scaphoid because their radiological mobility was different.

Taleisnik, in 1976, starting from Linscheid's work, modified Navarro's thesis. He demonstrated, like Bryce, that the scaphoid was not firmly attached to the trapezium or the trapezoid, and concluded that the two rotatory columns could be composed only of the scaphoid and the triquetrum. He retained the idea of a central column and imagined a sort of "T", the transverse limb of the T consisting of the entire distal carpal row of the carpus, while the longitudinal limb was defined by the capitate and lunate. This theory, like that of Navarro, can explain the axial stability of the carpus.

Lichtmann et al., in 1981, disputed Taleisnik's analysis, since the proximal row, in particular the lunate, is not closely bound to the capitate. They regard the proximal row of the carpus as a functional unit, bound to the distal row by the V ligaments. The arrangement they propose explains the radiological observations well. They support Gilford's theory explaining the ability of the carpus to withstand axial compression. In other words, they consider the scaphoid the key bone. We now know with certainty, on the basis of our dissections and the work of other authors (Bonnel and Allieu 1984), that no ligamentous system exists between the lunate and the capitate. The lunate is free in relation to the capitate, and thus Taleisnik's theory does not correspond to reality.

The theory of Lichtmann et al. satisfactorily explains the radiological observations and the mobility of the proximal row. It revives the theory of Gilford et al., and yet, on the mechanical level, it is hardly satisfactory. It is not realistic to imagine that the scaphoid, by itself, stabilizes the carpus while limiting its movements. Nevertheless, we have not found any other concepts to explain the spatial coherence of the carpus.

## The Radius and the Radio-carpal Joint

It is surprising to note that the theories of stability of the carpus summarized above do not account for the midcarpal instability observed after fracture of the distal radius. This instability, first described by Taleisnik and Watson in 1984, results from radio-carpal ligamentous insufficiency. Prior to this it had been thought that the malalignment of the carpal bones was no more than the result of mechanical disturbance secondary to malunion. Since the work of Pouteau and of Colles, fracture of the distal radius has been considered a separate entity, just like de Quervain's fracture-dislocation, which combines carpal lesions with those of the forearm. Officially, no real effort has yet been made to understand and define the factors linking these two conditions.

It is Mayfield et al. (1980) who deserve the credit for introducing the concept of lesional zones. They were able to demonstrate that it was possible, by varying the position of the hand and the traumatising force, to obtain different lesions localized either in the carpus, the radius, or in both structures at once. The distal radius, the ulna and the carpus thus become a morpho-pathological entity. The lesion can involve the whole or part of this entity, and the lesional combinations are almost unlimited. This is far removed from the ideas of Frykmann (1967) who distinguished between fractures of the radius with or without fracture of the ulnar styloid. Though based on analogous experiments, such a subdivision takes no account of the phylogenesis or the function of the wrist. Indeed, even if the ulnar styloid is no longer directly articulated with the triquetrum, as is still the case with certain species of monkeys, the ulna retains a fundamental part in the function of the radio-carpal joint, since it is intimately linked to the lunate, the triquetrum and the hamate by the triangular fibrocartilage complex (described in the chapter on functional anatomy). Lewis et al. (1970) and Kauer (1980), for their parts, have demonstrated that the most powerful ligamentous attachments are not to the tip of the styloid but to its base. Thus, to take the styloid itself as an index of the severity of a lesion is to ignore the fundamental role of the ligamentous system and its true attachments. The cardinal importance of these ligaments will be shown in the subsequent anatomical study. It is certainly possible to classify distal radial fractures from a therapeutic point of view, and we shall endeavour to do this, but without prejudging the extent of the associated lesions. To assess their true significance, one must define the radiological methods employed.

The presence of a ligamentous lesion raises the principle of the use of the external fixator to exploit the ligaments as distracting elements. According to the anatomy, this principle is invalid! We are far from condemning the external fixator, an excellent method of fracture retention, but it does call for further discussion of the principles and indications governing its use. It is asking too much of the external fixator if it is to pull on ligaments which are damaged, or whose axes are oblique, and on a bone which in the majority of cases has lost actual volume. Its use must be governed by the anatomy of the wrist and of the fracture.

Pouteau and Colles have the credit for having defined a previously unrecognized bony lesion. Radiology and our current knowledge no longer allow us to ignore the diversity of the lesions of the wrist, even if the obvious lesional mechanism, a forward fall and forced hyperextension, always seems the same. The detection and treatment of these recently recognized conditions calls for a profound modification of the approach to diagnosis and treatment.

Ignorance of this possible lesional multiplicity doubtless explains the diversity of opinions about the treatment and consequences of fracture of the distal radius. There cannot, in fact, be a perfect correlation between anatomical bony reduction, function and pain, since a fair number of ligamentous lesions, some of them critical, remain hidden from the eyes of the examiner. The inability of the physician to understand, and therefore to treat adequately, leads resigned patients to declare themselves content with their fates. Despite that, a good clinical result does not readily co-exist with malunion, and sooner or later the consequences of the abnormal constraints will become obvious. The studies of Castaing (1964), Frykmann (1967) and Cooney et al. (1979) argue in favour of this concept. We will prove in a subsequent chapter, and this has not been done before to our knowledge, that a statistical correlation exists between the quality of the clinical result and the radiological result. Naturally, ligamentous lesions, with their frequent sequelae even after perfect treatment, will always provide arguments for the defeatists. However, here, as elsewhere, it is clear that it is necessary to regularly obtain perfect anatomical results if one is to understand the precise role and importance of the residual ligamentous lesions. Once more, an overall view is essential. It is misunderstanding of the anatomy, bone physiology and biomechanics which has prevented the external fixator, though it has been known since the last world war, from taking its due place in the treatment of this fracture. If a new and valid idea takes 20 years to be accepted, will it not require even longer to get rid of an erroneous one? Is one generation enough for the distal radius, its problems being so very complex?

## References


Allieu Y (1984) Instabilité du carpe, principes thérapeutiques généraux. Ann Chir Main 3:317–321

Bonnel F, Allieu Y (1984) Les articulations radio-cubito-carpienne et médio-carpienne. Organisation anatomique et bases biomécaniques. Ann Chir Main 3:287–296

Bryce TH (1897) On certain points in the anatomy and mechanism of the wrist joint reviewed in the light of a series of Roentgen ray photographs of the living hand. J Anat 31:59–79

Castaing J (1964) Les fractures récentes de l'extrémité inférieure du radius. Rev Chir Orthop 50:581–696

Cooney WP, Linscheid RL, Dobyns JH (1979) External pin fixation for unstable Colles fracture. J Bone Joint Surg [Am] 61:840–845

Daremberg Ch (1854) Oeuvres anatomiques, physiologiques et médicales de Gallien. Baillière, Paris. Vol 1, pp 187–190

Destot E (1923) Traumatismes du poignet et rayons X. Masson, Paris

Fick R (1901) Über die Bewegungen in den Handgelenken. Abh Math Phys D Wissensch Math-Phys 26:419–468

Fisk GR (1970) Carpal instability and the fractured scaphoid. Ann R Coll Surg Engl 46:63–76

Frykmann G (1967) Fracture of the distal radius including sequelae of the shoulder-hand-finger syndrome, disturbance in the distal radio-ulnar joint and impairment of nerve function. Acta Orthop Scand 108 [Suppl]: 5–143

Gilford WW, Bolton RH, Lambrinudi C (1943) The mechanism of the wrist joint with special reference to fractures of the scaphoid. Guy's Hosp Rep 92:52–59

Henke W (1859) Über die Bewegung der Handwurzel. Ztschr F Rat Med R. Vol 7

Kauer JMG (1980) Functional anatomy of the wrist. Clin Orthop 1949:9–20

Lewis OJ, Hamschere R, Buck Nill TM (1970) The anatomy of the wrist joint. J Anat 106:539–552

Lichtmann DM, Schneider JR, Swafford AR, Mack GR (1981) Ulnar midcarpal instability – Clinical and laboratory analysis. J Hand Surg 6:515–523

Linscheid RL, Dobyns JH, Boabout JW, Bryan RS (1972) Traumatic instability of the wrist: Diagnosis, classification and pathomechanics. J Bone Joint Surg [Am] 54:1612–1632

Mayfield JK, Johnson RP, Kilcoyne R (1980) Carpal dislocations: Pathomechanics and progressive perilunar instability. J Hand Surg 5:226–241

Mouchet A, Belot J (1934) Poignet á ressaut (subluxation médio-carpienne en avant). Bull et Mem Soc Nat de Chir 31:1243–1244

Navarro A (1937) Anatomia y fisiologia del carpo. An Inst Clin Quir Chir Exp 1:162–250

Taleisnik J (1976) The ligaments of the wrist. J Hand Surg 1:110–118

Taleisnik J, Watson K (1984) Midcarpal instability caused by malunited fractures of the distal radius. J Hand Surg 9A:350–357

Trojan E, de Mourgues G (1959) Fractures et pseudarthroses du scaphoïde carpien. Etude thérapeutique. Rev Chir Orthop 45:614–677

Virchow H (1899) Das Skelett der ulnarwaerts abducierten und radialwaerts abducierten Hand. Ztschr f Morpholog u Anthropol 1(3):453–382
Weber ER (1980) Biomechanical implications of scaphoid waist fractures. Clin Orthop 149:83–89
Youm Y, McMurtry RY, Flatt AE, Gillespie TE (1978) Kinematics of the wrist. J Bone Joint Surg [Am] 60:423–431

CHAPTER I

# Anatomical Approach

The wrist joint, although extremely mobile in all three planes of space, is nevertheless able to support several times the body weight without damage. Its architecture, based on eight bones (Fig. I.1) and a special ligamentous bonding, is very complex but guarantees stability under all circumstances. If a single component should fail, whether it be bony or ligamentous, the articulation becomes unstable and painful. It may then develop progressive deformity and arthrosis.

The object of this presentation is to understand better the anatomy of the different ligaments of the carpus, in order to define their respective functions in the stability of this articulation. We shall deal with this under the following five headings:

A. Bony anatomy
B. Ligamentous anatomy
C. Kinematics
D. Functional ligamentous anatomy
E. The concept of stability

## A. Bony Anatomy

The architecture of the carpal bones can be considered globally or either vertically or horizontally.

*Global view.* The view shown in Fig. I.1 is a familiar one, and is found in every textbook of anatomy; it provides purely descriptive information. Such a representation is static and takes

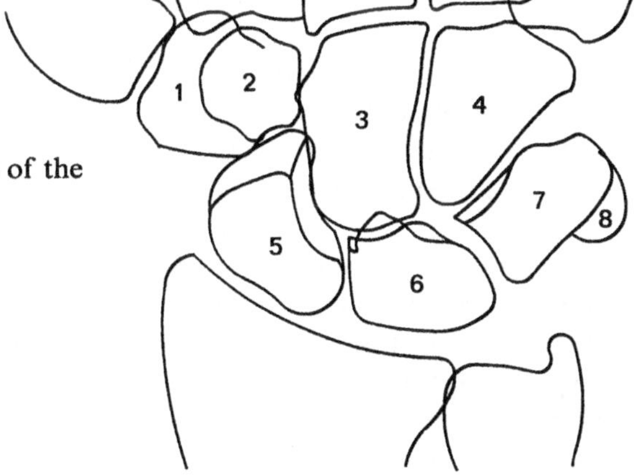


**Fig. I.1.** The eight bones of the carpus.
*1* Trapezium
*2* Trapezoid
*3* Capitate
*4* Hamate
*5* Scaphoid
*6* Lunate
*7* Triquetrum
*8* Pisiform

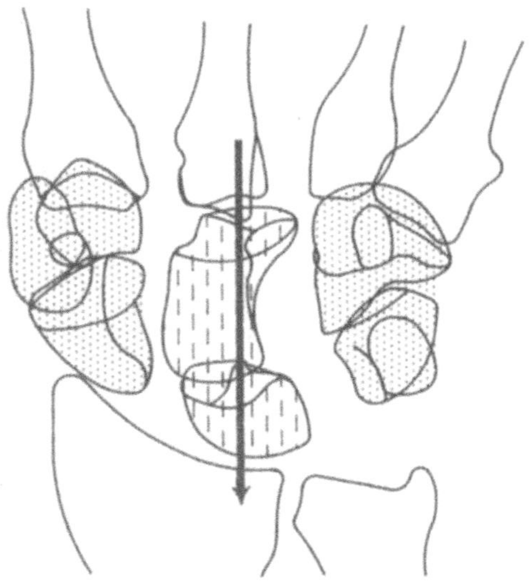

**Fig. I.2.** Vertical section; mechanical aspect (*arrow*, transmission of forces)

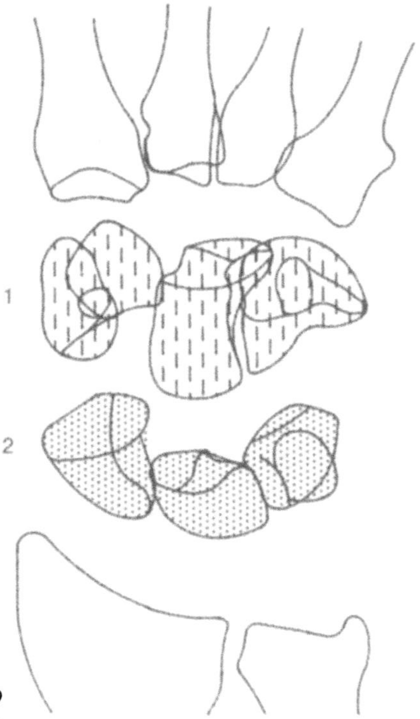


**Fig. I.3.** Horizontal section
*1* distal row
*2* proximal row
– dynamic
– intercalated

no account of function. Here the scaphoid seems to belong to both rows, forming a sort of bridge. Distally, it articulates with the trapezium and the trapezoid, and on its medial aspect with the capitate. The latter appears to be the centre of the carpus, and if it is considered to be associated with the lunate, it is possible to divide the carpus into three columns: radial, ulnar and central. However, the alignment of the axis of the central column is imperfect. The lunate is translated ulnarly in relation to the capitate, with a resultant overhang. The alignment of the lunate with the radius is likewise imperfect, since a third of this bone is supported by the ulnar ligamentous complex. The triquetrum, isolated on the ulnar aspect and flanked by the pisiform, seems to have no particular function: in this it is similar to the hamate, which is like a piece of a jig-saw puzzle serving to fill a gap between the capitate and the bases of the fourth and fifth metacarpals. These bones form the vault of the carpal tunnel, the floor of which is the flexor retinaculum stretching between the hook of the hamate and the trapezium. The function of this ligament is still only partly understood.

*Horizontal or transverse section.* This subdivides the carpus into two rows: proximal and distal. In this view, the proximal row appears as a distinct structure intercalated between the radius and the distal row of the carpus (Fig. I.3).

*Vertical or longitudinal section.* There are three columns as outlined above, which implies the existence of a mechanical axis of transmission of forces between the radius and the carpo-metacarpal complex (Fig. I.2). However, this mechanical view must take into account the architecture of the distal radius socket, which exhibits two particular structural features:

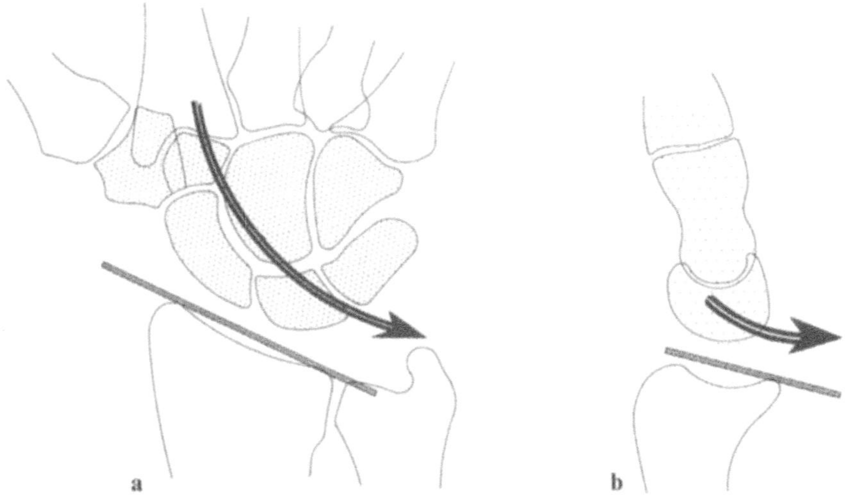


**Fig. I.4a, b.** Plane of articular gliding.
**a** frontal plane,
**b** sagittal plane

- In the frontal plane, the axis of the articulation forms an angle of 20° with the perpendicular to the longitudinal axis of the radius.
- In the sagittal plane, the articular axis varies between 10° and 20°.

Therefore, the distal radius appears to be a gliding plane, on which the carpus has a constant tendency to skid. In fact, this shift does not take place, thanks to the ligamentous complex (Fig. I.4).

## B. Ligamentous Anatomy

There are two issues to be resolved here. The first is purely semantic because of the different nomenclature employed by different authors. The second is related to the fact that the ligamentous system is actually double; an "articular" or deep system can be distinguished from an "extra-articular" or superficial system, namely the flexor and extensor retinacula.

### Nomenclature

Taleisnik (1976) distinguishes two types of ligaments, the intrinsic and the extrinsic. The intrinsic ligaments join the carpal bones to one another, while the extrinsics connect the carpus to the radius and to the metacarpus. This subdivision has the advantage of providing an overall view useful for understanding carpal function. Bonnel and Allieu (1984), on the other hand, subdivide the 33 ligaments of the carpus into three groups: intra-articular, intra-capsular and extra-capsular. Like Kuhlmann and Tubiana (1983), they define the extra-capsular ligaments as the anterior and posterior annular ligaments. The intra-articular ligaments join the different carpal bones together; these are the intrinsic ligaments of Taleisnik, though Bonnel and Allieu include the radio-scapho-lunate and triangular ligaments in this group. The third group, intra-capsular, unite the carpal bones to one another, as well as to the radius and the metacarpals.

### Classification

Each of these classifications has its advantages, but also has the drawback of standing in the way of a global functional concept. Stimulated by these three authors, we have adopted a practical anatomical classification which satisfies these functional criteria. We distinguish two ligamentous systems:
1. *The articular system*, comprising the interosseous and intracapsular ligaments
2. *The extra-articular system*, the ligaments of which are outside the joint

### 1. Articular Ligamentous System

The articular ligamentous system is subdivided into four anatomical and functional groups:
- The interosseous group: of the distal row
  of the proximal row
- The palmar V group: the distal V and the proximal V
- The ulnocarpal complex
- The dorsal group

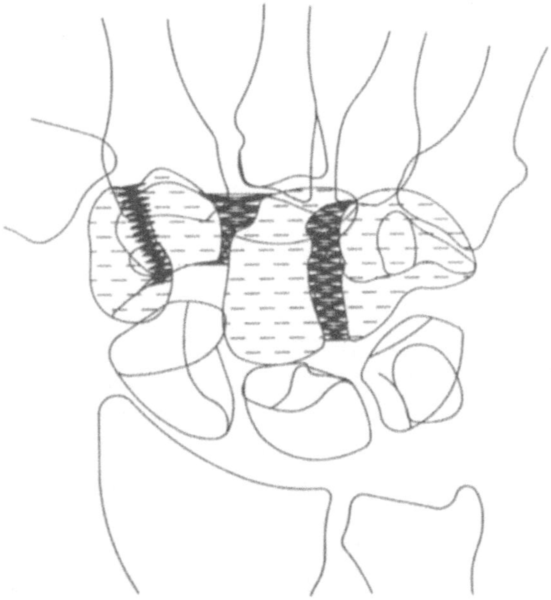

**Fig. I.5.** Distal interosseous ligaments
- no degrees of freedom
- distal row functions as a single unit

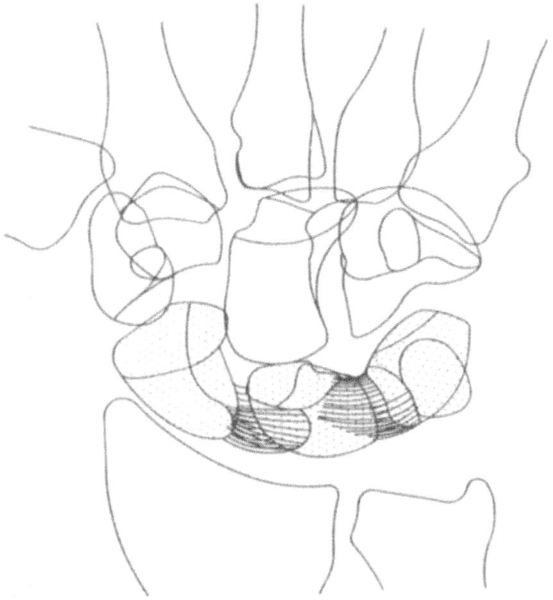

**Fig. I.6.** Proximal interosseus ligaments
- strong
- major degree of freedom
- modular functional unit

**Interosseous Group**

*Distal row.* This group consists of short, strong ligaments that allow no movement between the bones of the distal row they unite. These are the short ligaments of Taleisnik (1976), who considers this row as a functional monolith (Fig. I.5).

*Proximal row.* The two ligaments joining the three bones of the proximal carpal row are less taut than their homologues of the distal row. They allow some movement between the bones they unite. This makes the proximal row a semi-rigid modular unit, continuously and harmoniously adjustable to the constraints imposed on it by the two blocks between which it is interposed: the radius and the distal carpal row (Fig. I.6).

**The Palmar V Group**

*The proximal V.* Under this heading we include the different ligaments joining the radius, the lunate and the triangular fibrocartilage complex. Figures I.7 and I.8 will help in memorizing this information.

*The distal V.* This is composed of the ligaments joining the lateral border of the radius to the capitate; it is prolonged, via the hamate, to the triquetrum and the pisiform. This extension to the pisiform is the point of junction of the deep and superficial systems. In fact, the flexor retinaculum also exhibits ligamentous attachments extending to the pisiform.

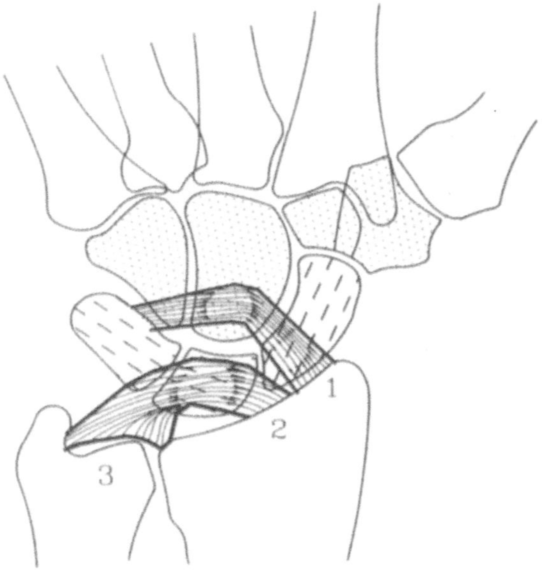


**Fig. I.7.** Palmar ligaments:
*1* distal V
*2* proximal V
*3* ulnocarpal complex

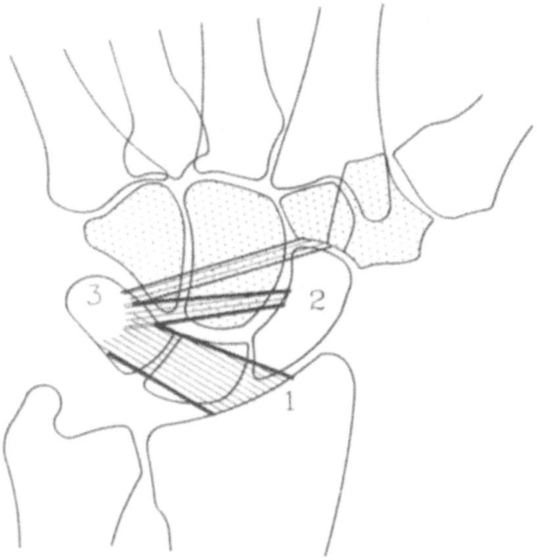


**Fig. I.8.** Dorsal ligaments:
*1* radio-triquetral ligament
*2* triquetral-scaphoid ligament
*3* occasional second band

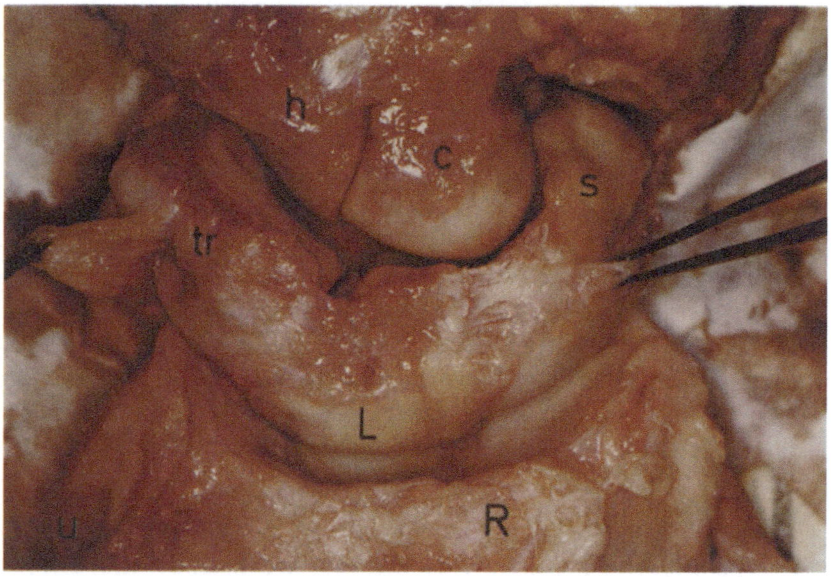


a

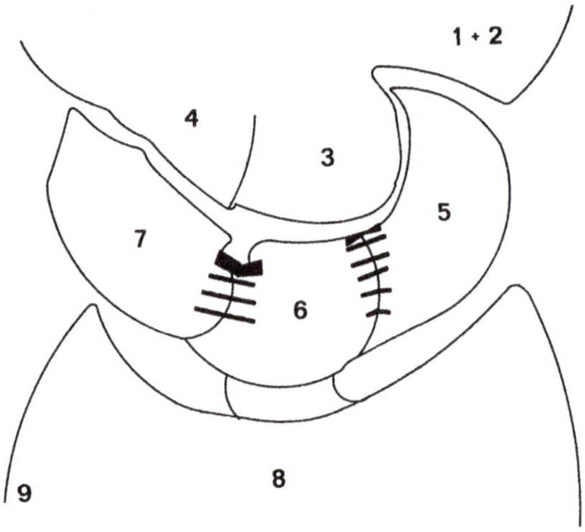


b

**Fig. I.9. a** Dorsal aspect of the proximal row after resection of the dorsal V, the proximal row is perfectly free. The scapho-lunate and triquetro-lunate ligaments are easily identified. The head of the capitate is situated between the lunate and scaphoid.
**b** Dorsal view of distal unit
*1* Trapezium
*2* Trapezoid
*3* Capitate
*4* Hamate
*5* Scaphoid
*6* Lunate
*7* Triquetrum
*8* Radius
*9* Ulna

## The Ulnocarpal Complex

This is the least known of the ligamentous systems of the wrist joint, the structures comprising it being difficult to separate from one another. Evolution seems to have played an important part in this anatomical complex, as demonstrated by Lewis et al. (1970). Palmer et al. (1981, 1984) divide it into five structures which we shall discuss in detail later; they join the distal radius to the ulnar styloid by a fibroligamentous complex which is itself attached to the carpus by the ulnar portion of the proximal V.

## The Dorsal V Group

A V may be distinguished that, unlike its palmar homologue, presents its apex towards the ulnar side and not distally; i.e. a transverse V (Fig. I.8). The proximal branch of the V unites the radius and the triquetrum. At this point the extensor retinaculum fuses with the articular ligamentous system in order to

Fig. I.10. Scapho-lunate ligament: a ligamentous semicircle, strongest on the palmar side, very resistant to traction, but less so to shearing stresses

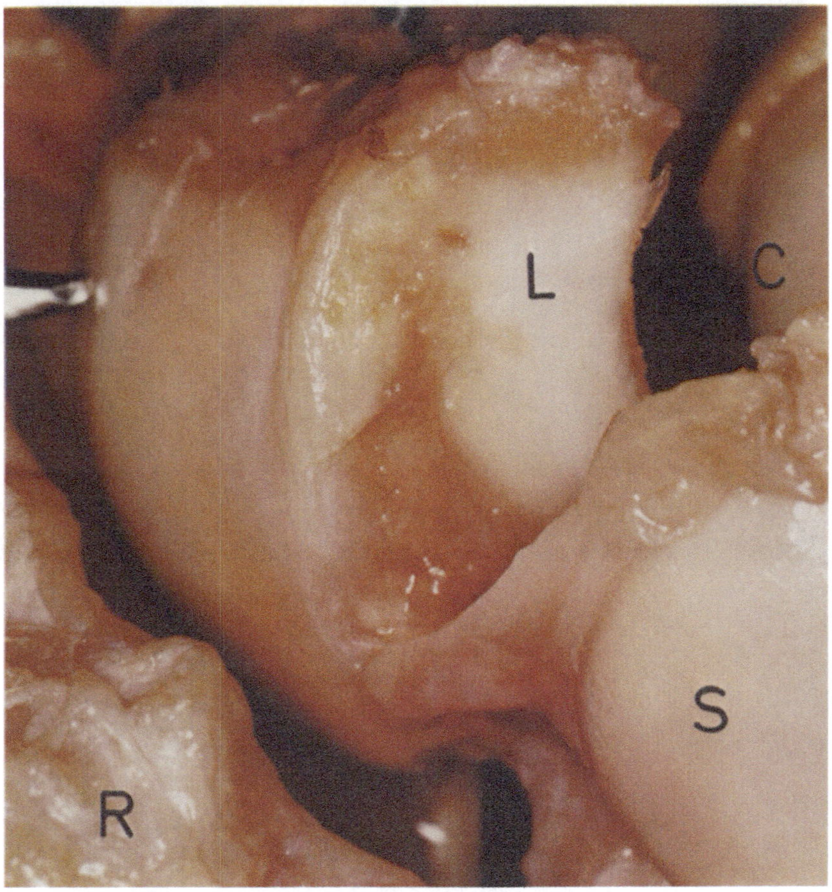


attach to the pisiform. Thus the pisiform becomes the unifying element of both the palmar and dorsal ligamentous systems, and also of the articular ligamentous and extra-articular systems.

The second branch of the V, the distal branch, unites the triquetrum with the scaphoid via the lunate. Occasionally, this branch is double; this distal strip courses from the triquetrum to the trapezium-trapezoid group. So the dorsal V runs horizontally from the radial to the ulnar side of the wrist as opposed to the vertically orientated palmar V.

## Systematic Analysis

### *The Group of Interosseous Ligaments*

There is no need to dwell on the function of the three interosseous ligaments of the distal row; the movements they allow between these bones are so minor that the distal carpal row acts as a functional unit; virtually an anatomical block comparable to the radius and firmly attached to the metacarpals distally. Between these two structures lies the proximal row (Fig. I.9) with the two remaining interosseous ligaments. These join the lunate to the scaphoid on the radial side and to the triquetrum on the ulnar side. They deserve a more extensive analysis.

a

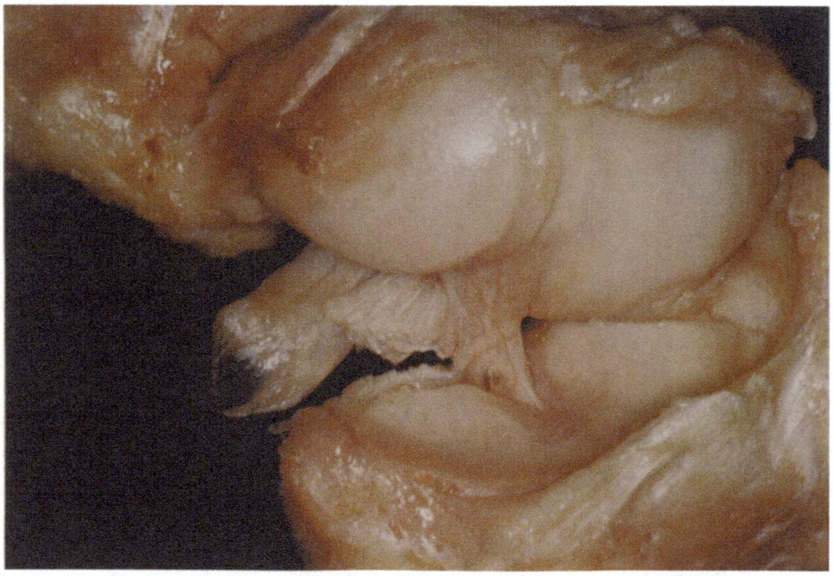

b

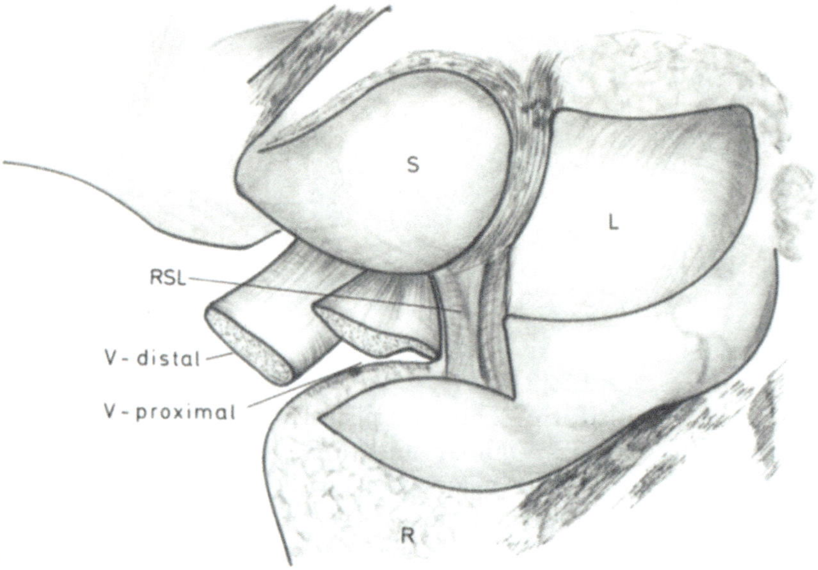


**Fig. I.11 a, b.** Radio-carpal joint. **a** The diameter of the scaphoid is plainly less than that of the lunate. The strong V ligaments have been divided at their attachment to the radius. The partial superimposition of the distal V and proximal V is well shown, and explains the difficulty of anatomical identification from the palmar aspect. The radio-scapho-lunate ligament is relatively weak compared with the two other ligaments; it serves to conduct vessels.
**b** distal and proximal V
*S* scaphoid
*L* lunate
*R* radius
*RSL* radio-scapho-lunate ligament

Kauer (1980) demonstrated that the complex movements observable between the scaphoid and the lunate are dependent on the peculiar morphology of the ligamentous semi-circle that joins them. On the palmar aspect the fibres of this semi-circle are longer and less dense, which is why palmar interosseous mobility is greater than dorsal; hence the movement of translation between these two bones during flexion-extension of the wrist. This translation between the two bones is indispensable for normal function, since the radius of rotation of the scaphoid is greater than that of the lunate (Fig. I.11). Mayfield and Williams (1979) demonstrated the strength of this ligament, which is resistant to traction but somewhat vulnerable to shearing stresses.

The ligament joining the lunate to the triquetrum is not as well known. Presumably its function is similar to that of its

**Fig. I.12a–c.** The palmar V ligaments.
**a** General appearance: between the capitate and lunate there are no fibres whose axis is longitudinal.
**b** The proximal V has been elevated; the lunate is exposed and easily recognizable.
**c** The distal V is clearly defined.
*R* radius
*S* scaphoid
*L* lunate
*Tr* triquetrum
*P* pisiform

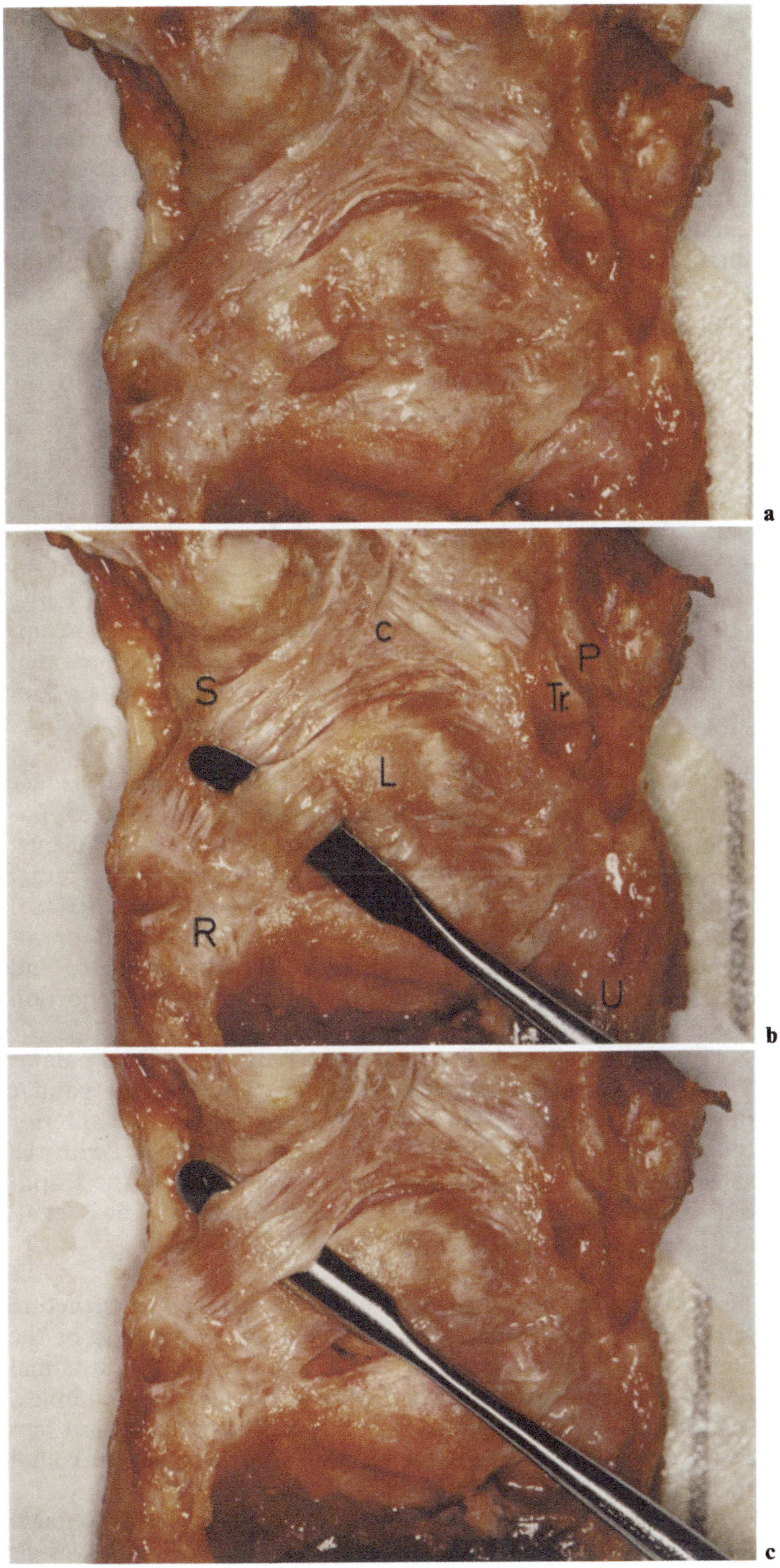

scapho-lunate homologue. However, rotational movements between these two bones are minimal, since the triquetrum does no more than glide by translation along the hamate. Likewise, the pressure it must bear is entirely different; the head of the capitate is essentially between the scaphoid and the lunate, so that the main thrust of the axial forces is concentrated on the scapho-lunate ligament. Thus, everything works to separate the scaphoid from the lunate. This is not the case for the triquetro-lunate articulation, where the stresses are fewer. This explains why scapho-lunate lesions are well known whereas triquetro-lunate lesions are rarely recognized. The triquetro-lunate ligament is essentially a linking element; the consequences of its rupture are difficult to assess, even if it is evident that, without it, the proximal row is no longer a functional unit.

### *The Palmar V Ligaments*

These are thick ligamentous structures. Their superficial fibres present an uninterrupted course which makes it possible to divide the palmar structures into two constituent elements. Firstly, a distal V, joining the radius to the distal part of the triquetrum-pisiform complex, via the capitate; and secondly, a proximal V, joining the radius to the ulnar styloid, via the lunate and the proximal pole of the triquetrum (Fig. I.12).

*The distal V.* Analysis of the deep fibres of the distal V shows that it can be split up into radio-scaphoid (Fig. I.13), scapho-capitate, capitate-triquetral and triquetral-pisiform ligaments. The distal V is thus an articulated system joining the radial styloid to the pisiform; the axis of its fibres, both superficial and deep, is oblique. The superficial layer is responsible for coherence, while the deep layer seems to act as a guidance and control system, especially as far as the radio-scaphoid portion is concerned.

The radial collateral ligament forms part of the distal palmar V, and is almost indistinguishable from this, since its palmar fibres are stretched between the radial styloid and the anterior tubercle of the scaphoid. Moreover, its dorsal bundle, with the same origin, but terminating on the lateral aspect of the scaphoid, is a weak structure with a limited function. Lewis et al. (1970) also concur with this opinion.

*The proximal V.* The superficial fibres of this massive structure join the anterior margin of the radial fossa to the base of the ulnar styloid via the palmar pole of the lunate, the proximal pole of the triquetrum and the triangular fibrocartilage complex. These fibres form a supporting strap, resisting the natural tendency of the lunate to palmar subluxation, and they surround the styloid like a sleeve.

The deep fibres of this sling form the radio-scapho-lunate ligaments (clearly visible with the nutrient radio-lunate vessels

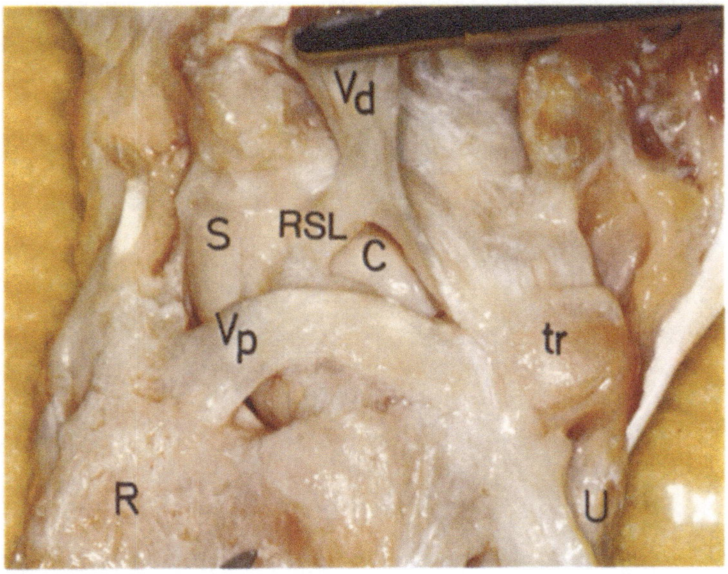


a

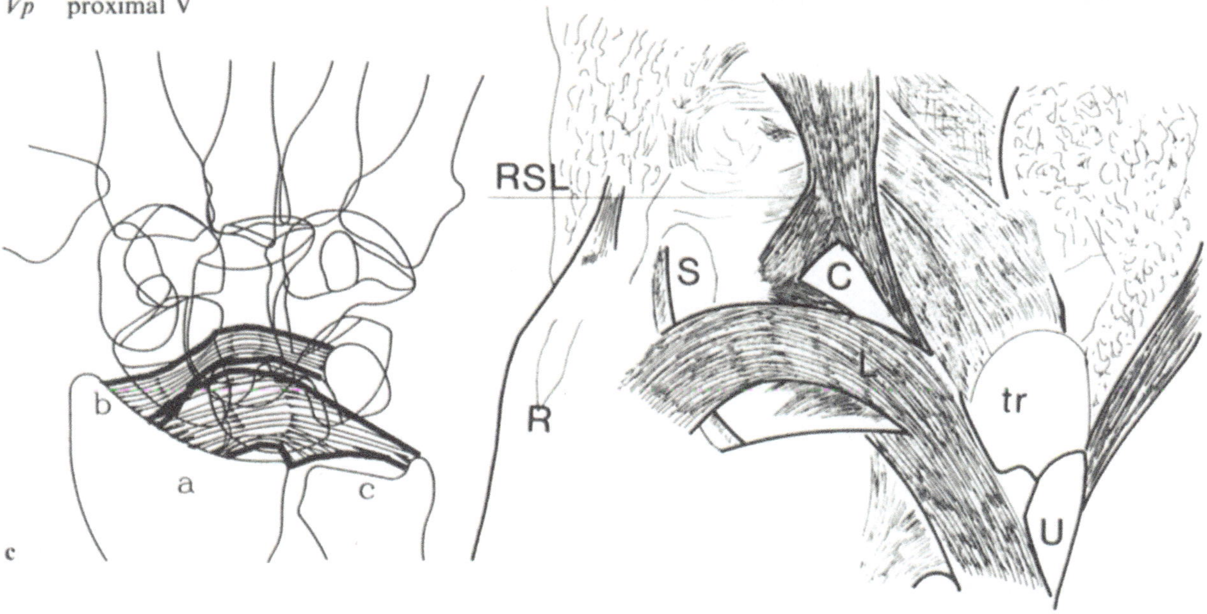


c

b

**Fig. I.13. a, b** Structure of distal V: detachment of the distal V from the radius displays the radio-scaphoid component and the rather loose attachment to the scaphoid. **c** Schema of palmar ligaments
*a* proximal V
*b* distal V
*c* triangular fibrocartilage complex
*C* capitate
*R* radius
*RSL* radio-scapho-lunate ligament
*S* scaphoid
*tr* triquetrum
*U* ulna
*Vd* distal V
*Vp* proximal V

in Fig. I.14) and ulno-carpal bundles going from the ulnar styloid to the triquetrum and lunate as part of the triangular fibrocartilage complex. The function of these deep fibres is difficult to determine; it may be to reinforce the intra-articular ligaments or to regulate tension. Their twisted appearance suggests the latter (see Fig. I.15). There is sometimes a capsular reinforcement binding the neck of the capitate to the ulnar styloid; this less-developed structure is known as the ulno-capitate ligament.

Three facts emerge from dissection: firstly, there is no ligament between the lunate and the capitate; secondly, the proximal V supports the lunate; and thirdly, there is no longitudinal ligamentous system.

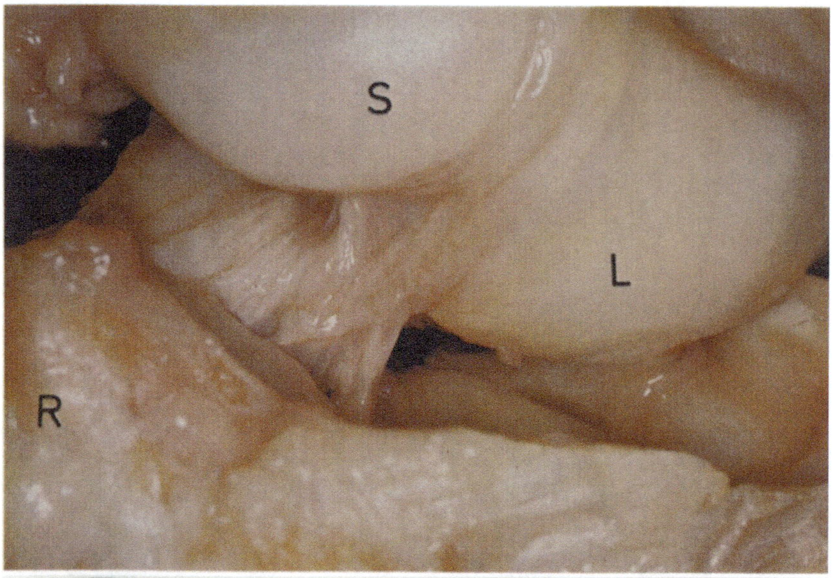


a

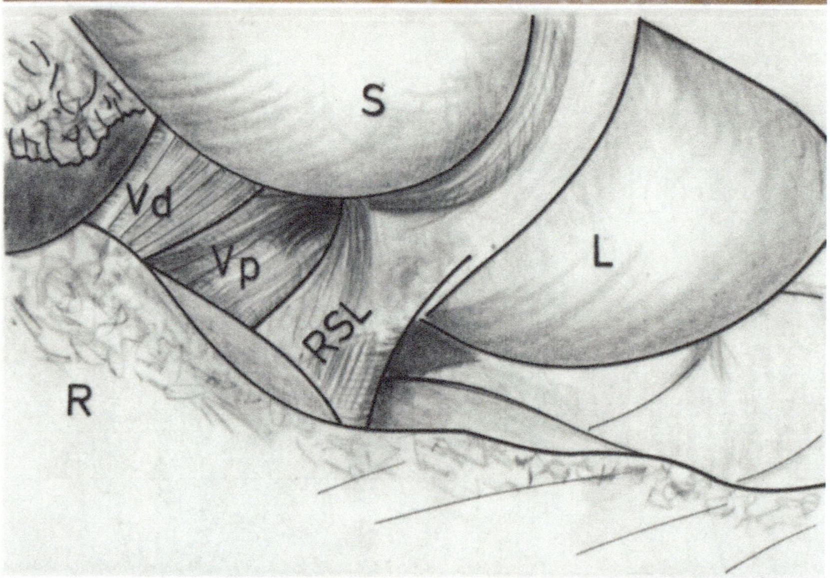


b

**Fig. I.14a, b.** Deep aspect of palmar V (compare with Fig. I.11). The vessels of the radio-scapho-lunate ligament can be seen opposite the radial socket, marked with a cross.
*Vd* distal V
*Vp* proximal V
*R* radius
*S* scaphoid
*L* lunate

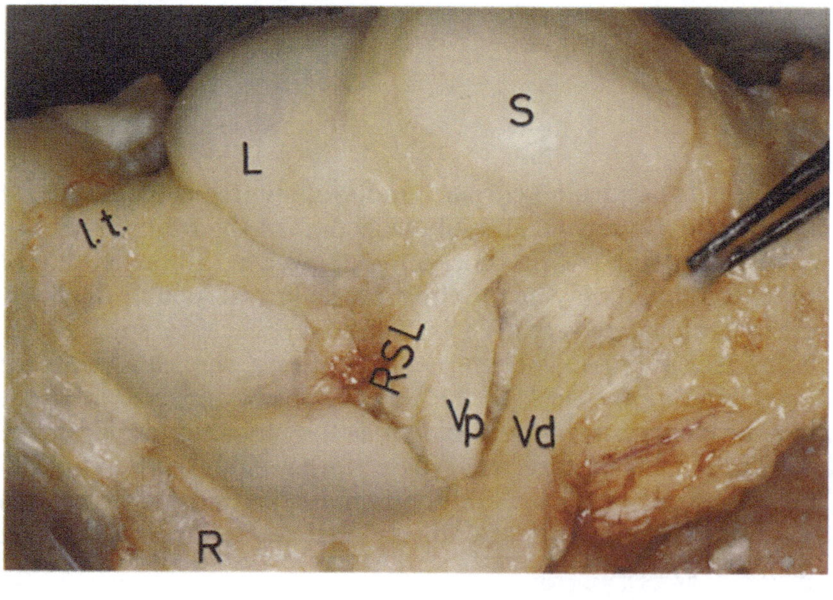


**Fig. I.15.** Deep aspect of palmar V ligaments: the radio-scapho-lunate ligament and the radial portion of the proximal V (RL ligament) are twisted. The triangular ligament cannot be studied in this photograph.
*Vd* distal V
*Vp* proximal V
*R* radius
*S* scaphoid
*lt* triangular ligament

*The Triangular Fibrocartilage Complex (TFCC)*

Palmer and Werner (1981) divided this complex into five structures virtually inseparable from one another:

1. The medial or ulnar collateral ligament
2. The triangular fibrocartilage (or articular disc) and its two dorsal and palmar capsular reinforcements
3. The ulno-carpal meniscus (or radio-triquetral ligament)
4. The ulno-lunate ligament: from our viewpoint the ulnar portion of the proximal V
5. The sheath of the extensor carpi ulnaris

*The medial ligament.* Bonnel and Allieu (1984) described two bundles stretching from the medial border of the ulnar styloid to the pisiform (anterior bundle) and to the triquetrum (posterior bundle). The anterior bundle is poorly developed, and hence its functional role appears negligible. The posterior bundle, plainly more powerful, may act as a brake, and indeed its oblique fibres tighten with radial deviation. However, as with its radial homologue, one may question its true identity. Is it rather, as described by Lewis et al. (1970), the most medial portion of the ulno-lunate ligament? Their phylogenetic arguments are convincing.

*The triangular fibrocartilage.* This originates from the margin of the sigmoid fossa of the radius and inserts into the base of the ulnar styloid (Taleisnik 1976). It is shaped like an asymmetrical bi-concave lens, its dorsal border being thicker than its palmar border. Its thickness varies from one individual to another and depends on the length of the ulna relative to that of the radius (Palmer et al. 1984); i.e. it is thicker when the ulna is short. In the fetus and the new-born child, this structure is impervious, and allows no communication between the radio-carpal and distal radio-ulnar joints (Kauer 1975). On the basis of 180 dissections, Mikic (1978) demonstrated that there are no perforations in the first two decades of life, these lesions being observed only after the third decade. They increase in frequency with age to reach 53% by the 60th year. Weigl and Spira (1969) disagree with the previous authors, and believe there are three types of perforation: congenital, traumatic and degenerative. However, the validity of their work is in doubt, as it is based on a heterogenous collection of wrists, some from cadavers and some from injured patients. In addition, they do not state whether a relationship exists between the type of perforation and the age-group, merely stating that perforations occur at all ages. The increased frequency of perforations with a long ulna argues in favour of a traumatic aetiology.

Two fibrous thickenings surround the cartilage. These are properly called the palmar and dorsal radio-ulnar ligaments.

*The ulno-carpal meniscus.* This has the same origin as the triangular fibrocartilage, at the medial side of the articulation of the radius. According to Taleisnik (1976), the meniscus immediately separates from the triangular fibrocartilage to become attached to the triquetrum, leaving a space between these two structures: the prestyloid recess. This cartilaginous structure, also known as the radio-triquetral ligament, is clearly separate from the triangular fibrocartilage.

Despite Palmer's work, the situation is far from being clear. Kauer (1975), who defined the origin of the triangular fibrocartilage ligament on the basis of embryological studies, reminds us that this structure is derived from the deep layers of the forearm fascia. This explains its peculiarity of connecting the ulnar styloid not only to the radius but also to all the adjacent structures, and in particular to the extensor carpi ulnaris. This peculiarity gives it an important stabilizing role. This concept, which does not emerge at all from Taleisnik's analysis, agrees perfectly with the phylogenesis described by Lewis.

According to Kuhlmann and Tubiana (1983), the triangular fibrocartilage ligament has three points of attachment to the ulna: firstly, in the small fossa situated between the styloid and the inferior surface of the ulnar head; secondly, on the lateral aspect of the ulnar styloid; and thirdly, on the deep aspect of the medial (ulnar collateral) ligament. They do not mention the meniscus as such.

Kapandji (1983) states that the radio-triquetral ligament corresponds to the meniscus of Lewis (1970). Thus it is a reinforcement of the capsule, but it is inconstant (Kuhlmann and Tubiana 1983) and therefore classed with the dorsal medial system. It is justified to differentiate the meniscus from the fibrocartilage, as does Taleisnik (1976), given the two functionally distinct parts of the structure involved. We are inclined to opt for this opinion in view of the embryology.

*The ulno-lunate ligament.* This is part of the ulnar portion of the palmar proximal V, a bundle joining the volar pole of the lunate to the ulnar styloid. It does not seem justified to include this perfectly recognizable and identifiable ligament in the TFCC, even if its deep fibres are intimately blended with the fibrocartilage to form a whole.

*The sheath of the extensor carpi ulnaris.* This cannot be separated from the complex, with which its fibres are intimately blended. Fig. I.16 gives some idea of its very considerable thickness.

It may be concluded that the functions of the TFCC are multiple: to stabilize the two forearm bones, to stabilize the lunate, and to buffer and transmit force from the carpus to the ulna.

### *The Dorsal V*

The number and size of the ligaments of the dorsal aspect are clearly less important than those of the ligaments on the palmar

**Fig. I.16.** The very thick sheath of extensor carpi ulnaris, closely blended with the ulnar complex, seen here under the *forceps*.
*tr* triquetrum

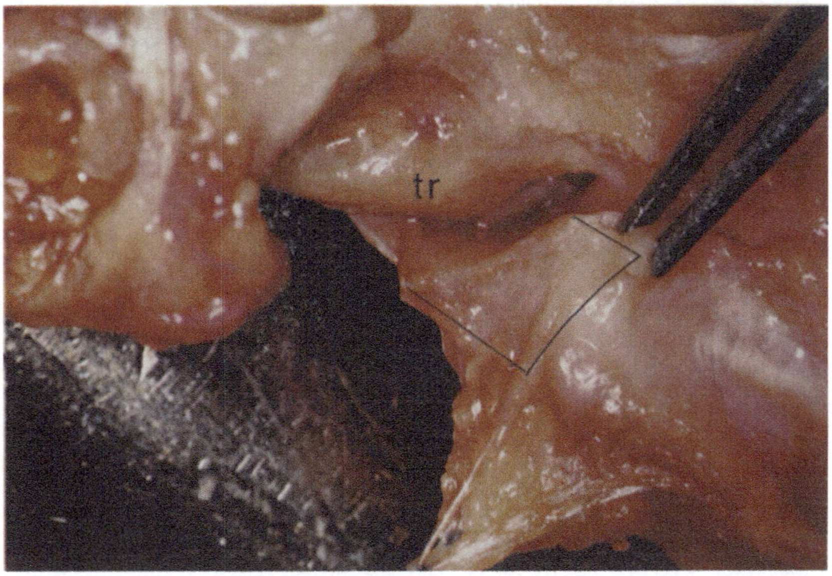


aspect, and their structural analysis is correspondingly simplified. The dorsal V is composed of two bundles of unequal importance:

– The radio-triquetral ligament, a relatively strong structure, stretches between the posterior margin of the articular surface of the radius and the posterior aspect of the triquetrum. In its course, it fixes the posterior pole of the lunate, which it helps to stabilize, along with its palmar homologue (the proximal V). There it joins with the distal part of the dorsal annular ligament (extensor retinaculum), the whole complex extending like a lasso around the triquetrum as far as the pisiform. The distal palmar V and the radio-triquetral ligament literally clasp the carpus, and prevent it from gliding along the radial socket; i.e. they provide the brake to ulnar translation.

– The scapho-triquetral ligament is the second part of this V; it takes its origin at the meeting-point of the two previously described ligaments (radio-triquetral and extensor retinaculum), and is attached to the distal pole of the scaphoid. Its size and development are variable. Sometimes a second band is found also originating from the triquetrum and extending to the trapezium and trapezoid (Fig. I.17).

## 2. Extra-articular Ligamentous System

This term relates to those ligaments without any direct articular contact. They are the extensor and flexor retinacula.

### Extensor Retinaculum

The average breadth of this specialized thickening of the dorsal fascia of the forearm varies between 3 and 8 cm. It is easily recognizable (Fig. I.18), and extends from the dorsal aspect of

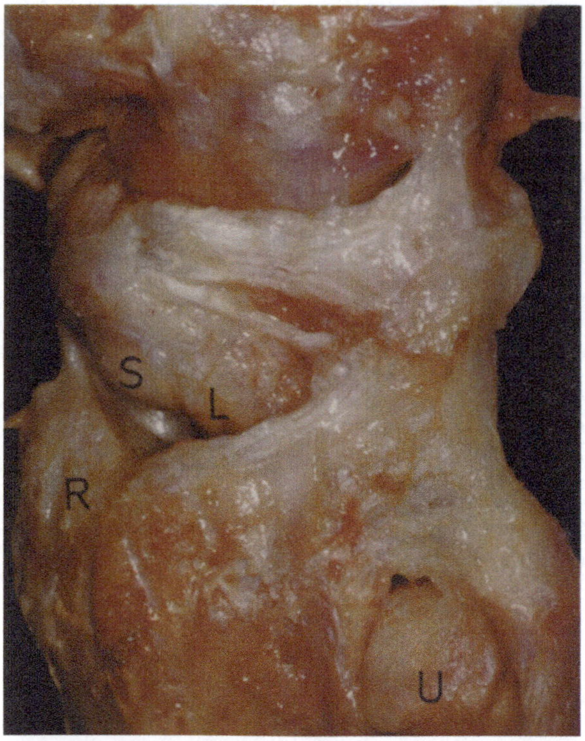


a

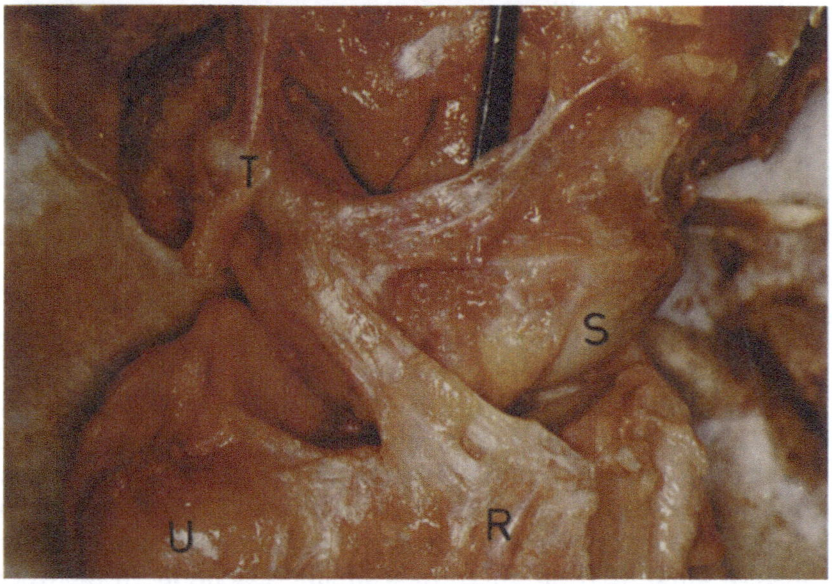


b

**Fig. I.17 a, b.** Two different views of the dorsal V. **a** Right wrist, dorso-ulnar view. **b** Left wrist, dorso-radial view. On the *left*, the triquetro-scaphoid ligament extends to the trapezium and trapezoid; on the *right* this is not the case. Note that the *head of the ulna* is free from attachments; note also the relative weakness of the *dorsal ligaments* compared with the *palmar structures*

the radius in an oblique course to be attached, mainly, to the triquetrum. When viewed under magnification (Fig. I.19) it is often possible to detect an interlacing of its constituent fibres (Palmer et al. 1985). It forms six dorsal compartments, and the different extensor tendons which traverse these are endowed with synovial sheaths. Table I.1 shows the position of each tendon. Taleisnik et al. (1984) consider that each compartment is formed by the splitting of the retinaculum into two sheets, superficial (or supratendinous) and deep (or infratendinous). Situated between each compartment are points of anchorage; these are bony on the radial side, and essentially ligamentous on the ulnar side.

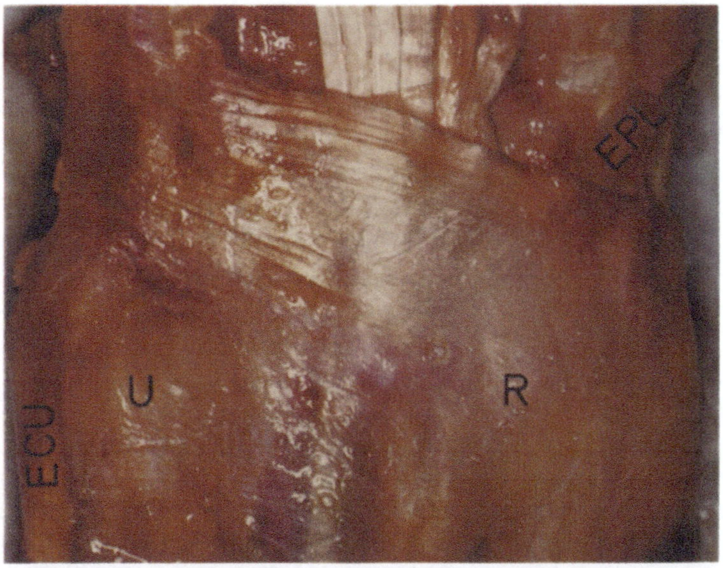


**Fig. I.18.** The extensor retinaculum, which is easily recognized, is not attached to the ulna but mainly to the triquetrum, and has an oblique course.
*EPL* extensor pollicis longus
*ECU* extensor carpi ulnaris
*R* radius
*U* ulna

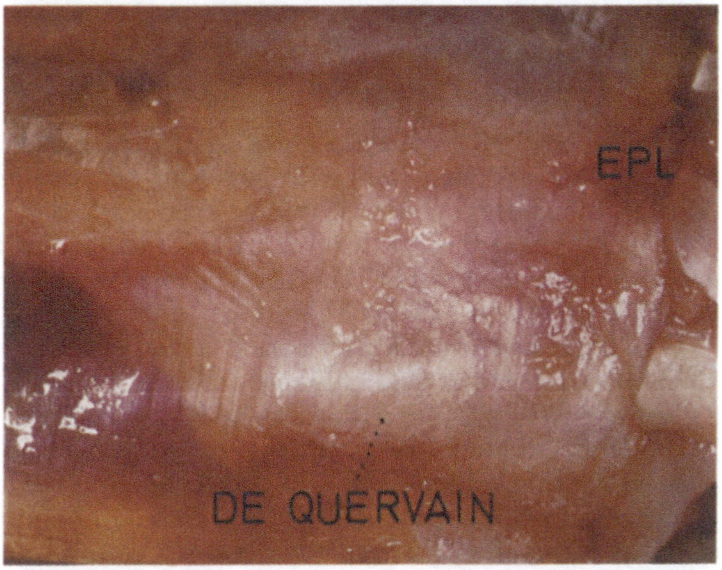


**Fig. I.19.** Close-up of the extensor retinaculum: interlacing fibres are visible in places.
*EPL* extensor pollicis longus

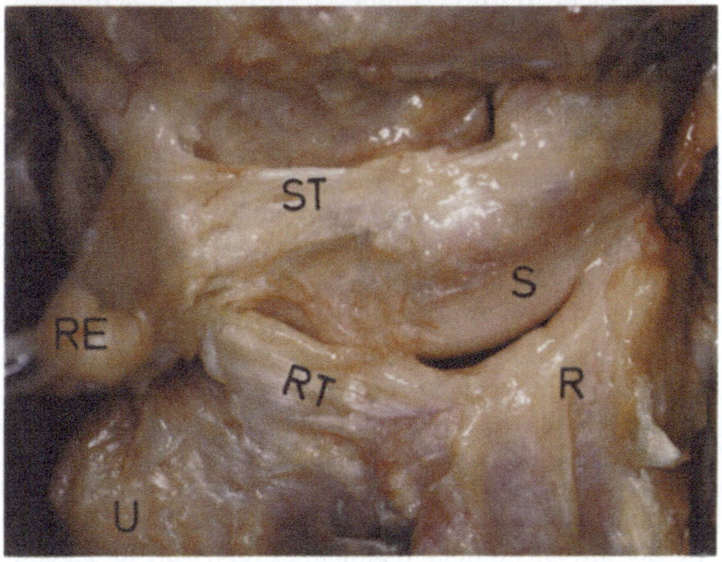


**Fig. I.20.** Point of altered orientation of fibres of extensor retinaculum at the triquetrum.
*RE* extensor retinaculum
*RT* radio-triquetral ligament
*ST* scapho-triquetral ligament
*R* radius
*S* scaphoid
*U* ulna

**Table I.1.** Extensor retinaculum with six compartments

| Compartment | Tendons enclosed |
|---|---|
| 1 (De Quervain's) | Abductor pollicis longus<br>Extensor pollicis brevis |
| 2 | Extensor carpi radialis longus<br>Extensor carpi radialis brevis |
| 3 | Extensor pollicis longus |
| 4 | Extensor proprius indicis<br>Extensor communis (4 tendons) |
| 5 | Extensor proprius digiti V |
| 6 | Extensor carpi ulnaris |

Numerous variations characterize the first compartment, e.g. there are often three tendons (the abductors being duplicated) and a septum (often partial) may separate the long abductor from the short extensor

### *The Ulnar Points of Anchorage*

On the medial side there are three points of fixation, none of which is on the ulna itself. The extensor retinaculum can be divided into thirds: proximal, middle and distal.

- The proximal third is formed by the merging of the fibres of the retinaculum and the sheath of the flexor carpi ulnaris (FCU). Together, they lock the ulna to the radius.
- The fibres of the middle third are attached to the dorsal aspect of the triquetrum and prolonged to the pisiform. Once at the triquetrum, some of them make a 180° turn and fuse with the radio-triquetral ligament (Fig. I.20). The middle third has a course that is parallel to the underlying radio-triquetral ligament, an analogous function and a common point of attachment.
- The distal third is composed of fibres attaching partly to the aponeurosis of the abductor digiti minimi and partly to the base of the fifth metacarpal.

### *The Radial Points of Anchorage*

These three massive points of attachment are to be found between the radial compartments. Only the fibres of the middle third are involved. The fibres of the proximal third fuse with the palmar antebrachial fascia after having surrounded the flexor carpi radialis. Those of the distal third disappear into the aponeurosis of the thenar eminence. Taleisnik et al. (1984) stated that the point of anchorage between the fifth and sixth compartments is situated on the dorso-medial aspect of the radius and not on the ulna, which must be left free. As a result, the extensor carpi ulnaris (ECU) has a very special structure. Unlike the other extensor tendons, it is not contained within a reflection of the dorsal annular ligament, which can be elevated without baring the tendon. It remains fixed to the ulna by its own sheath, distinct from the retinaculum. This applies not only to the dorsal aspect of the distal ulna, but also the triquetrum. Because of this, the tendon of the ECU acquires a particular function: placed under tension, it aligns the dorsal surface of the triquetrum with that of the distal ulna, transfers this tension to the ulnar portion of the annular ligament, stabilizes the proximal row of the carpus and pronates the carpus. Kuhlmann and Tubiana describe it as an anti-torsion device, and it is indeed a dynamic stabilizer. This concept of the functional anatomy has been confirmed by electromyography: Bordes (1970) and Sirvente (1978) have shown that the extensor carpi ulnaris is the only extensor of the wrist to possess electrical activity during palmar flexion. This anatomical peculiarity also explains how the tendon may subluxate despite an intact extensor retinaculum. Burkhardt et al. (1981), as well as Eckhardt and Palmer (1982), demonstrated this clinically, and also proposed a treatment plan based on the aetiology.

*Note*. It may be asked whether it is appropriate to use the classical term "septum" to define the partitions separating the different compartments, and therefore the different points of anchorage of the retinaculum. In fact, the term is probably incorrect given the fact that the retinaculum is really composed of two sheets, as suggested by Taleisnik et al. (1984).

**Flexor Retinaculum**

This is the anterior annular ligament of the carpus, well-known to surgeons operating for carpal tunnel syndromes. This structure is revealed after resection of the centre of the palmar aponeurosis. It gives the impression of being a reinforcement of the superficial aponeurosis of the forearm, but one may wonder whether it is not truly a structure of the wrist. It supports and stabilizes the carpal tunnel and its division results in laxity of this bony arch. Fisk (1984) showed this by comparing a hundred wrists operated unilaterally for carpal tunnel syndrome: the distance between the pisiform and the scaphoid, measured at the most palmar point using an axial carpal tunnel view, was 3 mm greater on the operated side.

The flexor retinaculum also serves as a point of origin of the different thenar and hypothenar muscles (Table I.2). It is a strong fibrous arch and Razemon (1983) has pointed out that its average thickness is 2–3 mm. It inserts at the margins of the carpal tunnel of which it forms the roof, the hook of the hamate and the tubercle of the trapezium being the two principal points of attachment.

On the ulnar side, the annular ligament forms the floor of the canal of Guyon, whose roof is formed by the fibrous expansion of the flexor carpi ulnaris muscle, the palmaris brevis muscle (or its fibrous equivalent), and by some fibrous expansions de-

Table I.2. Palmar muscles attached to flexor retinaculum

| Muscles | Origin | Insertion |
|---|---|---|
| **a** Radial side | | |
| *Abductor pollicis brevis* | Tubercle of trapezium<br>Transverse carpal ligament | Radial sesamoid at MP I<br>Base of 1st phalanx |
| *Flexor pollicis brevis* | Superficial part: transverse carpal ligament<br>Deep part: trapezium, trapezoid, capitate | Ulnar sesamoid at MP I |
| *Opponens pollicis* | Tubercle of trapezium<br>Transverse carpal ligament | Radial aspect MC I (entire length) |
| *Adductor pollicis* | MC III (entire length), trapezium and trapezoid | Ulnar sesamoid at MP I (as for flexor pollicis brevis) |
| **b** Ulnar side | | |
| Superficial layer | | |
| *Palmaris brevis* | Palmar aponeurosis | Subcutaneous fascia of hypothenar eminence |
| Deep layer | | |
| *Abductor digiti minimi* | Pisiform<br>Transverse carpal ligament | Ulnar side base 5th proximal phalanx |
| *Flexor digiti minimi brevis* | Transverse carpal ligament | Common insertion with abductor digiti minimi |
| *Opponens digiti minimi* | | Ulnar aspect 5th metacarpal |

MC, metacarpal; MP I, first metacarpophalangeal joint

rived from the flexor retinaculum itself. French authors speak of the "volar ligament".

It may be appropriate to recall, with Fahrer (1980), that the FCU is not inserted only into the pisiform, which seems to act as a sesamoid bone, but that it sends further expansions to:
- the annular carpal ligament
- the piso-hamate ligament
- the base of the fifth metacarpal
- the extensor retinaculum

The exact role played by the flexor retinaculum in maintaining the relationships between the carpal bones remains to be determined. Patients in whom the carpal tunnel has been decompressed do not seem to suffer any dynamic functional disabilities, despite the widening of the carpal arch that results. The intra-articular and capsular ligamentous systems of the distal row maintain their integrity and the bones of the proximal row are not directly linked with the flexor retinaculum.

## 3. Anatomical Study: Conclusions (see also Table I.3)

Eight points emerge from this study:

1. The ligamentous system of the wrist is subdivided into two complementary parts: articular and extra-articular.
2. Each system has a dynamic component, the mechanism of which can be direct or indirect. The articular system is directly affected by the dynamic action of the FCU, which is attached to the pisiform. There is also an indirect mechanism involving the extra-articular system, because of the action of the extensor carpi ulnaris on the extensor retinaculum.
3. The general orientation of the fibres of the two ligamentous systems is oblique.
4. The proximal V, a massive, strong supporting band, maintains the lunate in place, and with it the proximal row of the carpus.
5. The distal V joins the radius to the centre of rotation of the carpus (the head of the capitate); it stabilizes the distal and ulnar portions of the proximal row and guides the scaphoid, which it straddles. It acts as a guidance system.
6. The fibres of the superficial and deep systems converge on the triquetrum and the pisiform in a sort of anti-glide lasso, preventing any ulnar displacement.
7. The cohesion of the carpal bones depends only on the articular system; it is true that the extra-articular system reinforces certain functions, but it cannot compensate for deficiencies in the articular system.

**Table I.3.** The two ligamentous systems of the carpus

| Articular System | Extra-articular System |
|---|---|
| Interosseous ligaments (proximal and distal) | Flexor retinaculum<br>Flexor carpi ulnaris |
| Pisiform<br>Triquetrum | |
| Palmar V (proximal and distal)<br>Dorsal V<br>Ulnar complex | Extensor retinaculum<br>Extensor carpi ulnaris |
| Static | Dynamic |

The articular (deep) system has no dynamic components. The extra-articular (superficial) system is influenced by the flexor carpi ulnaris (attached to the pisiform) and the extensor carpi ulnaris (attached to the triquetrum)

8. The distal radio-ulnar joint is a phylogenetic unit united by the ulnocarpal complex.

## C. Kinematics

Radiological analysis of the three-dimensional motion of the carpal bones in relation to the position of the wrist leads to the following conclusions:

1. The bones of the distal carpal row behave as a single unit. Flatt et al. (1983) calculated that, during active motion of the wrist, the relative mobility between the capitate and the third metacarpal, and between the trapezoid and the second metacarpal, did not exceed 2°.
2. The centre of rotation of the carpus is situated in the head of the capitate, an observation made by Fick in 1901. Youm et al. (1978) confirmed this analysis, but went on to state that this point is different in the frontal plane and sagittal plane. It is important to recognize that this point is actually situated on an ellipse, since the position of the capitate is modified by the movements of the proximal row.
3. Although the distal row, including the metacarpals, acts as a single block, the proximal row of the carpus functions more like a chain of ossicles interposed between the radio-ulnar complex and the hand. Harmonious movement of the wrist depends on the cohesion and guidance of this assembly. Therefore it is essential to observe the carpus in motion to understand how it functions and define the roles of the various groups of ligaments.

### 1. Analysis of the Mobility of the Proximal Row in the Frontal Plane

**Ulnar Deviation** (Fig. I.21)

With adduction, the scaphoid assumes an elongated appearance. Its long axis becomes parallel to that of the radius as it becomes more horizontal and its proximal pole glides in a palmar direction. It also exhibits a shift in relation to the lunate; in fact, the proximal pole of the scaphoid is markedly more distal than that of the lunate and the space between these two bones seems to increase. The lunate likewise undergoes a palmar shift, combined with a tilting motion evidenced radiologically by the appearance of a rounding-off. The palmar lip of the lunate, the prominence of which is projected on the shadow of the capitate, appears bulbous. The triquetrum follows the lunate in its movement of palmar shift, and glides under the hamate; the triquetrohamate joint is now no longer parallel to the X-rays, and the articular cleft diminishes or disappears. The triquetrum presents its smallest diameter. The pisiform is projected between the triquetrum and the ulna, its projection indicating the position of

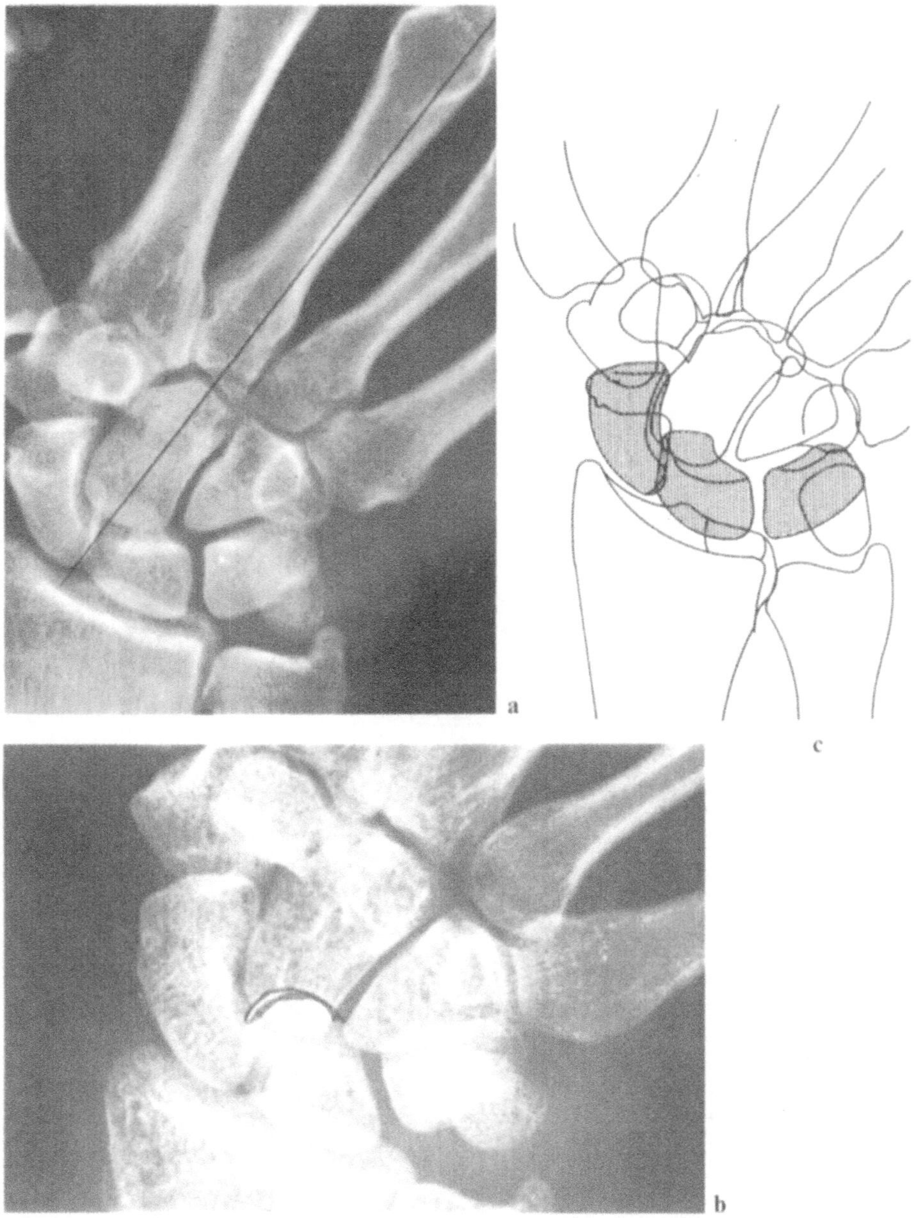

**Fig. I.21 a–c.** Intercarpal relationship in ulnar deviation. **a** Axis of the third metacarpal projected between the scaphoid and lunate. **b** Close-up specifying the exact position of the bones of the proximal row (as shown in **c**). The scaphoid is elongated, with its axis parallel to that of the radius. The palmar translation of the lunate is indicated by its swollen appearance. The triquetrum is short, and the articular cleft between the triquetrum and hamate diminishes or disappears

the triquetrum; it serves as a landmark. The axis of the capitate projects exactly between the scaphoid and the lunate; the body of the latter rests entirely against the radius. The distance between the proximal pole of the capitate and the palmar lip of the radius, measured in the prolongation of the axis of the third metacarpal, is 12 mm in our specimen X-ray.

**Radial Deviation** (Fig. I.22)

The scaphoid now presents its smallest diameter with its axis perpendicular to the longitudinal axis of the radius. With this vertical orientation the proximal pole is drawn upwards and it seems to approximate the proximal pole of the lunate in a distinct shift. The lunate likewise undergoes a movement of as-

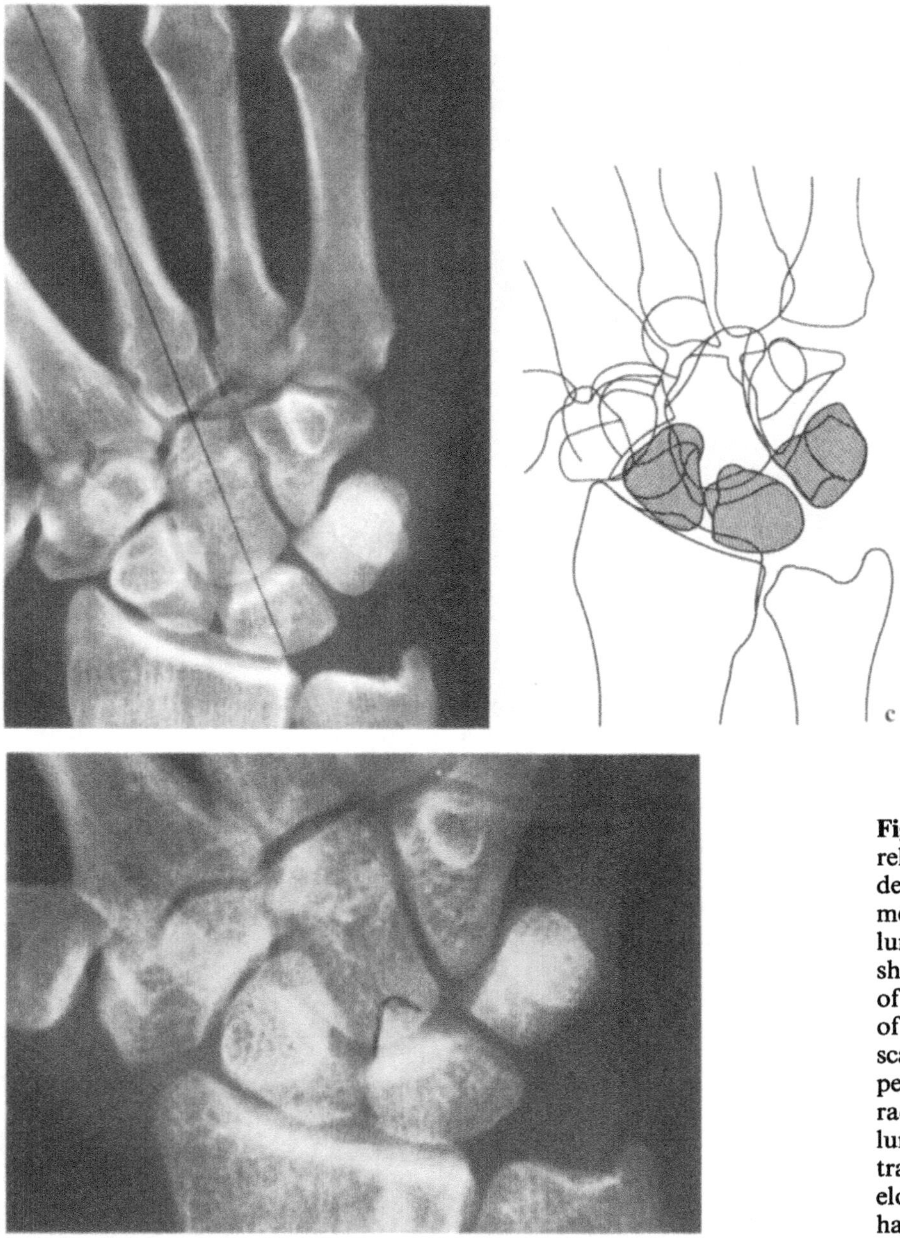

**Fig. I.22 a–c.** Intercarpal relationship in radial deviation. **a** Axis of third metacarpal prolonged through lunate. **b** Close-up clearly shows the pointed appearance of the lunate. **c** Interpretation of the radiograph: the scaphoid is short, with its axis perpendicular to that of the radius. The point of the lunate indicates its dorsal translation. The triquetrum is elongated, and the triquetro-hamate interspace is widened

cent; this is why its pointed dorsal lip is now projected onto the capitate, which it caps slightly. The lunate, in line with the axis of the third metacarpal, abuts partly against the radius and partly against the TFCC. The triquetrum, closely bound to the lunate, also undergoes a dorsal shift. It now presents its greatest diameter, the opposite of the behaviour of the scaphoid. The triquetro-lunate articulation seems wider (orthograde projection?). The pisiform is projected exactly onto the distal pole of the triquetrum, and appears to be very distant from the ulna. The distance between the proximal pole of the capitate and the palmar margin of the radius along the axis of the third metacarpal is 14 mm. This increase in distance corresponds to an increase in diameter of the lunate, an increase in diameter associated with the combined see-saw movement and dorsal shift (bear in mind its asymmetrical shape).

These statements are in agreement with the work of Youm et al. (1978). They demonstrate that the centre of rotation is not identical in the frontal and sagittal planes. Thus, it must be recognized that these two points are located on an ellipse, and that the movements of the carpus are ellipsoidal. The synchronous mobility of the bones of the proximal row make of it an anatomic-pathophysiological unit formed of three modules interdependent on each other. Abnormality of one element has repercussions on the whole complex.

#### Neutral Position

In this projection attention must be focused on the lunate (Fig. I.23). It exhibits a pointed dorsal lip projecting onto the capitate. This triangular lip is evidence of a normal palmar flexion of 5°. In this position, the ulnar third of the lunate rests on the triangular fibrocartilage, and the axis of the capitate is situated between the scaphoid and the lunate.

### 2. Analysis in the Sagittal Plane

Flexion and extension of the wrist depend on the mobility of the radiocarpal and midcarpal articulations. Therefore there are two centres of rotation in the sagittal plane:
- a centre of rotation in the lunate,
- a centre of rotation in the capitate.

The combination of flexion-extension with radial or ulnar deviation implies three points of rotation, mobile in relation to each other. In view of the magnitude of the problems this poses for analysis of carpal movements, it is not surprising that our knowledge is still limited. The solution will undoubtedly be found using three-dimensional analysis, but this calls for considerable financial resources, extremely sophisticated software and powerful computers such as are available in the aerospace industry. Access to these systems is limited, and requires information specialists able to make very costly modifications to existing programs. Hopefully the near future will bring developments that allow us to progress on smaller computer systems. The result of this is that, while the studies of Youm et al. (1978) are still valuable, it is necessary to be aware of their limitations, related to their experimental method.

Our kinematic study allows us to state:
1. The three bones of the proximal carpal row form a functional modular unit.
2. The wrist joint has both rotational and translational components to its motion and therefore does not have a single centre of rotation. The pathways of these centres remain to be defined.

a

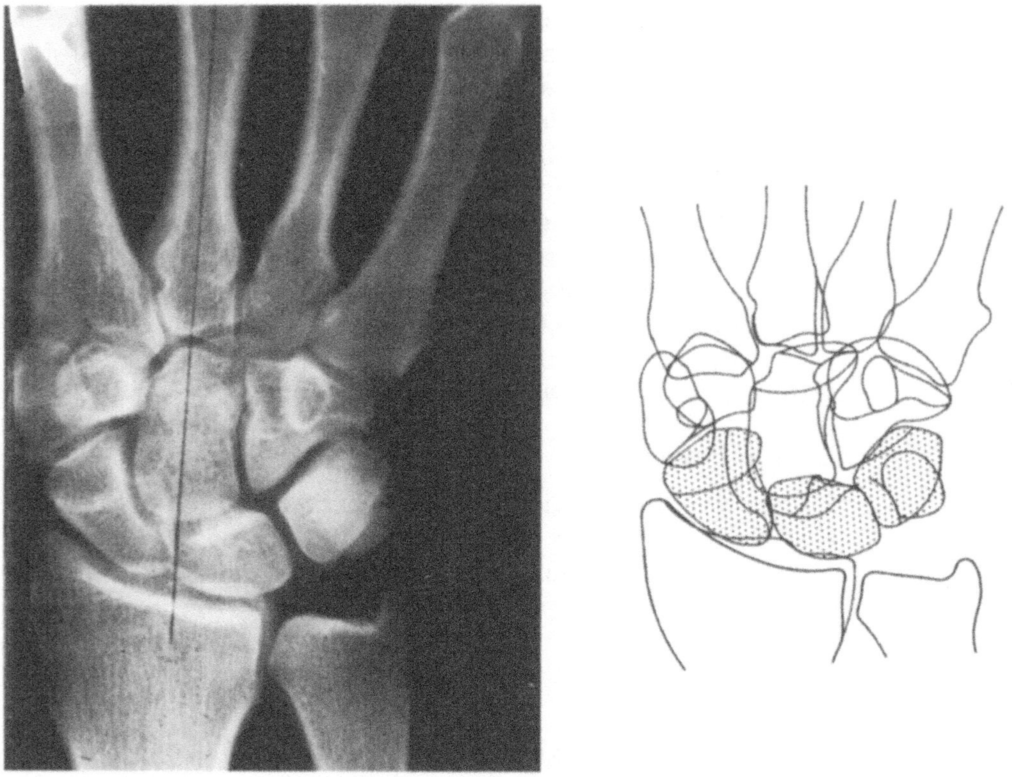

b

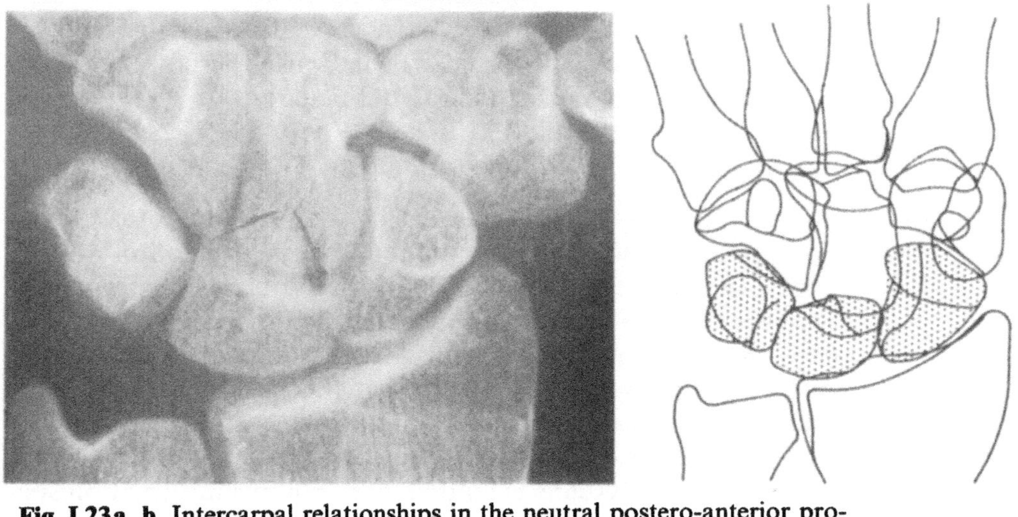

**Fig. I.23a, b.** Intercarpal relationships in the neutral postero-anterior projection. **a** shows that the *axis of the third metacarpal* may be prolonged through the radial third of the lunate. The close-up **b** shows the triangular shape of the dorsal lip of the lunate overhanging the large palmar lip. The pisiform is centred on the triquetrum and the cleft between the scaphoid and the lunate is virtually absent

## D. Functional Ligamentous Anatomy

The proximal row is intrinsically unstable since the centre of rotation of the carpus is located outside the row. This is compounded by the fact that the lunate is not fixed to the capitate and the distal attachments of the scaphoid and the triquetrum are eccentrically placed. Furthermore the lunate itself must be supported against a sloping joint. This support is critical since it is the keystone of two systems:

- a transverse intercalated system, the mobile proximal carpal row;
- an axial mechanical weight-bearing system, transmitting the loads from the hand to the forearm.

This requires that the ligaments simultaneously restrain, stabilize and guide the movements of the carpal bones so they work as a coordinated unit. Therefore we propose to distinguish three types of ligament:

- "restraining" ligaments,
- "stabilizing" ligaments,
- "guiding" ligaments.

### "Restraining" Ligaments

These ligaments allow no motion between the bones they unite and are characteristic for the distal carpal row. Therefore the distal row acts as a single block that may be compared to the radius, and the mobile proximal row is an intercalated system.

### "Stabilizing" Ligaments

These ligaments must allow motion but still maintain the correct spatial relationships between the bones; functions that may appear contradictory! In this category we find:

- the interosseous ligaments of the proximal carpal row,
- the deep layers of the proximal and distal V.

The oblique orientation of the fibres of the interosseous ligaments of the proximal carpal row allows for coordinated, differential motion between the bones they unite.

This principle of obliquity is found in the two V ligaments. The spiral orientation of the deep part of these two ligaments – as seen in Fig. I.15 – allows differential application of tension to the distal and proximal Vs. Part of the ligament system is always under tension and this alternation ensures cohesive, coordinated movement of the bones of the wrist, in the absence of active elements.

The result is a continuous and progressive transfer of tension between the distal V and proximal V systems. The distal V, which ensures the position of the capitate, is attached beyond the centre of rotation, and is therefore placed under tension during ulnar deviation. The resulting pressure modifies the position of the lunate in relation to the scaphoid, which is possible thanks to the concomitant relaxation of the proximal V. This relaxation allows the lunate to glide palmarwards and dorsiflex.

Conversely, during radial deviation, the distal V relaxes, since the distance between its insertion and the radial styloid decreases, while the proximal V becomes taut, raising the lunate and scaphoid, which palmarflex. Furthermore, the spiral arrangement of the ligaments limits the amplitude of these movements. Obviously the system functions properly only with an intact ligamentous system and normal bony architecture.

### "Guiding" Ligaments

This role is allotted to the superficial fibres of the distal V for they keep the distance between the radius and the capitate constant. The superficial fibres of the proximal V, stretched between the ulnar styloid and the outer third of the radius, have a similar role since they keep the lunate in place. These "guiding" ligaments simultaneously centre both the capitate and the lunate.

### Conclusion

Each carpal ligament is integrated into a complex system which controls the excursion and smoothness of motion between the carpal bones. Such a sophisticated mechanism is susceptible to an infinite variety of lesions. This is why the development of arthrosis, though inevitable in cases of instability, occurs at such a variable rate.

## E. The Concept of Stability

### History

In 1919 Navarro (1937) proposed dividing the wrist joint into three functional columns (Fig. I.24), a central column for flexion and extension and two lateral columns for rotation. The central column was formed by the hamate, capitate and lunate, thanks to the strong ligamentous system which unites them. The radial rotatory column consisted of the scaphoid, trapezium and trapezoid, while the ulnar rotatory column was represented by the triquetrum alone.

Based on the fact that the scaphoid seems to bridge the two carpal rows, and stating that the mechanism of the wrist joint can be compared to a single link, Gilford et al. (1943) defined the scaphoid role:

- it stabilizes the proximal row in relation to the distal,
- it limits the movements of the proximal carpal row thanks to a triangular system.

Fisk, in 1970, used this work as the basis for his explanation of the collapse of the carpus after scaphoid fractures. Taleisnik, in 1976, modified Navarro's concept (Fig. I.25). Like Bryce, he stated that the scaphoid is not firmly fixed to the trapezium or the trapezoid, and concluded that the two rotatory columns consist only of the scaphoid and the triquetrum. Thus, the central column of flexion-extension becomes a "T", whose transverse limb consists of the entire distal row, and whose longitudinal limb is the capitate and lunate.

Lichtmann et al., in 1981, disputed Taleisnik's analysis. According to them, the proximal row, the lunate in particular, is not joined to the capitate; there cannot therefore be a stabilizing longitudinal limb. On the contrary, the lunate moves with the scaphoid and triquetrum. For these authors the proximal row must be considered as a functional unit, and its stability is explained according to the concept proposed by Gilford et al. (Fig. I.26).

We may conclude by stating that two theories of stability currently exist:

- The first postulates a central flexion-extension column and two lateral mobile rotatory columns. This is the concept of longitudinal stability.
- The second conceives of the proximal row as an intercalated row, stabilized by the scaphoid as a link, due to its privileged position.

### Discussion

Taleisnik's theory is unsatisfactory on an anatomical basis. In fact, no ligament of any significance exists between the lunate and the capitate. As described by Bonnel and Allieu (1984), this region represents an area of weak ligaments. Our own dissections have led us to similar conclusions. Thus, the anatomy is not consistent with the theory of a central column of flexion-extension.

Lichtmann's theory is attractive. Radiological examination of the wrist in radial and ulnar deviation demonstrates the mobility of the bones of the proximal row of the carpus; motion that is certainly complex, but synchronous. But the theory does not account for stability. The slope of the radial socket and the axial forces act to sublux the lunate palmarwards. This subluxation occurs as soon as the attachments between the lunate and the radius are cut. Thus, a theory which makes the scaphoid the only factor stabilizing and controlling the proximal row is inexact. We therefore regard Lichtmann's theory as incomplete, and that of Gilford as superseded. Thus, no satisfactory concept to explain the stability and cohesion of the carpus yet exists.

### Ligamentous Anatomy

Let us recall the essential conclusions from our dissections, in order to elaborate a concept of stability:

- the absence of a ligament between the lunate and capitate,
- the existence of the massive proximal V, a strap supporting the lunate,
- the absence of a longitudinal ligamentous system,
- the cohesion of the carpal bones, depending only on the articular ligaments (the extra-articular ligaments may reinforce certain functions, but cannot replace them).

Fig. I.24. Navarro

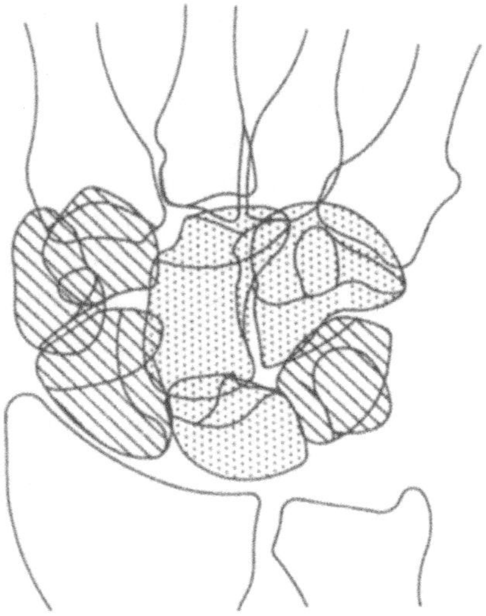

*Rotation:*
scaphoid
trapezium
trapezoid
triquetrum

*Stability:*
hamate
capitate
lunate

**Fig. I.24.** Navarro's concept: *cross-hatched areas* constitute the rotatory columns, the lunate-capitate joint carries out flexion-extension

**Fig. I.25.** Taleisnik's concept: the rotatory column consists of the scaphoid and triquetrum only. The lunate-capitate joint carries out flexion-extension; the distal row is a single unit

**Fig. I.26.** Lichtmann's concept: the distal row acts as a single unit; the proximal row is mobile, stabilization of the proximal row occurs according to Gilford's principle

**Fig. I.25.** Taleisnik

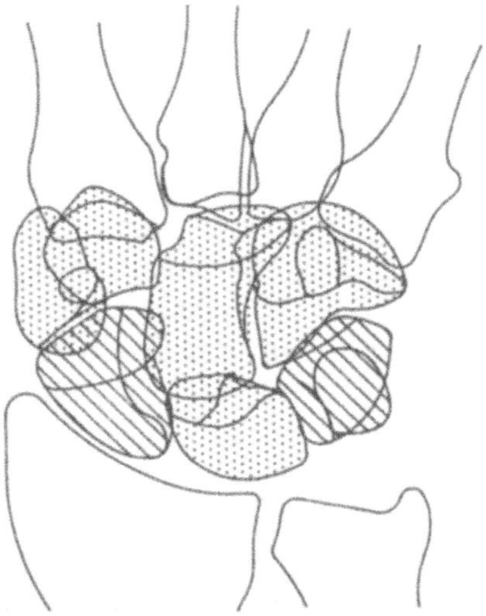

*Rotation:*
scaphoid
triquetrum

*Stability:*
hamate
capitate
lunate
trapezium
trapezoid

**Fig. I.26.** Lichtmann

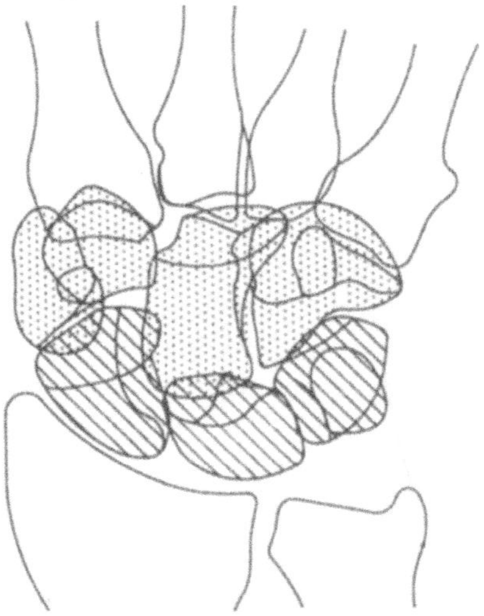

*Rotation:*
scaphoid
lunate
triquetrum

*Stability:*
hamate
capitate
trapezium
trapezoid

**Observation of the Stretched Carpus** (Fig. I.27)

Observation of the radiological image obtained by stretching a normal undissected wrist with an external fixator raises three interesting points:

- the lunate remains close to the radius,
- the scaphoid is fixed to the capitate in its distal portion,
- the triquetrum tends to remain with the hamate-capitate group.

**Concept of Stability** (Fig. I.28)

The centres of rotation of the wrist are situated within the head of the capitate, and thus in the rigid part of the carpus, for this bone is solidly attached to the adjacent hamate, trapezium and trapezoid. The mobile portion, i.e. the proximal row, is intrinsically unstable because of the eccentric distal centre of rotation. Furthermore, because of the slopes of the radial socket, against which it rests proximally, there is a tendency to sublux palmarly and ulnarly. The result is a modular articular chain in the form of a semicircle, exhibiting a double instability that is:

- dynamic, because of its centre of rotation,
- anatomic, because of the double inclination of the radial glenoid socket.

To stabilize such a system, proximal and distal anchorage are required. The proximal system must neutralize the anatomic factors and the distal system, the dynamic. Axial stabilization is impossible, since the central anatomical structures are oblique, and there are no elements directly attaching the lunate to the capitate. Thus, there cannot be a central axis as Navarro and Taleisnik propose. The absence of any ligamentous structure

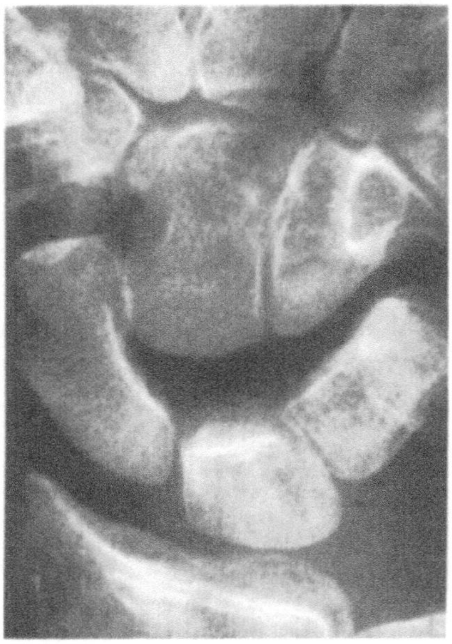

**Fig. I.27.** View of stretched carpus: the lunate is adherent to the radius, the distal part of the scaphoid is fixed to the capitate, and the triquetrum is attached to the hamate

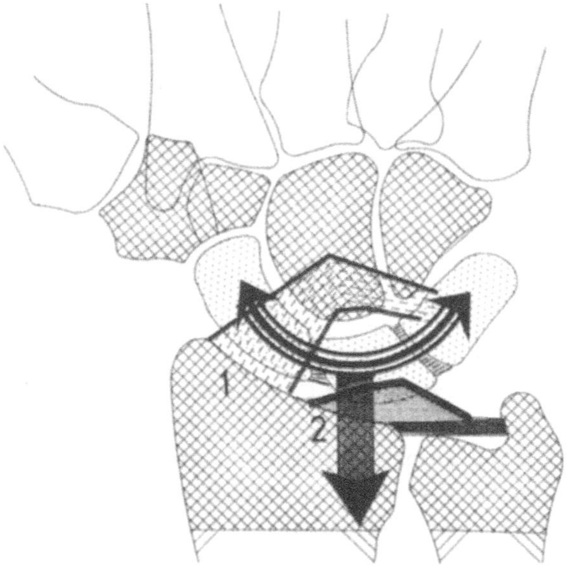


**Fig. I.28.** Concept of stability: the proximal V stabilizes the lunate, which becomes a load-bearing component; the proximal interosseous ligaments maintain the relationships of the proximal row, a unit with differential mobility; the distal V is a guidance and control system for the wings of the proximal row.
*1* distal V
*2* proximal V

between the scapho-lunate couple and the capitate likewise vitiates Gilford's theory, and renders Lichtmann's schema inexact.

In fact, we have established that there exists a strong ligamentous structure stretched between the middle third of the radius on the palmar side and the ulnar styloid. This massive structure supports the lunate, and resists its gliding along the slope of the radial articular surface. The orientation and disposition of its fibres allow the mobility required during the different movements of the wrist. It is worth stressing that this proximal V not only fixes the proximal pole of the lunate, but also sends ramifications to the proximal pole of the scaphoid and triquetrum thus reinforcing the interosseous ligaments.

Dorsally, the lunate is fixed to the distal bundle of the dorsal V, which supports and reinforces the scapho-triquetral interosseous ligaments. Thus, the lunate acts as the keystone of the wrist. It is the centre of two systems: on one hand, it is the intermediate element transmitting the forces of axial pressure and on the other, it is the central stabilizing element of the mobile proximal row.

However, the mobility of this modular system calls for precise guidance. This role is played by the distal V. It stabilizes the two ends of this intercalated unit at the centre of rotation of the carpus. Furthermore, on the radial side, it maintains a constant distance between the head of the capitate and the radius, which implies an extremely mobile and intact scaphoid. Loss of the mobility of the scaphoid or disharmony in its movements gives rise to excessive local pressure, which may lead to degenerative changes.

## Conclusions

The lunate is the keystone of the carpus:

1. It stabilizes the transverse intercalated unit, which is mobile and unstable.
2. It withstands the axial mechanical forces transmitted from the hand to the forearm.

This double role is guaranteed by the proximal interosseous ligaments, responsible for maintaining spatial relationship, and by the V ligaments, responsible for guidance of these intercalated elements.

## References

Bonnel F, Allieu Y (1984) Les articulations radio-cubito-carpienne et médio-carpienne. Organisation anatomique et bases biomécaniques. Ann Chir Main 3:287–296

Bordes JP (1970) La prono-supination. Etude anatomique. Restauration chirurgicale dans la polyarthrite chez l'adulte. Thesis, Toulouse

Burkhardt SS, Wood MB, Linscheid R (1981) Posttraumatic recurrent subluxation of the extensor carpi ulnaris tendon. J Hand Surg 6:629–631

Eckhardt WA, Palmer AK (1982) Recurrent dislocation of extensor carpi ulnaris tendon. J Hand Surg 7:1–3

Fahrer M (1980) L'éminence hypothénar. In: Tubiana R (ed), Traité de chirurgie de la main, vol 1. Masson, Paris, p 294

Fick R (1901) Ueber die Bewegung in den Handgelenken. Abh Math Phys D Wissensch Math-Phys 26:429–468

Fisk GR (1970) Carpal instability and the fractured scaphoid. Ann R Coll Surg Engl: 46:63–76

Fisk GR (1984) Influence du ligament annulaire antérieur du carpe (flexor retinaculum) sur la stabilité du carpe. Ann Chir Main 3:297–299

Flatt AE, Youm Y, Berger RA (1983) Les mécanismes des mouvements du poignet humain. In: Razemon JP, Fisk GR (eds) Le poignet. Expansion Scientifique Française, Paris, pp 53–61

Gilford WW, Bolton RH, Lambrinudi C (1943) The mechanism of the wrist joint with special reference to fractures of the scaphoid. Guy's Hosp Rep 92:52–59

Kapandji IA (1983) L'articulation radio-cubitale inférieure, anatomie fonctionnelle. In: Razemon JP, Fisk GR (eds) Le poignet. Expansion Scientifique Française, Paris, pp 42–52

Kauer JMF (1975) Note sur le développement du ligament triangulaire chez l'homme. Bull Assoc Anat 59:893

Kauer JMF (1980) Functional anatomy of the wrist. Clin Orthop 149:9–20

Kuhlmann JN, Tubiana R (1983) Mécanisme du poignet normal. In: Razemon JP, Fisk GR (eds) Le poignet. Expansion Scientifique Française. Paris, pp 62–71

Lewis OJ, Hamshere R, Buck Nill TM (1970) The anatomy of the wrist joint. J Anat 106:539–552

Lichtmann DM, Schneider JR, Swafford AR, Mack GR (1981) Ulnar midcarpal instability – Clinical and laboratory analysis. J Hand Surg 6:515–523

Mayfield JK, Williams WJ (1979) Biomechanical properties of human carpal ligaments. Orthop Trans 3:143

Mikic DZ (1978) Age changes in the triangular fibrocartilage of the wrist joint. J Anat 126: 367–384

Navarro A (1937) Anatomia y fisiologia del carpo. Ann Inst Clin Quir Chir Exp 1:162–250

Palmer AK, Werner FW (1981) The triangular fibrocartilage complex of the wrist – Anatomy and function. J Hand Surg 6:153–162

Palmer AK, Glisson RR, Werner FW, Mech ME (1984) Relationship between ulnar variance and triangular fibrocartilage complex thickness. J Hand Surg 9A:681–683
Palmer AK, Skahen JR, Werner FW, Glisson R (1985) The extensor retinaculum of the wrist: anatomical and biomechanical study. J Hand Surg 10B:11–16
Razemon JP (1983) Traitement chirurgical du syndrome du canal carpien (à propos de 520 observations). In: Razemon JP, Fisk GR (eds) Le poignet. Expansion Scientifique Française, Paris, p 175
Sirvente C (1978) Contribution à l'étude de l'anatomie fonctionnelle du cubital postérieur. Thesis, Toulouse
Taleisnik J (1976) The ligament of the wrist. J Hand Surg 1:110–118
Taleisnik J, Gelbermann RH, Miller BW, Szabo RM (1984) The extensor retinaculum of the wrist. J Hand Surg 9A:495–501
Weigl K, Spira E (1969) The triangular fibrocartilage of the wrist joint. Reconstr Surg Traumatol 11:139–153
Youm Y, McMurthry RY, Flatt AE, Gillespie TE (1978) Kinematics of the wrist. J Bone Joint Surg [Am] 60:423–431. PN 41

CHAPTER II

# Diagnosis of Osteo-ligamentous Lesions of the Carpus

The evaluation of wrist pain is based on a thorough knowledge of regional anatomy and pathological conditions. However, before thinking of some subtle, difficult to demonstrate lesion of a complex ligamentous system, the clinician has to take a careful, systematic and complete history. It is important to exclude congenital and metabolic disorders (diabetes, gout, chondrocalcinosis), avascular osteonecrosis of the lunate, rheumatic diseases, snapping tendon syndrome (especially the extensor carpi ulnaris), tenosynovitis (de Quervain) or carpal tunnel syndrome. A minor traumatic event may cause a microscopic cyst, a carpal boss or a pre-existing arthrosis to become symptomatic. It may also produce a tenosynovitis or allow detection of pre-existing intra-osseous bone cysts or ligamentous lesion.

## History

When investigating trauma from sport or work, the history is one of the essential steps in the intellectual process; the events must be clearly defined with an attempt to determine whether there has been:

1. Swelling, and its time of onset (a haematoma causes early, and oedema more delayed swelling), site and extent
2. Treatment, including its nature and duration
3. A latent period without pain or discomfort
4. Other previous injury

It is then necessary to analyse the type of disturbance, especially with regard to:

1. Pain; whether at rest or only on exertion, diurnal variation (maximal at the end of the day or minimal on rest days), or associated with certain movements (dorsi- or palmar flexion or pronation-supination)
2. Reduced mobility, jolting phenomenon
3. Reduced strength with giving way
4. Swelling, and its timing and severity
5. Sensory disturbance, such as occurs in carpal tunnel syndrome

However, usually everything is vague, diffuse and indefinable. An exception is the snapping and "click" typical of a scapholunate dissociation as seen in the patient of Fig. III.4.

*Note.* One should bear in mind that lesions of the elbow or shoulder are always evident on the day of the accident; these too result from a fall broken by the hyperextended wrist. So, in the presence of an injury of the elbow or shoulder, one must give some thought to the wrist, which may have minor symptoms by comparison. It is by no means rare to encounter patients treated for the elbow who subsequently complain about their wrists.

## A. Physical Examination

This requires complete relaxation and begins with careful inspection for specific areas of swelling, warmth or obvious deformity. Palpation then seeks to localize precisely, to a specific anatomic structure if possible, any swelling or tenderness in order to exclude a carpal boss, an ordinary cyst, an entrapment syndrome, a rheumatic disease or neuritis. Phalen's test, i.e. holding the wrist in forced flexion for at least 2 min, should be done routinely, to rule out a carpal tunnel syndrome.

Finally, having performed this examination, the wrist is moved passively in the search for an abnormal "snapping", "clicking" or "drawer" sign. This mobilization is accompanied by palpation of the different bones of the proximal row, which may reveal abnormal mobility or a tender point (particularly in the anatomical snuffbox or in the articular clefts separating the lunate from the scaphoid and triquetrum). One should conclude by endeavouring to obtain the radiographs made on the day of injury, since the X-rays are decisive in the diagnosis; the ability to compare serial film is valuable in assessing the course of the lesion.

## B. Radiology

This assumes major importance in view of the frequent paucity of clinical findings. However, it is laborious, and the value of the different techniques varies so it is important to define its possibilities and limitations. Techniques that are currently available are classical radiography, arthrography, CT scanning, xerography, scintigraphy and cineradiography. Interpretation of these various examinations calls for a comprehensive understanding of anatomy and function. Their limitations are due to the fact that we are dealing with an analysis of Chinese shadows. In the final analysis it is up to the doctor to interpret them and to decide whether the lesion is bony or ligamentous or a combination of the two. An eclectic approach is therefore essential.

### Routine Projections

These are the postero-anterior (frontal) and lateral views. However, if the radiological examination is intended to confirm a ligamentous lesion, it must be reproducible in order to determine:

- the angles of inclination of the radius (frontal dorsal and frontal palmar)
- the sagittal angle of inclination of the radius
- the carpal height ratio (Youm)
- the carpal-ulnar distance ratio
- the positions of the bones of the proximal row and the width of the joint-spaces (Figs. I.21, I.22 and I.23)
- the radio-lunate, scapho-lunate and capitate-lunate angles

This requires precise conditions. The hand must always be in the neutral position, as the least deviation provokes a see-saw movement of the bones of the proximal row. Valid conclusions can only be drawn from a defined position:

1. The axis of the third metacarpal must be aligned with the prolongation of the axis of the radius, i.e. the natural rest position (Fig. II.1).
2. The transverse axis of the hand must always be parallel to the axis of the humerus, i.e. in a position intermediate between pronation and supination, as shown in Fig. II.2a and b; this is the zero position. It is rare for a patient to be unable to place the hand in this position; however, it is common for pronation-supination to be restricted; thus all the patients would be excluded from possible studies if radiographs in full supination or pronation were required.
3. The metacarpophalangeal (MP) joints must be seen on all the films, both in the frontal and lateral views. It is essential to know the length of the third metacarpal in order to calculate Youm's index from the postero-anterior view and to analyse the axes in the lateral film (Figs. II.1 and II.2).

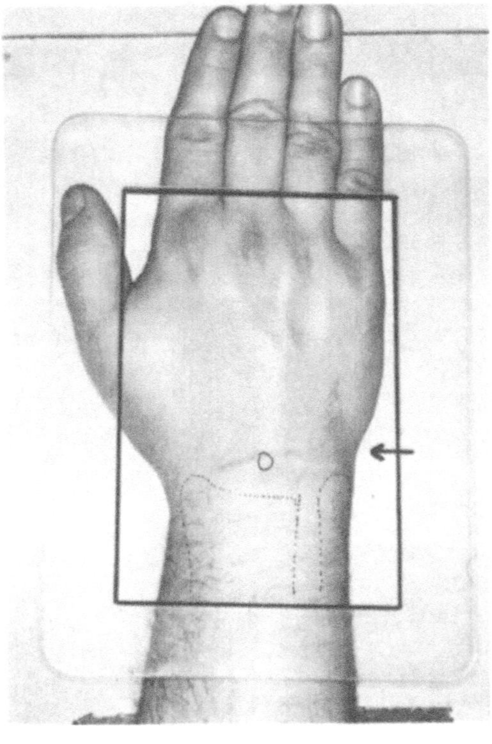

**Fig. II.1.** Radiographic technique. The hand is flat, fingers straight (MP joints at 0°), axis of third metacarpal (MC) is aligned with radius. Beam is centred on lunate but includes MC heads

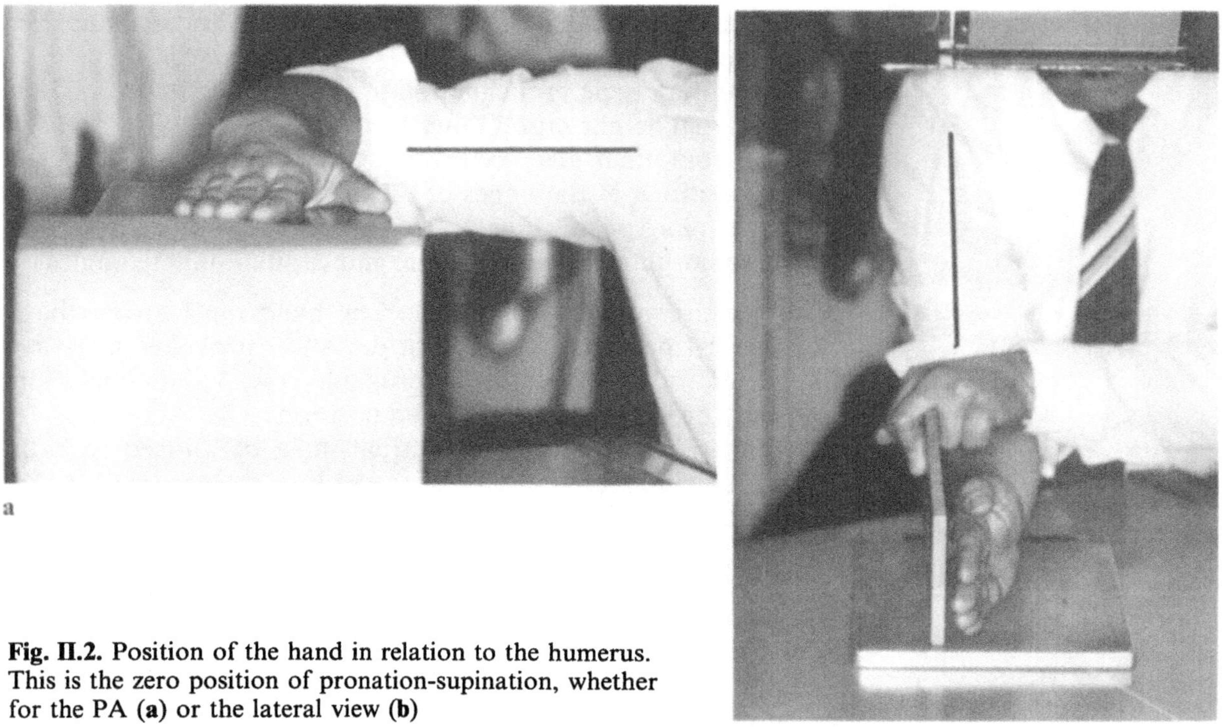

a

b

**Fig. II.2.** Position of the hand in relation to the humerus. This is the zero position of pronation-supination, whether for the PA (**a**) or the lateral view (**b**)

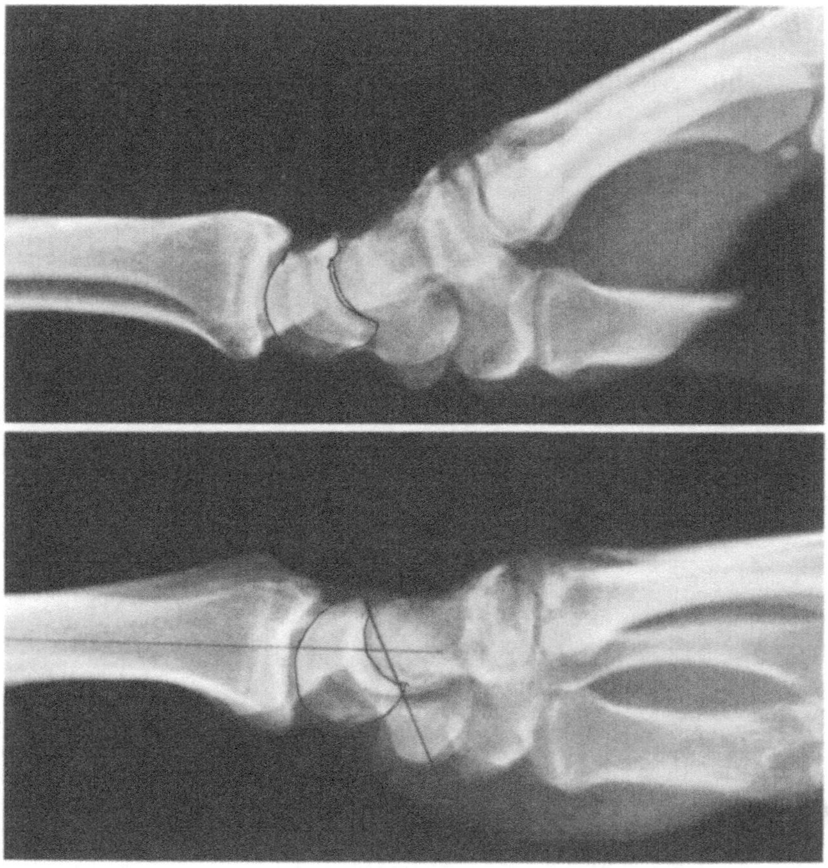

a

b

**Fig. II.3. a** View without the use of a guide. The position of the lunate appears normal. **b** With a guide: palmar subluxation of the lunate is now evident

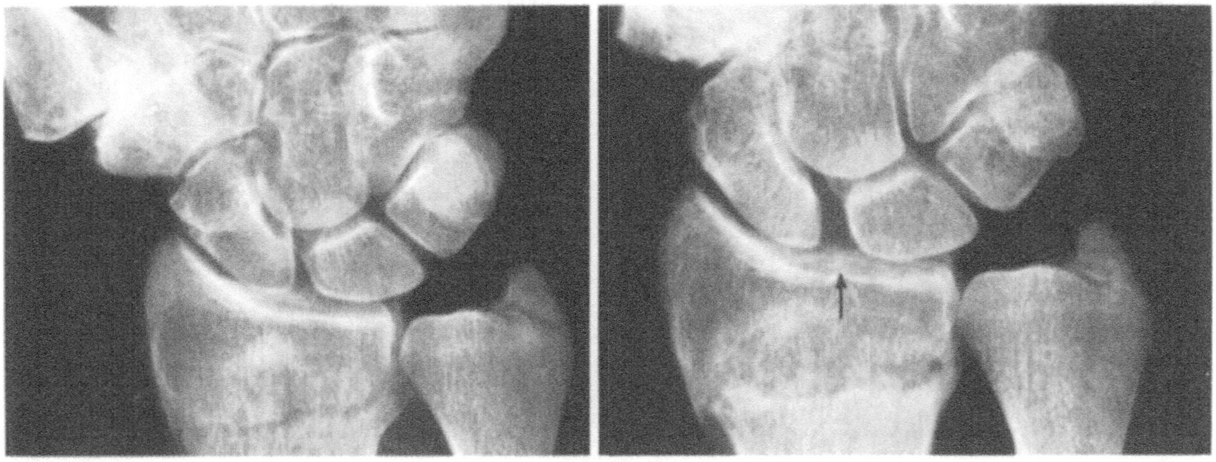

a b

**Fig. II.4. a** Classical view with the hand flat. The scapholunar cleft appears normal. **b** With a 20° upward tilt of the ulnar border of the hand, the scapho-lunate dissociation becomes evident (see Fig. III.3b for line of lesion)

4. The films must be centred on the lunate (Fig. II.1).
5. The presumably normal wrist must be X-rayed at the same time and in the same manner, to provide a reference. This prevents simple anatomical variants from being regarded as abnormal (ligamentous laxity may vary with the individual and the sex).
6. The routine lateral view is worthless unless it is taken with the use of a guide exactly aligning the axis of the radius with that of the capitate and third metacarpal (Fig. II.3).
7. It is sometimes useful to raise the ulnar border of the hand by 20°. The articular faces of the lunate and scaphoid are then parallel to the X-ray beam, and the space between these two bones can be measured easily (Fig. II.4), as noted by Moneim (1981).

Having standardized the projections, we can now define the different parameters required for the recognition of a static instability, first in the postero-anterior and then in the lateral views.

*Postero-anterior View*

In the neutral position, i.e. with the hand placed flat on the X-ray table, we can determine:

1. *The frontal inclination of the distal radial epiphysis.* The frontal angle of inclination is defined by the intersection of the perpendicular to the axis of the radius and the line drawn between the most distal medial and lateral points of the distal radial epiphysis. Normally, this defines the dorsal frontal angle, which is less than the palmar frontal angle. In cases of fracture, when comparative measurements are required, it is necessary to precisely define the dorsal and palmar reference points on the medial side of the radial epiphysis. With fracture impaction and dorsal angulation, the dorsal medial corner will become proximal to the apex of the palmar medial corner. Failure to recognize this trap results in underestimation of the actual degree of tilt (see Fig. II.5a, b).

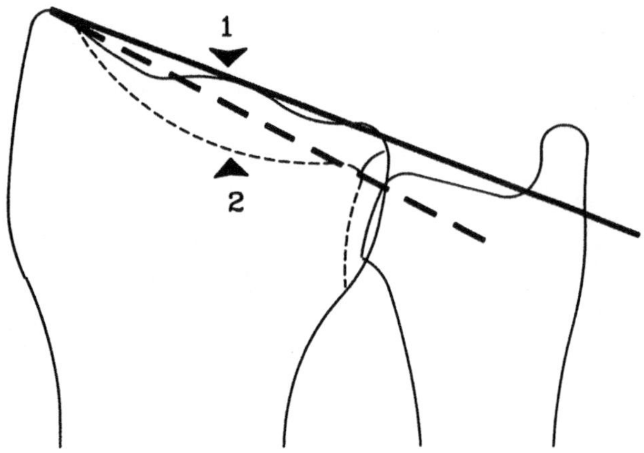


**Fig. II.5a.** Articular axes of distal radius, frontal plane:
*1* dorsal margin and dorsal frontal axis
*2* palmar margin and palmar frontal axis

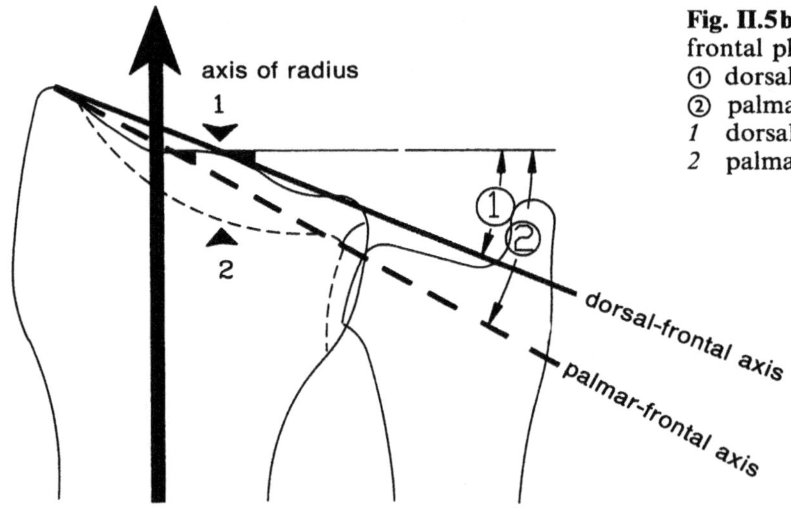


**Fig. II.5b.** Angles of inclination; distal radius, frontal plane:
① dorsal frontal angle
② palmar frontal angle
*1* dorsal lip of radius
*2* palmar lip of radius

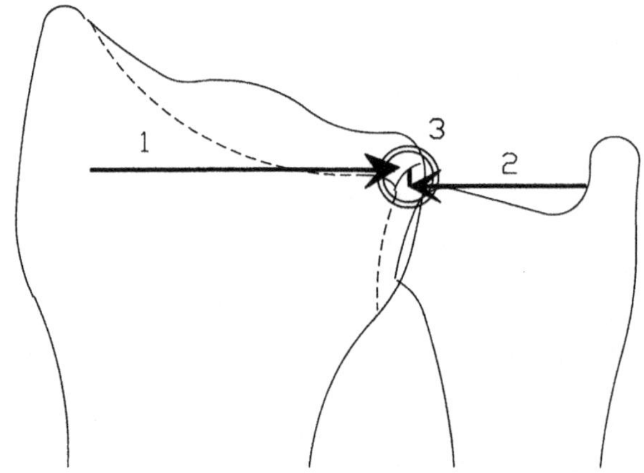


**Fig. II.5c.** Measurement of radio-ulnar index:
*1* radial point of measurement
*2* ulnar point of measurement
*3* radio-ulnar index

**Fig. II.6.** Carpal height ratio defined as:
$L2/L1 = 0.54 \pm 0.03$

**Fig. II.7.** Carpal-ulnar distance ratio:
$L3/L1 = 0.30 \pm 0.03$
*1* axis of the ulna drawn through its middle

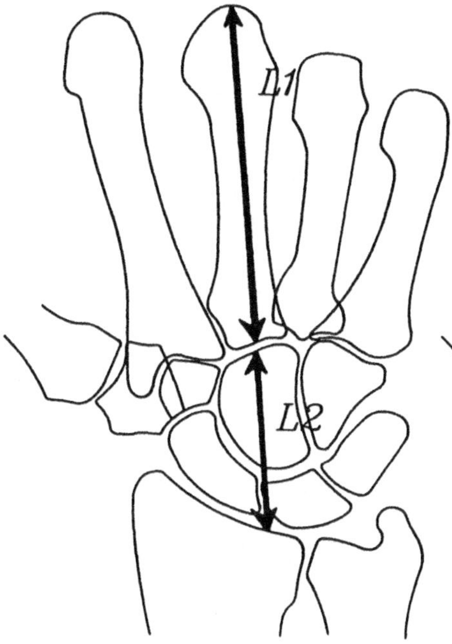


**Fig. II.6**

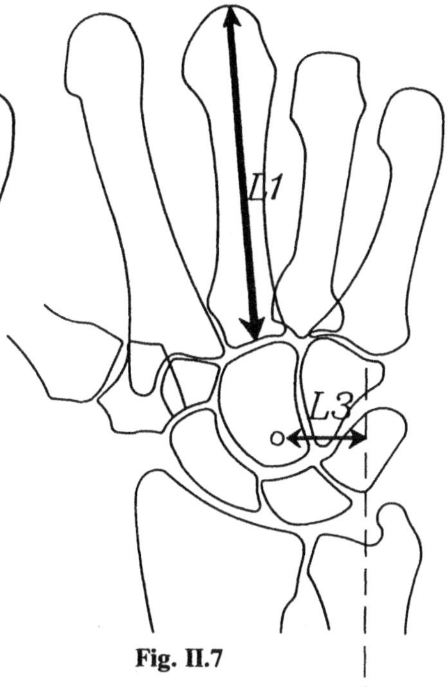


**Fig. II.7**

2. *The radio-ulnar index.* This is defined as the distance separating two straight lines perpendicular to the longitudinal axes of the two forearm bones: the first is defined by the most distal point of the radius on its ulnar side, while the second corresponds to the distal articular surface of the ulna. However, this classical definition is imprecise; to be more exact on the distal radius, one must choose the point situated equidistant between the two medial corners, palmar and dorsal, of the radial socket (Fig. II.5c).

3. *The carpal height ratio.* This index is defined by ratio $L2/L1$; where $L1$ is the radiological length of the third metacarpal, and $L2$ the distance between the edge of the radius and the joint between the capitate and the third metacarpal; it is measured on the line that prolongs the axis of the third metacarpal. Normally, this index amounts to $0.54 \pm 0.03$ (Fig. II.6). Unfortunately, $L2$ is an uncertain measurement, Youm speaks of the "distal" edge of the radius without stating whether this is palmar or dorsal. The values of his index correspond to the palmar margin. A similar uncertainty exists for the proximal and distal points of $L1$.

4. *The carpal-ulnar distance ratio.* This is defined by the formula $L3/L1$, where $L3$ is the horizontal distance from the centre of rotation of the carpus (head of capitate) to the straight line obtained by prolonging the axis of the ulna, drawn through its middle. This index amounts to $0.30 \pm 0.03$ (Fig. II.7).

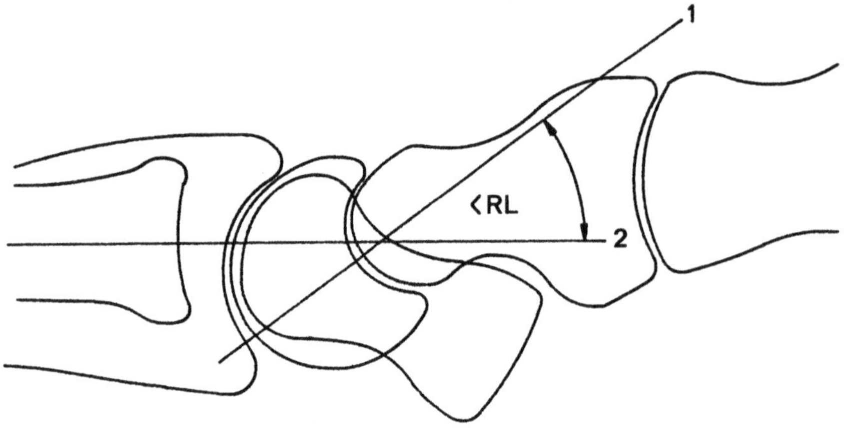


**Fig. II.8.** Radio-lunate angle (< RL):
normal = $-5°$
DISI $> +10°$
PISI $> -20°$
*1* lunate axis
*2* radial axis

*Lateral View*

This must be a strict lateral, with superimposition of the heads of the second and third metacarpals and projection of the head of the ulna on the radius (Fig. II.3b). The beam is centred on the lunate. In order to obtain the alignment of the axis of the metacarpals, one must have the help of a guide, and observe the neutral position of the hand. Under these conditions, it is possible to verify the sagittal inclination of the radius and to analyse the radio-lunate, capitate-lunate and scapho-lunate angles.

1. *Sagittal inclination of the distal radius.* This is defined by the intersection of the perpendicular to the axis of the radius with the straight line drawn between the two most distal points, palmar and dorsal, of the distal radial epiphysis.

2. *Radio-lunate angle.* This is determined by the intersection of the axis of the radius and the axis of the lunate. The angle is said to be in dorsiflexion when the two lips of the lunate point to the dorsal surface of the hand (see Fig. II.8). According to Meyrueis (1984), the normal angle of the lunate is 5° of palmar flexion, i.e. $-5°$. Instability is said to be diagnostic of "dorsal intercalated segmental instability" (DISI) as soon as the angle of dorsiflexion exceeds 15° (Linscheid et al.

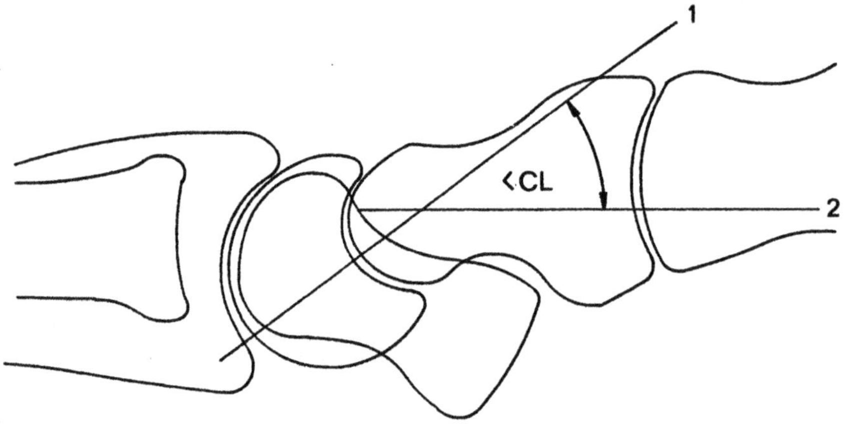


**Fig. II.9.** Capitate-lunate angle (< CL):
*1* axis of lunate
*2* axis of capitate

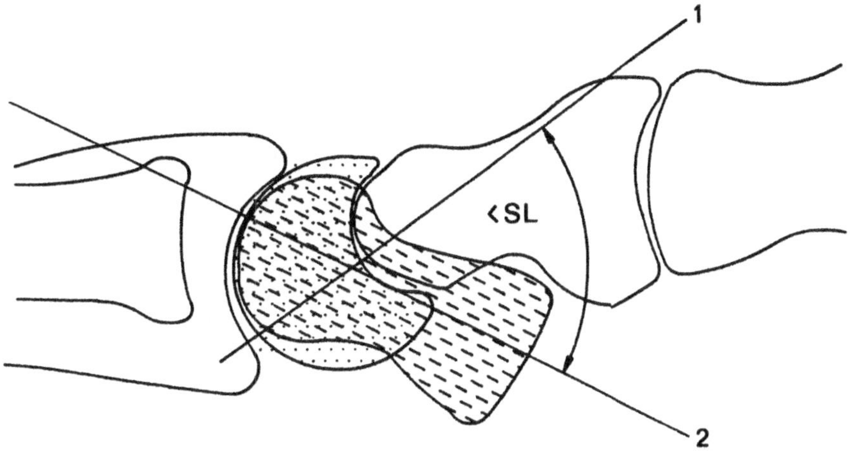


**Fig. II.10.** Scapho-lunate angle (<SL):
For the SL angle
mean value 47°
norm 30°–60°
values above 70° are abnormal
*1* axis of lunate
*2* axis of scaphoid

1972), and to be "palmar intercalated segmental instability" (PISI) as soon as the angle of palmar flexion exceeds −20°. The radio-lunate angle is essentially an index of the state of the ligaments of the proximal V. The greater the disruption of the deep fibres of the proximal V, the more pathological this angle becomes.

3. *The capitate-lunate angle*. This is defined by the intersection of the axis of the lunate with the axis of the capitate (Fig. II.9).
   In principle, the axis of the capitate is parallel to that of the radius, so that the capitate-lunate angle should be the same as the radio-lunate angle. However, Sarrafian et al. (1977) showed this was not always the case. In the presence of instability a certain degree of participation of the capitate in the deformity is possible and this makes interpretation of the measurements difficult; dorsal subluxation, as evident in Fig. II.3b, indicates the difficulties in interpretation, and we should add that the axis of the capitate is not as easy to define as the axis of the radius.

4. *The scapho-lunate angle*. This is determined by the intersection of the axis of the scaphoid and the axis of the lunate (Fig. II.10).
   Its normal value lies between 30° and 60° according to Dobyns et al. (1975), with an average of 47°. Values above 70° are definitely abnormal. It is important to know this angle, as it permits an assessment of the state of the scapho-lunate ligament. However, it is sometimes difficult to determine the axis of the scaphoid as the contours of the bones are blurred by the lunate.

*Note*. Before concluding study of these X-rays, one should follow the example of Bellinghausen et al. (1983) in seeking a break in the arcs defining the concavity and convexity of the three bones of the proximal row.

Tables II.1 and II.2 summarise the data provided by standard radiology.

**Table II.1.** Compilation of radiographic values

**a.** PA view

| | Normal values | Anatomical variations |
|---|---|---|
| Frontal inclination | 25° | 13–30° |
| Radio-ulnar index | $0 \pm 2$ mm | $\pm 2$ mm |
| Youm's index: | | |
| 1. Carpal height | $L2/L1 = 0.54$ | $\pm 0.03$ |
| 2. Carpal-ulnar distance ratio | $L3/L1 = 0.30$ | $\pm 0.03$ |
| Space between bones | $<2$ mm | $\pm 1$ mm |
| 3 Bony arcs | Congruent | – |

**b** Lateral view

| Angles | Normal values | Pathological |
|---|---|---|
| Radio-lunate | $-5°$ Palmar flexion | $> +10°$ (DISI)<br>$> -20°$ (PISI) |
| Capitate-lunate | $-5°$ Palmar flexion | |
| Scapho-lunate | 47° (30°–60°) | $>70°$ |

**c** Dynamic films

| Mobility (%) | Flexion | Extension |
|---|---|---|
| Radiocarpal | 40% | 60% |
| Intercarpal | 60% | 40% |

$L1$, length of axis of third metacarpal; $L2$, length of carpal prolongation of this axis; $L3$, horizonal distance from mid-carpal point to prolongation of ulnar axis

**Table II.2.** Value of radiological features

| View | Criteria | Compartment | | |
|---|---|---|---|---|
| | | Radial | Central | Ulnar |
| Lateral | <RL (CL) | (+) | + | – |
| | <SL | + | – | – |
| Frontal | "Gap" | + | – | (+) |
| | Carpal height | (+) | + | – |
| | Carpal-ulnar distance ratio | (+) | (+) | – |
| | Arc | + | + | (+) |
| | Dynamic/stress | + | + | (+) |
| | Arthrography | + | – | – |

The lateral views in flexion and extension allow detection of pure SL lesions; + (+), (relatively) easy diagnosis; –, diagnosis difficult to establish; diagnosis of lesions of the ulnar compartment usually requires arthrography

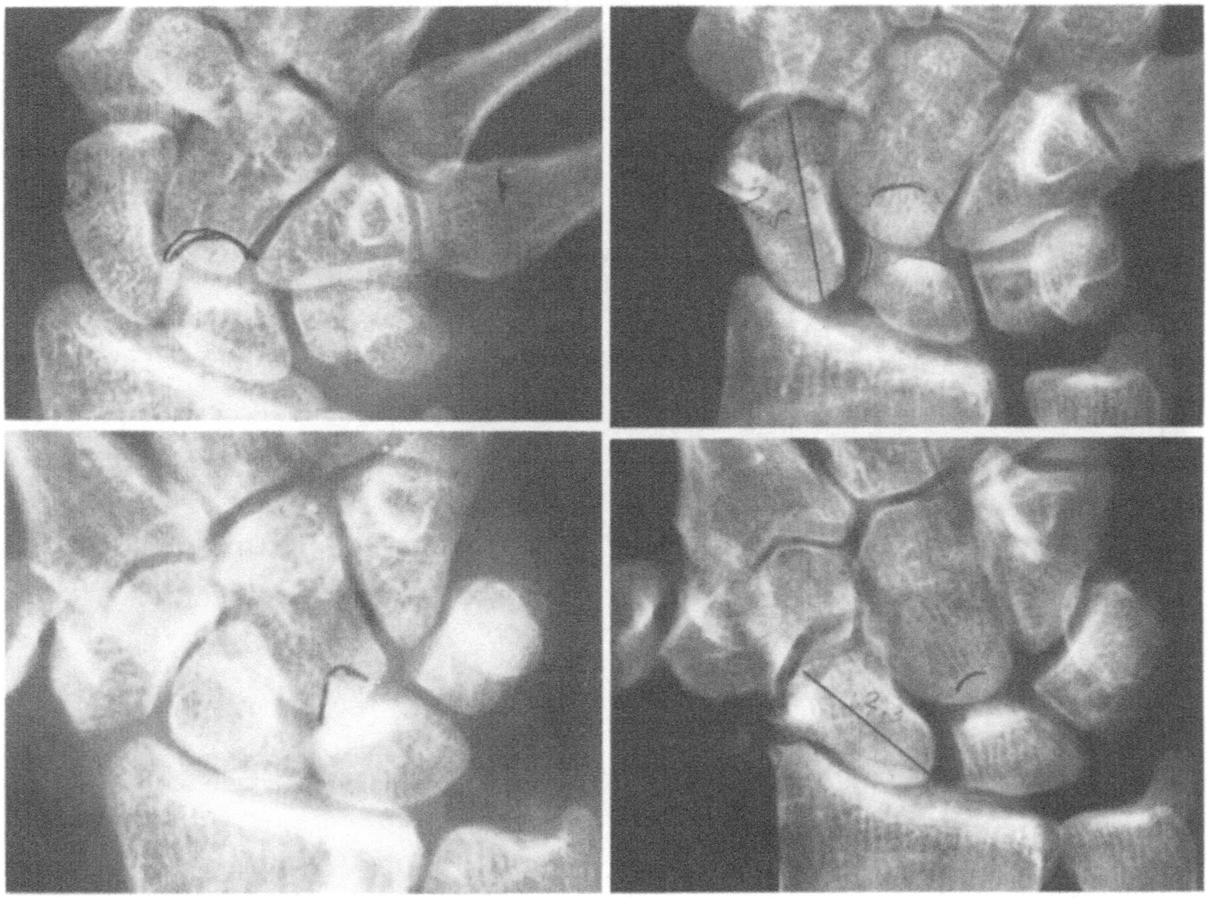

a¹ a² b¹ b²

**Fig. II.11 a, b.** Comparison of mobility of proximal row, abnormal on *right*, normal on *left*; the injured side (**a²**, **b²**) shows arthrosis of the radial compartment and abnormal mobility of the scaphoid, lunate and triquetrum, whether in radial or in ulnar deviation

### "Dynamic" View

Here, the principle of the examination is different, since it is not the rest position but the position of maximal deviation that is desired. Therefore, these views are made in forced radial, ulnar, palmar and dorsal flexion in order to analyse the effects of these stresses on the relationship of the bones to one another (by comparing with the normal side).

Figure II.11 illustrates this. The reference wrist is on the left, the damaged wrist on the right. The injured side shows (see also Fig. III.5) minimal arthrosis of the radial compartment, especially in relation to the radial styloid and the scapho-trapezoid articulation. In ulnar deviation (Fig. II.11 a), the "horizontalization" of the scaphoid is only minor; the bulging lunate has its palmar pole emphasized with a pencil stroke. In radial deviation (Fig. II.11 b), the length of the scaphoid is hardly modified; the lunate is in dorsiflexion with its dorsal pole hidden. The projection of the pisiform onto the triquetrum is only slightly modified.

A similar approach is used with the lateral films. Schuhl et al. (1985) suggested a calculation of the range of movement of the lunate and scaphoid and then measured the difference of angular motion between the two bones. The range of move-

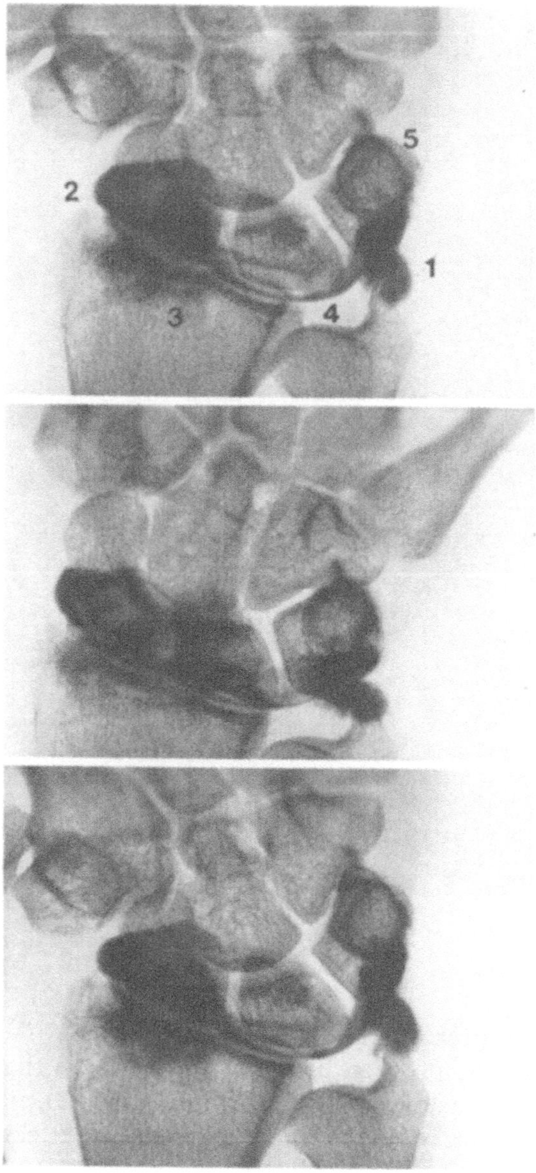


a
b
c

**Fig. II.12a–c.** Normal arthrogram. **a** The different recesses. *1* prestyloid recess *2* prescaphoid recess *3* radial recess *4* triangular fibro-cartilage *5* piso-triquetral joint **b** Ulnar deviation. **c** Radial deviation

ment of the lunate was 51° and the scaphoid 87°, a difference of 36°. They stated that experimental section of the scapholunate ligament causes this difference to increase, significant if greater than 15°. Berger et al. (1982) were unable to demonstrate the role of this ligament in a similar experiment using static views.

It is difficult, currently, to comment on drawer sign views obtained by shearing stresses. One hand fixes the forearm of the wrist to be studied while the other exerts either palmar or dorsal pressure on the metacarpus. This examination is painful in disease states, and the necessary muscular relaxation is not reliable. It is difficult to ensure the position of the hand and, according to Gérard et al. (1984), dorsal angulations of 25° and palmar angulations of 45° are normal. Although we have not

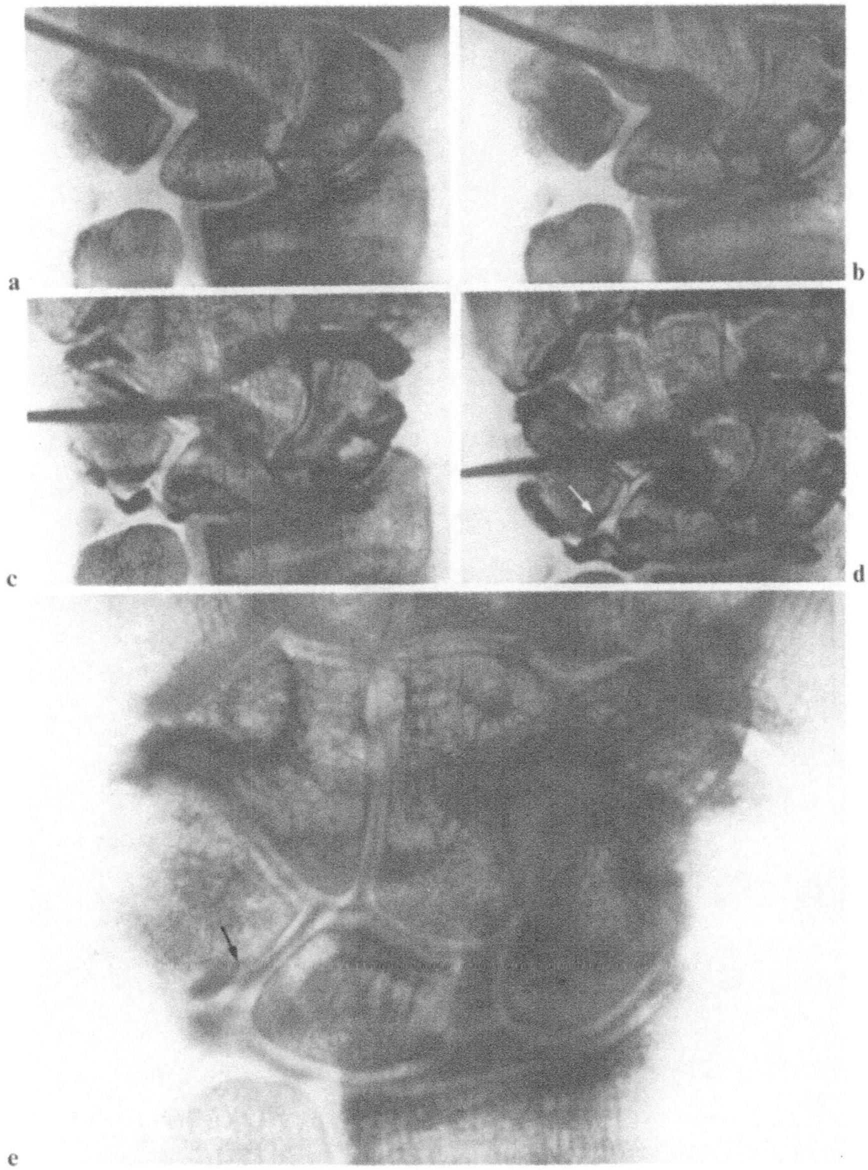

**Fig. II.13 a–e.** Injection of contrast medium into the intercarpal joint.
**a** Scapho-lunate dissociation, radial recess beginning to opacify.
**b** Radial recess clearly defined, opacification of scaphoid recess.
**c, d** Progressive filling of ulnar compartment, with demonstration of triquetro-lunate lesion.
**e** Despite avulsion of the ulnar styloid, the fibrocartilage is intact

abandoned testing for the drawer sign of the wrist under the image intensifier, we no longer do so except during arthrography, a procedure which has proved indispensable when the static and dynamic films do not adequately explain the patient's symptoms.

### Arthrography

The injection of a water-soluble tri-iodinated contrast medium into the radio-carpal joint is a well accepted procedure. Normally, the radio-carpal joint does not communicate with the distal radio-ulnar (Mikic 1978) or the midcarpal joints. After the age of 30 years, and sometimes earlier in cases of elongated ulna (Palmer et al. 1983), a communication appears between the

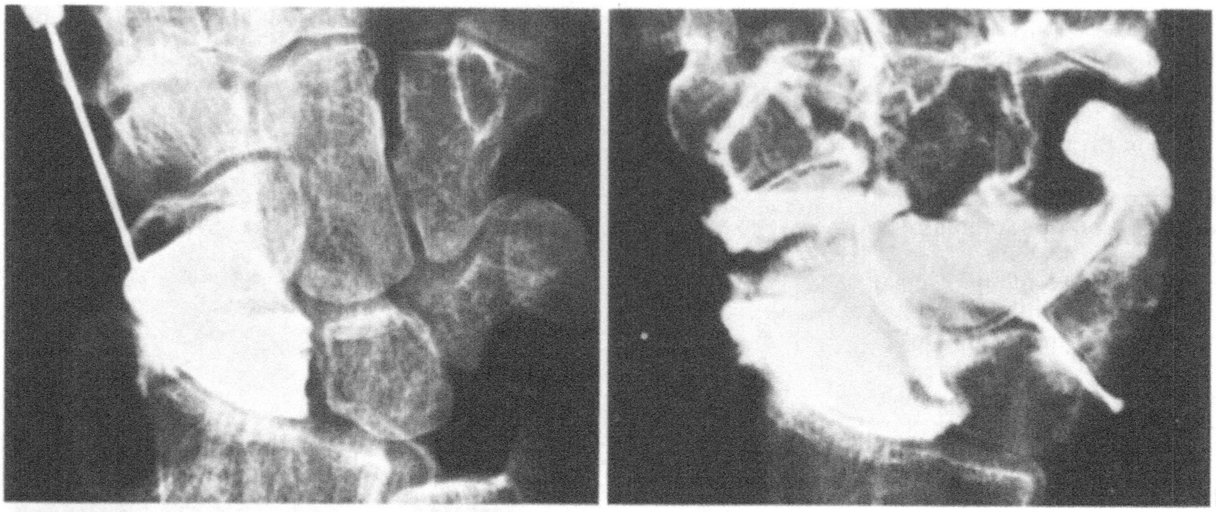

a b

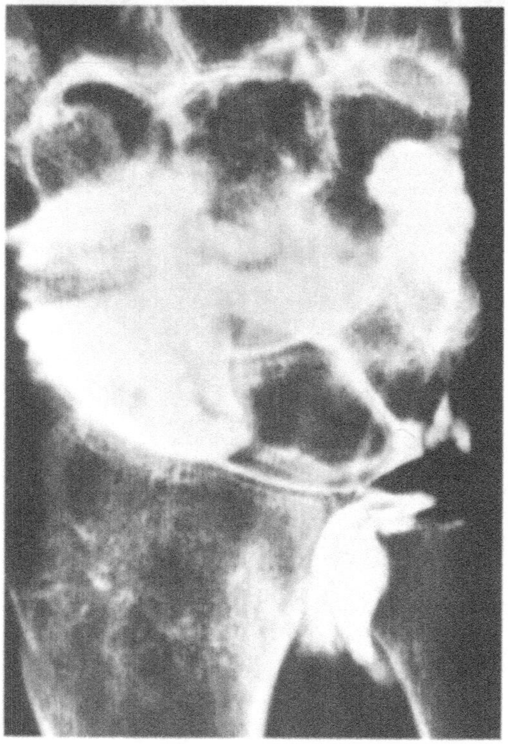

c

**Fig. II.14. a** First injection: synechiae in the region of the RSL ligament; the contrast medium shows only the radial compartment. **b** Second injection: demonstration of the intercarpal joint; the scapho-lunate and triquetro-lunate ligaments are impervious. **c** Third injection: spread into the distal radio-ulnar joint demonstrates incompetent fibrocartilage

radio-carpal and distal radio-ulnar joints. This is a consequence of wear and tear of the fibrocartilage, which is constantly acting as a shock-absorber between the carpus and the ulna. On the other hand, a communication between the piso-triquetral and radio-carpal articulations is the rule: 80% of cases according to Mansat et al. (1983) and 73% in the findings of Palmer et al. (1983). A communication between the radio-carpal and mid carpal joint is always pathological.

*Technique*

The technique is relatively simple. Injection of the contrast medium into the radio-carpal articulation, as described by Palmer, is adequate in the majority of cases. The wrist is flexed over a foam-rubber wedge, and the space bounded by the radius and the scapho-lunate joint is visualized under the image intensifier. The site of injection having been defined, the contrast medium is injected under local anaesthesia on the radial border of the radio-scaphoid joint. The speed of injection is slow, and the spread of the medium is constantly monitored. This spread provides useful information as to the presence of synechiae or about the routes of communication between the different articulations and their importance. The radiographical angles employed depend on the pathology and are selected under the image intensifier.

Figure II.12 shows a normal arthrogram. The triquetro-hamate articulation is visible, the triangular fibrocartilage is perfectly outlined and the prestyloid recess is plainly shown; on the other hand, neither the prescaphoid recess nor the radial recess are clearly in evidence.

*Special Techniques*

The standard technique is excellent in the majority of cases. Sometimes it is preferable to inject the contrast medium into the intercarpal joints or the distal radio-ulnar joint. This is illustrated by two examples:

1. Figure II.13a and b are from G.E., aged 27. The injury and the clinical findings suggest a combined lesion of the triangular fibrocartilage and the triquetro-lunate ligament, the radiological interval between the lunate and triquetrum exceeding 2 mm. Injection of the contrast medium into the intercarpal articulation permits better observation of the spread of the fluid and appreciation of the distribution of the lesions and their severity.
   The inadequacy of the scapho-lunate ligament is evident at the start of the injection. The slow progress of the contrast medium allows successive study of the opacification of the radial recess (a), the pre-scaphoid recess (b) and finally of the ulnar compartment. The fibrocartilage is intact, despite the avulsion of the ulnar styloid; on the other hand, triquetro-lunate lesion is plainly evident. Figure II.13 leaves no doubt as to the lesion.
2. Figure II.14a, b and c are from Y.Y., aged 35, with wrist pain after a distal radius fracture. The differential diagnosis was a ligamentous lesion of the proximal row or involvement of the fibrocartilage. The routine injection opacifies only the radial compartment; synechiae prevent any diffusion into the ulnar compartment. The second injection, into the intercarpal space, allows verification of the integrity of the interosseous ligaments. The third injection, into the distal radio-ulnar

joint, demonstrates the involvement of the fibrocartilage and the consequent opacification of the proximal row.

This arthrography demonstrates a condition that is still not widely known, namely deranged mobility of the proximal row secondary to tethering of the lunate by synechiae. Palmer and Mansat make no reference to such lesions or derangements.

*Note.* Tomographic arthrography may prove necessary to define the position of the lesions. This does not replace dynamic examination and careful observation of the movements of the carpal bones, which must be carried out before and after arthrography, the latter sometimes emphasising the pathological movement under investigation.

### CT Scanner

Mino et al. (1983) have demonstrated in the cadaver the value of this technique in detecting subluxation of the distal radioulnar joint. Weeks et al. (1985) have endeavoured to obtain images of the carpal bones in three dimensions. Rapid progress is being made in this area, and certainly in the near future it will also be possible to visualize the ligaments simultaneously.

### Xerography

This technique permits enhancement of detail when contrasts are poor. We do not use it, the position and relationship of the different carpal bones being the key elements in diagnosis.

### Isotope Scintigraphy

This allows localization of inflammatory, infectious or traumatic lesions and also a better definition of the nature of unexpected findings in routine roentgenographic views, i.e. an intraosseous cyst.

### Costs and Chronology of Radiographical Examinations

We agree that it may appear excessive to perform a complete battery of examinations routinely for fractures of the scaphoid or radius. That is why it is essential to do them in a logical sequence. It is desirable that dorso-palmar radiography, including the heads of the metacarpals, should be a routine film. It permits immediate assessment of the position of the different carpal bones and serves as a baseline for assessment of the evolution of the case.

The lateral view, taken using a guide, is essential and it, too, should be routine, for it really determines the subsequent examinations. Also, the radio-lunate and scapho-lunate angles provide essential information about the state of the ligaments stabilizing the lunate, the keystone of the carpus. Dynamic films are needed only in old cases, and only if the persistence of symptoms leaves some doubts.

The inclusion of two routine films does not represent an excessive financial burden, given the advantages of early diagnosis of instability leading to adequate treatment: i.e. reduction and ligamentous suture in recent cases, and the Matti-Russe procedure with ligamentoplasty or partial carpal arthrodesis for unstable pseudarthroses.

## References


Bellinghausen HW, Gilula LA, Young LY and Weeks PM (1983) Posttraumatic carpal subluxation. J Bone Joint Surg [Am] 65:998–1006

Berger RA, Blair WF, Crownischield RD, Flatt AE (1982) The scapholunate ligament. J Hand Surg 7:87–91

Dobyns JH, Linscheid RL, Chao EY, Weber ER, Swanson GE (1975) Traumatic instability of the wrist. AAOS instructional course lectures, Mosby, St Louis, 24:182

Gérard Y, Meyrueis JP, Schernberg F (1984) Techniques radiologiques du poignet. Bilan radiographique dans les instabilités du carpe. In: Tubiana R (ed) Traité de chirurgie de la main. Masson, Paris, pp 482–496

Linscheid RL, Dobyns JH, Boabout JW and Bryan RS (1972) Traumatic instability of the wrist: diagnosis, classification and pathomechanics. J Bone Joint Surg [Am] 54:1612–1632

Mansat M, Mansat C, Martinez C (1983) L'exploration arthrographique du poignet. In: Razemon JP, Fiks GR (eds) Le poignet. Expansion Scientifique Française, Paris, pp 196–203

Meyrueis JP (1984) Instabilité du carpe, circonstances de diagnostic et étude clinique. Ann Chir Main 3:313–316

Mikic ZD (1978) Age changes in the triangular fibrocartilage of the wrist joint. J Anat 126:367–384

Mino DE, Palmer AK, Levinsohn ME (1983) The role of radiography and computerized tomography in the diagnosis of subluxation and dislocation of the distal radio-ulnar joint. J Hand Surg 8:23–31

Moneim MS (1981) The tangential postero-anteroanterior radiograph to demonstrate scapho-lunate dissociation. J Bone Joint Surg [Am] 63:1324–1326

Palmer AK, Levinsohn EM, Kuzma GR (1983) Arthrography of the wrist. J Hand Surg 8:15–23

Sarrafian SK, Melamed JL, Gosgarian GM (1977) Study of the wrist motion in flexion and extension. Clin Orthop 126:153

Schuhl JF, Leroy B, Comtet JJ (1985) Etude radiologique de la mobilité relative du scaphoïde et du semi-lunaire. Ann Chir Main 4:143–148

Weeks PM, Vannier MW, Stevens WG, Gayou D, Gilula LA (1985) Three-dimensional imaging of the wrist. J Hand Surg 10A:32–39

CHAPTER III

# Hyperextension Injuries of the Wrist: Pathomechanics and Clinical Approach

## A. Pathomechanics

### Introduction

Frykmann (1967), Mayfield et al. (1980) and Weber and Chao (1978) all applied themselves to understanding the pathophysiology of hyperextension, although from differing points of view. Frykmann was essentially concerned with fracture of the radius and does not seem to have fully appreciated the problem of the associated lesions of the intracarpal ligaments. Mayfield was the first to speak of lesional zones; he suggested defining the order of appearance of the lesions in four stages:

1. Stage I defines a fracture of the scaphoid or an equivalent lesion of the scapho-lunate ligament, with or without a lesion of the radial styloid.
2. Stage II corresponds to an extension of the ligamentous tears between the lunate and the capitate.
3. Stage III further indicates a rupture of the structures binding the lunate and triquetrum.
4. Stage IV marks the completion of the sequence with rupture of the remaining attachments of the lunate.

This lesional sequence may deserve to be made known, but we question its validity; in reality the lesions are more complex and various, as we shall endeavour to show in our clinical examples.

The experimental studies of Weber and Chao (1978) demonstrated the importance of the degree of dorsiflexion of the wrist. Below 95° they induced only fractures of the radius, no matter how much force was applied; as soon as dorsiflexion exceeded this value it was the scaphoid that fractured.

### Pathophysiology of Lesions

This is very difficult to analyse, for, while the position of the wrist may determine the type of lesion, in practice it is unknown. Moreover, the position is not the only factor; other very important factors must be taken into account, such as:

- the violence of the impact,
- the axis of the force applied,
- the zone of its application (radial, ulnar or central) and the resultant torsions,
- the mineralization of the bone,
- muscular power and reflexes,
- the buffer zone or shock absorption.

To consider the last factor as an example, shock absorption is markedly more effective when falling forward. In a backward fall the hand is already in maximum dorsiflexion and the muscles are no longer in a position to absorb part of the kinetic energy.

The roles of these various factors have not yet been clarified. Fracture of the scaphoid is known to become less common with age, though the precise reasons for this are not clear; are the consequences of injury modified by greater prudence, or by demineralization, or both? Theoretically, absorption of energy by the fracturing bone should spare the ligaments. Thus, Colles' fractures in women should exhibit a decreasing frequency of ligamentous lesions with age and severity of impaction. To verify this hypothesis statistically the techniques for radiography of the wrist would need to be standardized. Standardization is one of the aims of this work; and without it these issues will remain unresolved.

The reflexes and muscle power also play an important part; rapid reflexes and considerable muscular power will absorb the impact before the wrist reaches the end of its excursion; only at these extremes are the ligaments, and then the bone, placed under palmar tension and dorsal compression. Hence, from Weber's experiments, fractures of the scaphoid should become commoner with age, when, with diminishing strength and reflexes, the dorsiflexion produced by a fall increases. And yet, it is the opposite that occurs.

The traumatic event as experienced by the patient has generally been so rapid that the physician cannot draw any useful conclusions from the patient's recollection of it. He must therefore be aware of the entire spectrum of possible lesions and, above all, the methods of detecting them. Indeed, where the wrist is concerned, he must transform himself into a Sherlock Holmes, and study the biological, mechanical and, above all, radiological indices.

The purpose of this clinical review is to emphasise

- the importance of radiology
- the need to be familiar with the concepts of carpal stability
- the coupling of radius and carpus as an anatomical-pathological unit
- the different stages leading to perilunate dislocation (De Quervain fracture dislocation).

## Clinical Cases

1, B.B., a 60-year-old woman (Fig. III.1), presented to the emergency room following an ordinary fall on the hyperextended wrist, with minimal pain and disability. The undisplaced marginal radial fracture is evident in the PA film and gives rise to no anxiety. Despite the unsatisfactory view one can suspect a scapho-lunate dissociation. The lateral view made with a guide at our request confirmed the presence of a ligamentous lesion. The DISI is very marked: approximately 18°.

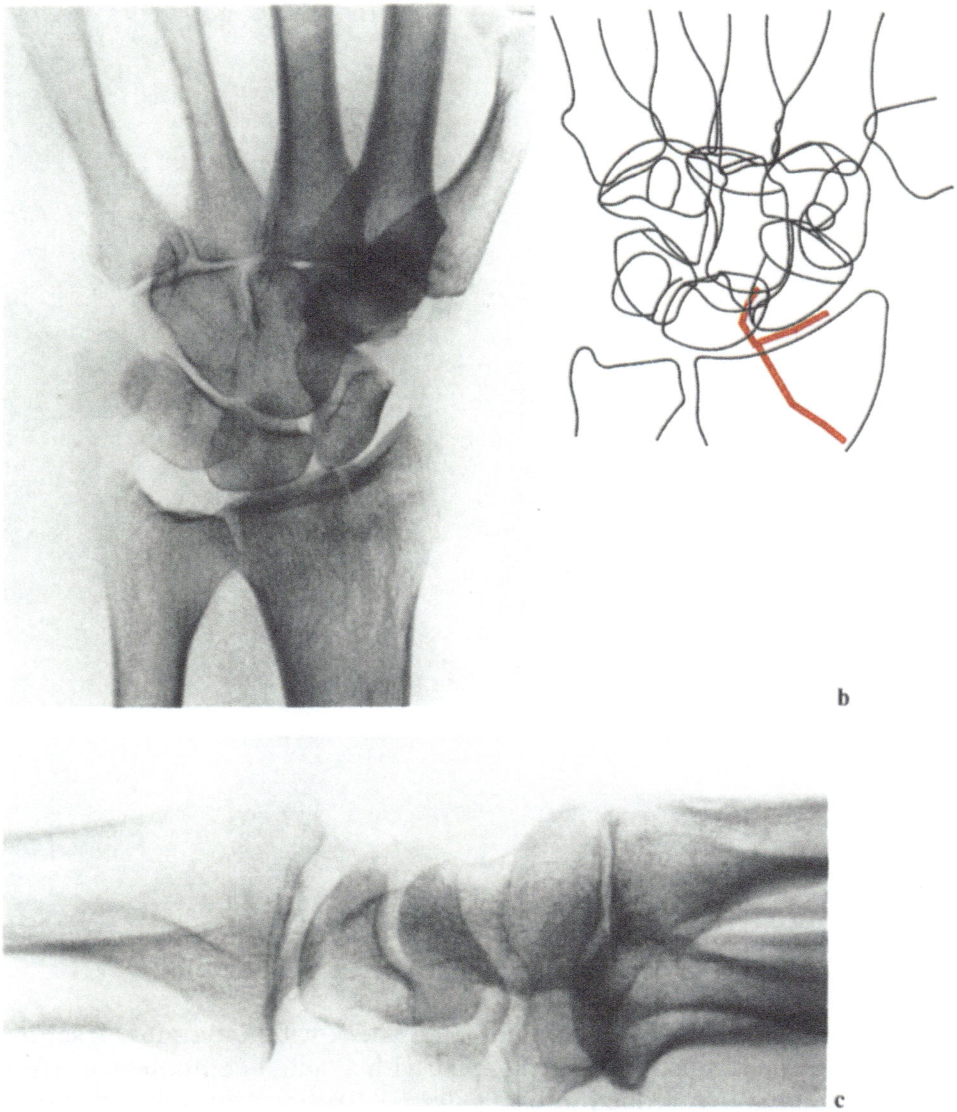

**Fig. III.1.** **a** PA: marginal fracture of radius. **b** Diagram: the line of injury corresponds to the radiographic appearance. The lesion involves the bone, the SL ligament and part of the proximal V. A lesion of the ulnar complex is possible, though uncertain, hence the *stippled line*. **c** Lateral: marked DISI, evidence of the SL lesion

*Discussion.* Contrary to appearances, it is not a simple marginal Barton's fracture, but a radius fracture combined with carpal instability. A lesion of the scapho-lunate ligament cannot be appreciated in the routine view and requires dynamic flexion-extension views. While a practised eye may perceive the abnormal position of the scaphoid, only the lateral view allows real assessment of the extent of ligamentous damage. On the basis of these views we may conclude that the lesion involves the bone, the scapho-lunate ligament and part of the proximal V. Figure III.1 b indicates the line of injury diagrammatically, corresponding to Mayfield's type I.

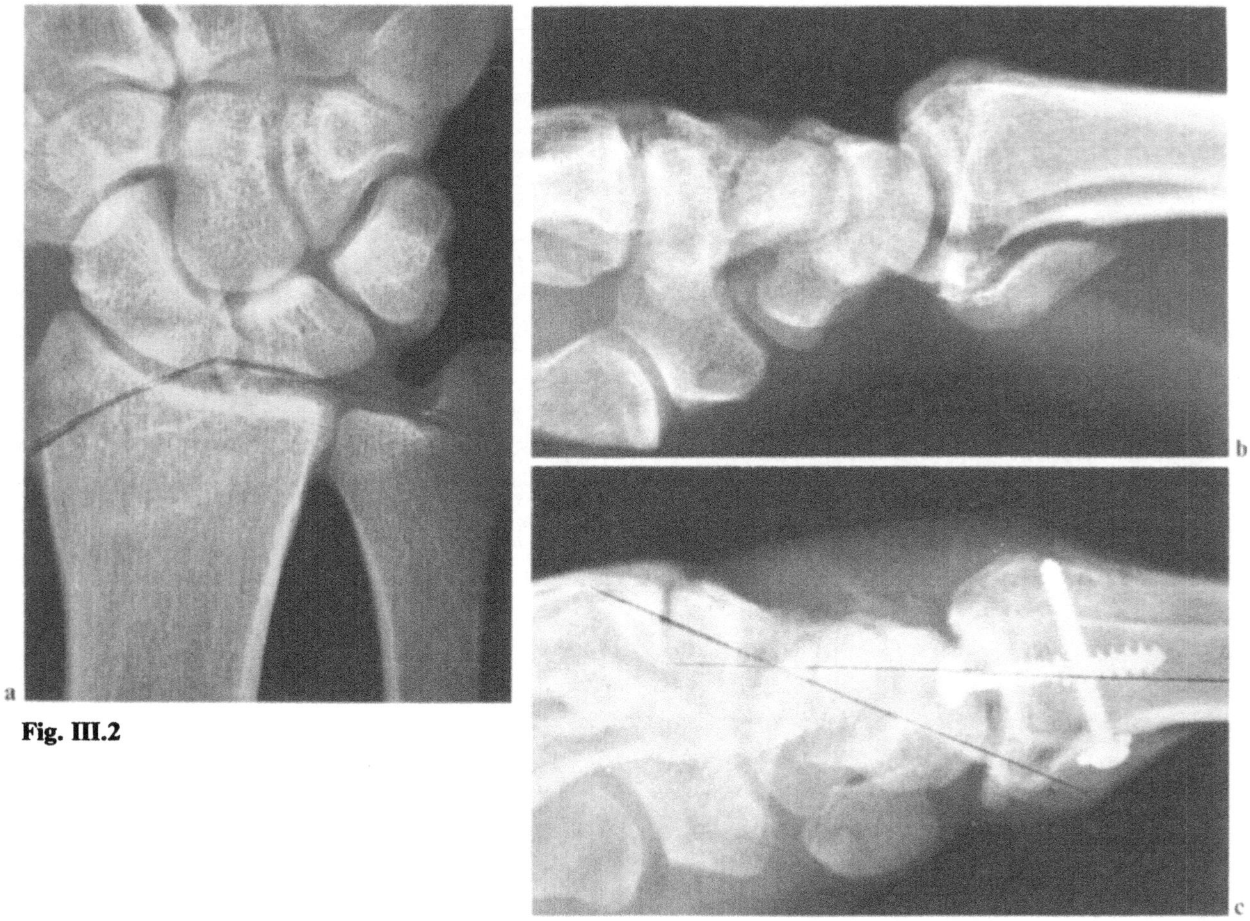

Fig. III.2

2. G.R., a 24-year-old man (Fig. III.2), with a marginal fracture of the radius (palmar fragment with a radial component). After anatomical reduction and internal fixation, the DISI position of the lunate persists.

*Discussion.* The line of the anatomical lesion is clearly defined: partial rupture of the proximal V and avulsion of the ulnar styloid have occurred. The physiological outcome is clear: the lunate, no longer held tightly, glides in a palmar direction and ends in DISI. This is not a so-called adaptive deformity of the lunate since the reduction is anatomical. This case confirms that fracture of the distal radius may be combined with major intracarpal ligamentous lesions. The lesional line does not correspond to the schema proposed by Mayfield, which is not surprising since he takes no account of the functional anatomy.

3. N.E., a 65-year-old woman (Fig. III.3a), presented with a single block fracture of the radius, with demineralized bone and massive impaction. However, the DISI deformation of the lunate is more marked than the angular deformity of the radius would suggest.

**Fig. III.2 a, b.** Marginal fracture of radius. **c** Osteosynthesis with perfect bony reduction: the residual lunate tilt indicates associated ligamentous lesions. The *line* in **a** indicates the line of the lesion: partial detachment of the proximal V and fracture of the ulnar styloid

**Fig. III.3 a, b.** Two fractures of the radius with a single block epiphysis. **a** DISI. **b** SL dissociation. In case **a** damage to the ulno-carpal complex seems as important as in case **b** despite the intact styloid. The marked lunate tilt indicates inadequacy of the proximal V

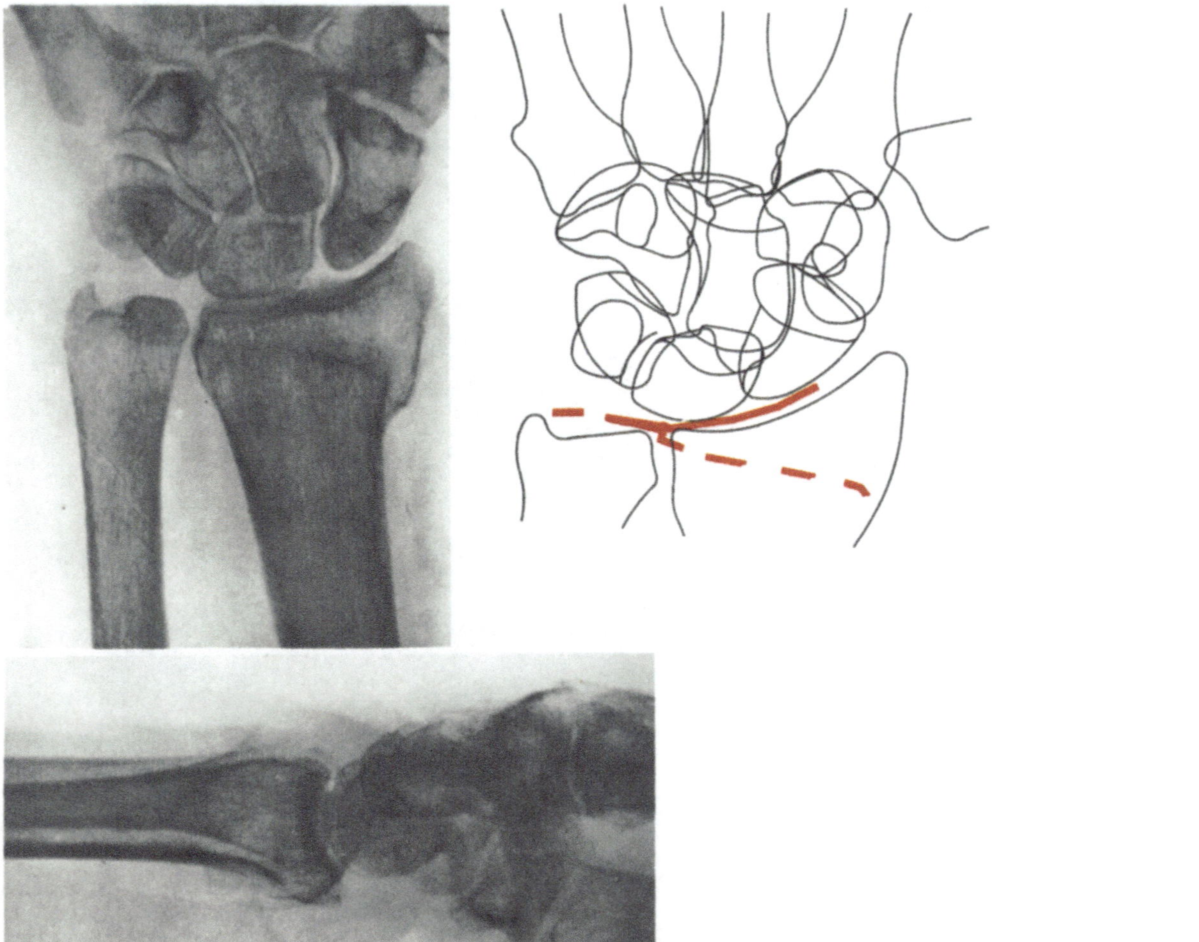

a

b

Fig. III.3

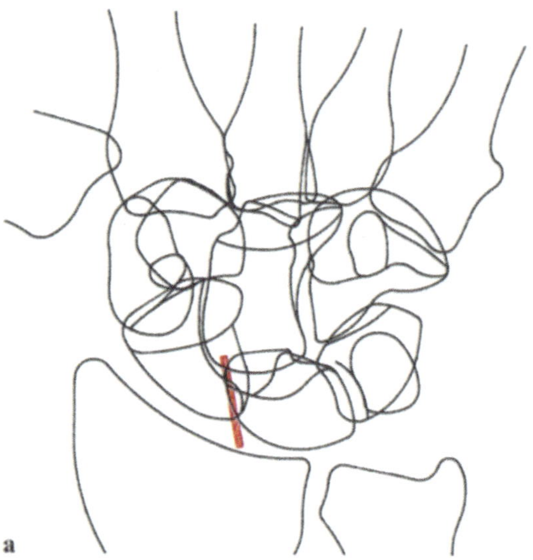

a

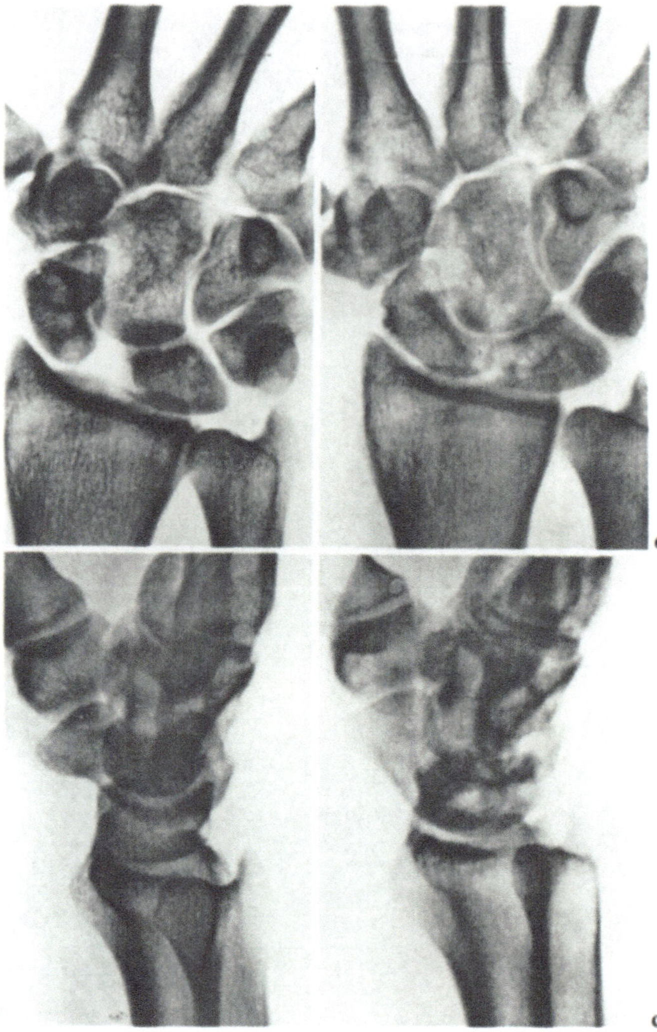

b[1] c[1] b[2] c[2]

**Fig. III.4. a** Schematic view of lesion in **b**[1]. **b**[2] Minimal lunate tilt: the proximal V is still mainly functional. **c**[1], **c**[2] Two years after reconstruction of the ligaments, a good subjective and objective result has been achieved

*Discussion.* The radial tilting implies stretching, and possibly a rupture of the proximal V. It is this associated ligamentous lesion that explains the importance of the observed DISI. The suggested lesional schema cannot be convincingly demonstrated even if the ligamentous lesion is present.

4. S.R., a 60-year-old man (Fig. III.3b), presented with a single block fracture of the radius, in demineralized bone, and scapholunate dissociation. The schema beside the radiograph traces the supposed line of the lesions, rather like a star.

*Discussion.* Here again is a difficulty to schematically represent the supposed outline of the lesions, torsional movements occurring during the injury can modify and complicate the trace of the lesional line.

5. S.F., a 30-year-old man (Fig. III.4), suffered a hyperextension injury 7 months previously and was left with permanent discomfort and a wrist "clunk". The click was easy to reproduce on

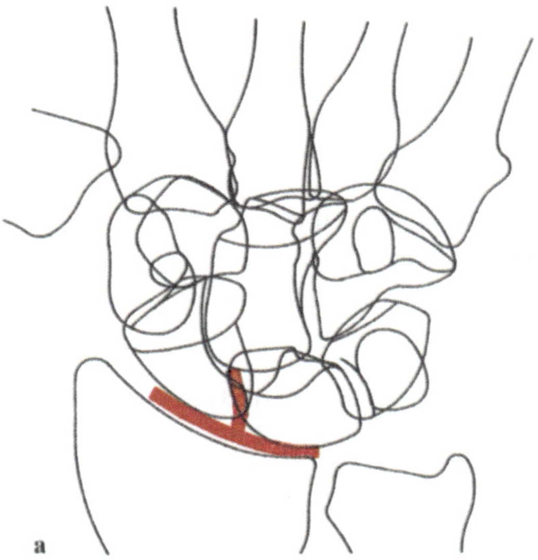

a

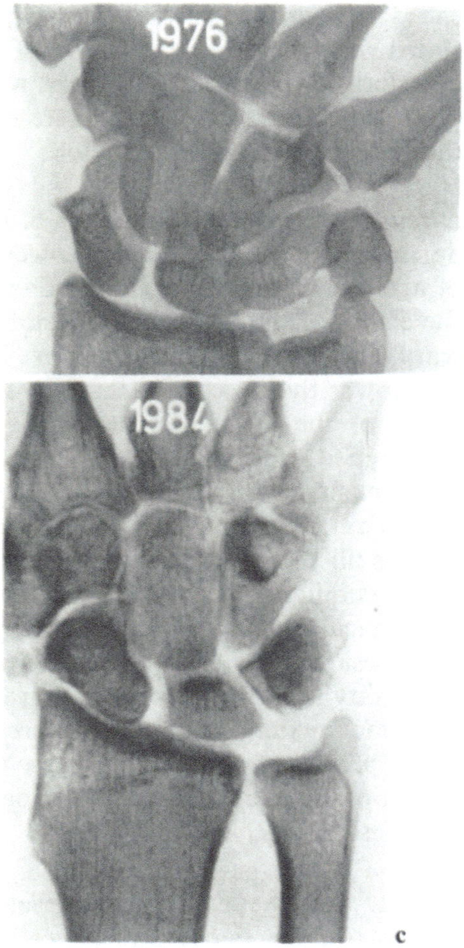


b

c

**Fig. III.5a–c.** Lesion of SL ligament, with partial lesion of proximal V. **a** Diagram of *line of lesion.* **b** Initial film showing scapho-lunate dissociation. **c** Post-traumatic arthrosis

physical examination and on the routine X-ray view (Fig. III.4b) the scapho-lunate dissociation is evident. Yet the lunate is in a normal radiological position. This stability indicates that the proximal V is functional, and therefore largely intact. Thus, a scapho-capitate-lunate plasty of the Linscheid type is suitable to restore a functional proximal row. Three years after operation, the wrist is painless and its function normal.

*Discussion.* This lesion is equivalent to a stable fracture of the scaphoid, i.e. not involving the proximal or distal V. The scaphoid, no longer guided by the lunate, moves jerkily during the movements of radial or ulnar deviation. Hence the clunk phenomenon when it is forced to change position by the pressure variation. Arthrosis is bound to occur, but after a very variable interval; it may take 15 years or more to note marked degenerative changes.

6. E.O., a 41-year-old man (Fig. III.5), had a hyperextension injury at the age of 30. No diagnosis was made, even though the initial films demonstrate scapho-lunate dissociation. Though the lesion resembles the previous case, the patient never experi-

enced any wrist click and sought advice because of pain associated with progressive arthrosis of the radial compartment. The deterioration was rather abrupt, a phenomenon we have often observed, but cannot explain. As opposed to the previous case, the DISI of the lunate is obvious.

*Discussion.* The natural history of this lesion is similar to pseudarthrosis of the scaphoid. However, the rate of development of arthrosis remains very unpredictable, probably depending on the extent of the ligamentous lesions. Without proof to the contrary, it would seem that the more limited the extent of a lesion, the slower the onset of arthrosis. Other factors, such as natural laxity of the ligaments, also play a role which has yet to be determined. The absence of wrist click may be explained by the persistence of part of the radio-scapho-lunate ligament and of the capsular portion of the proximal V. It is unrealistic to discuss all the possible hypotheses, especially as there is always the possibility of anatomical variations to explain the exceptions or atypical outcomes. Schematically, it may be argued that the basic lesion leads to abnormal constraints which aggravate the instability and thus promote arthrosis. The present lesion seems to be more extensive than in the previous case but this is impossible to prove retrospectively. These examples make us more conscious of our actual limits in understanding these problems at the present time.

7. D.L., a 17-year-old man, presented with a scaphoid fracture evident on the initial film (Fig. III.6a). Thanks to the plaster of Paris, the hand, wrist and forearm are aligned as they should be for a lateral X-ray, and now the palmar shift and the dorsiflexion of the lunate are obvious. The scaphoid fragments are not displaced and show no evidence of instability. The palmar subluxation of the lunate is evidence of an associated ligamentous injury. Thus, a fracture that is considered stable may be associated with a major ligamentous lesion. Prognostically, the precise diagnosis seems important since, despite treatment as advocated by Verdan (above-elbow plaster and 16 weeks of immobilization), the fracture did not heal.

*Discussion.* This scaphoid fracture is accompanied by a lesion of the radial portion of the proximal V. The failure of the supporting sling has led to DISI, and this instability and the resultant constraints are the cause of the pseudarthrosis that developed despite correct treatment. The fragment is of normal size, no vascular disturbance is detectable and there is no bony angulation. Failure can only be attributed to the ligamentous instability.

8. S.M., a 21-year-old man (Fig. III.7) who injured himself during karate training, was unable to explain exactly the circumstances of the accident. The scaphoid fracture diagnosed did

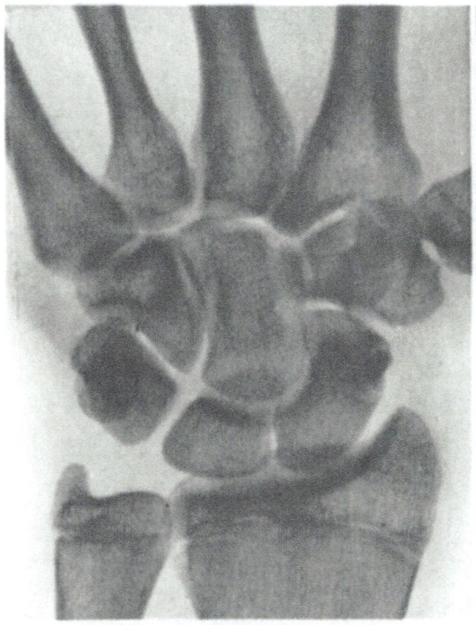

a

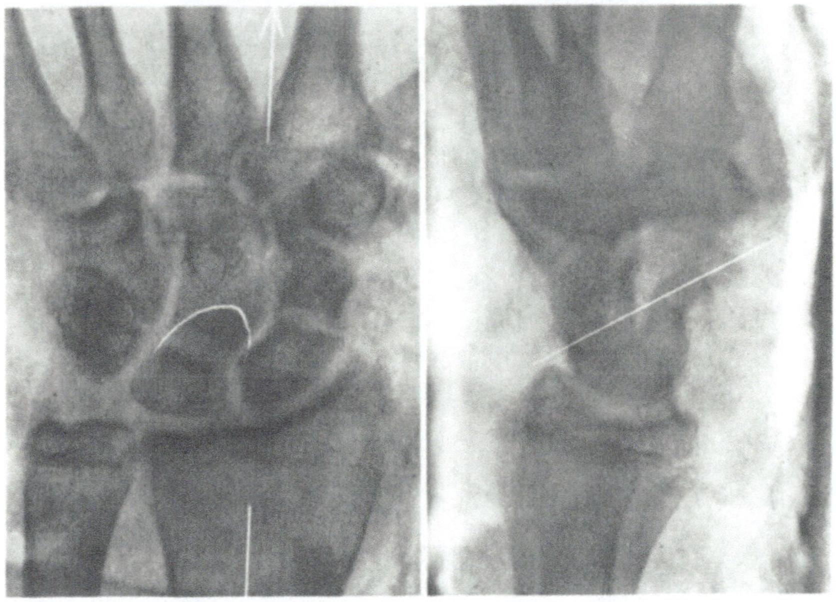

b

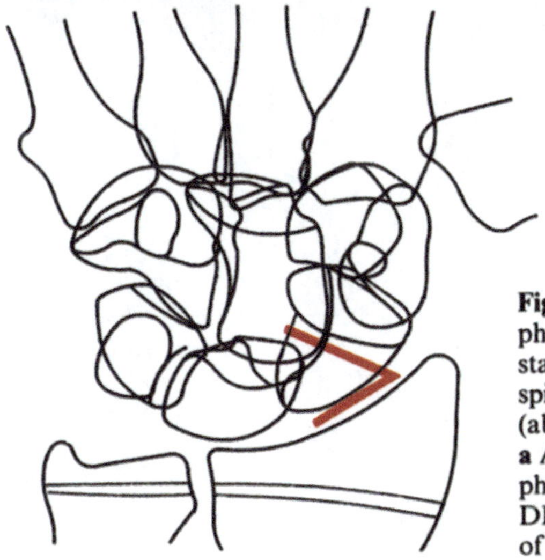

**Fig. III.6a, b.** Fractured scaphoid, unrecognized lunate instability, pseudarthrosis despite 16 weeks in plaster (above-elbow for 8 weeks). **a** Admission view, evident scaphoid fracture. **b** In plaster, DISI now obvious; *diagram* of lesion of proximal V

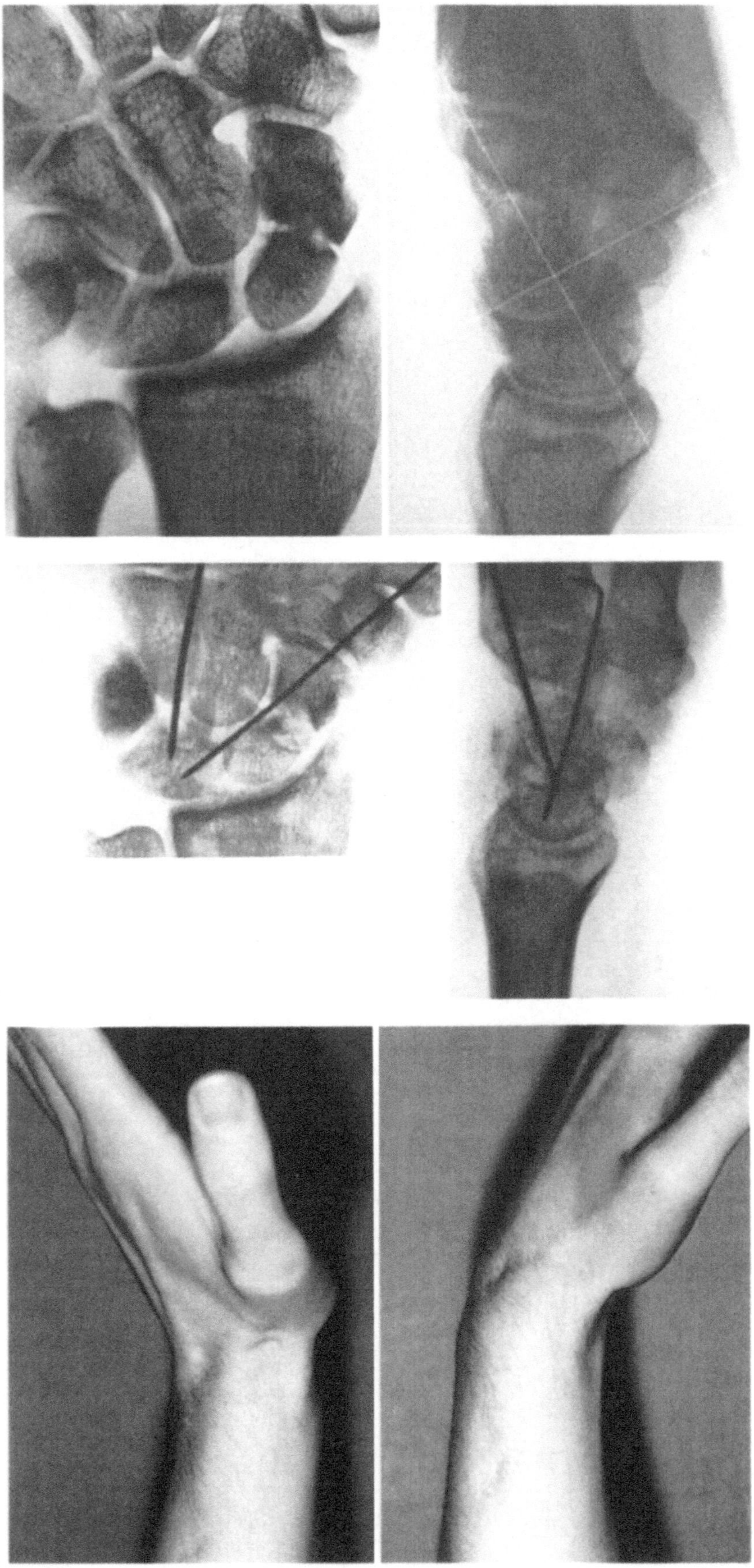

a b c

**Fig. III.7 a–c.** Fracture of scaphoid with unrecognized lunate instability and non-union, treated by Matti-Russe graft and dorsal Linscheid-type ligamentoplasty not unite, despite correct treatment (similar to that in the previous case). Eight months after injury routine radiological views showed a pseudarthrosis of the scaphoid without displacement, but combined with major DISI (radio-lunate angle: +22°, Fig. III.7a). We performed a Matti-Russe repair and added a Linscheid type of ligamentoplasty. The Kirschner wires (Fig. III.7b) stabilizing both the scaphoid and lunate were removed after 10 weeks, and the wrist was left free after 12 weeks. Two years after operation the wrist is painless and the patient has resumed karate. Flexion and extension (Fig. III.7c) are satisfactory.

*Discussion.* These last two cases are comparable regarding both the lesion and its course. These observations confirm the thesis of Weber (1980) that ligamentous instability associated with a scaphoid fracture is often the basis of a pseudarthrosis despite correct treatment. Recognition of these lesions is essential to the application of correct treatment: reduction and wiring, possibly revision and ligamentous suture. However, such recognition again requires standard radiological technique.

9. V.F., a 27-year-old man (Fig. III.8), could not precisely describe his fall, but ever since he has experienced vague pain on exertion, without being able to localize the discomfort. Clinical examination was unremarkable. The dynamic views do not

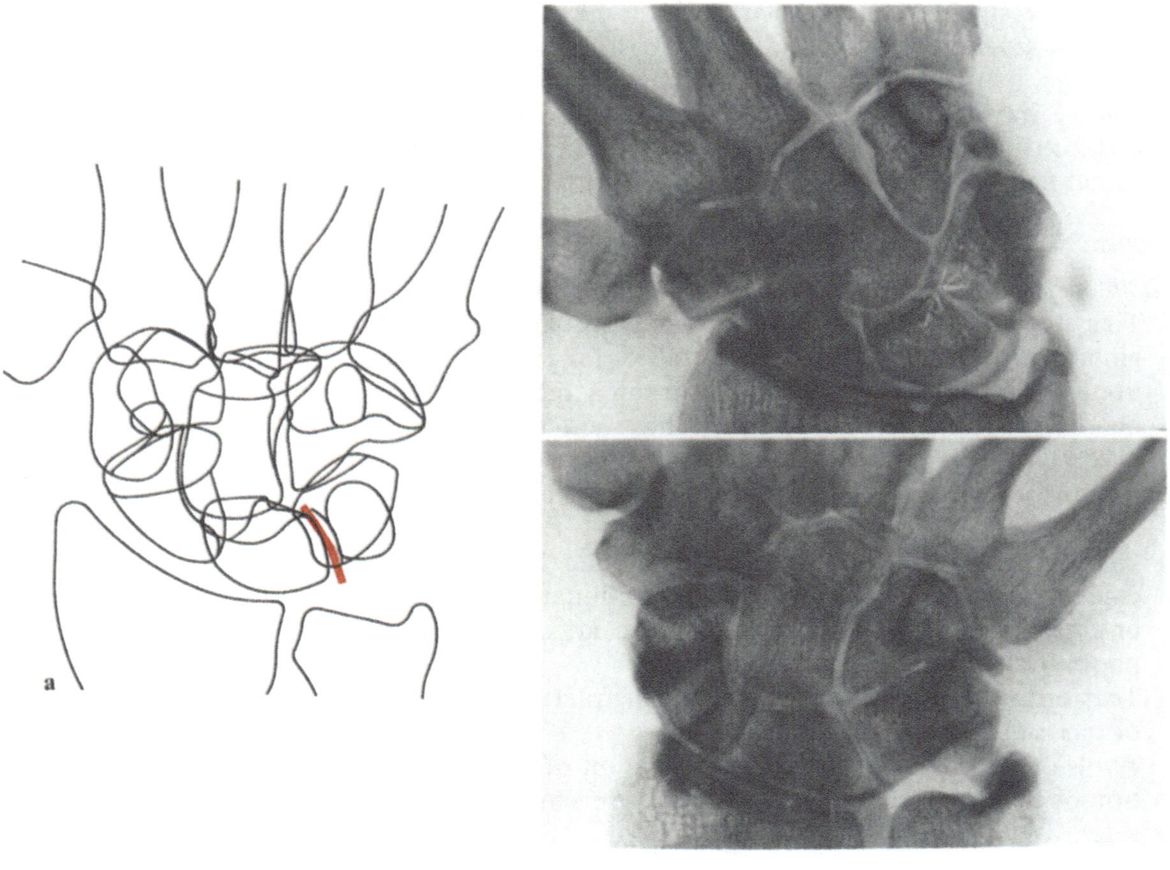

a b c

**Fig. III.8a–c.** Only arthrography enables diagnosis of failure of the triquetro-lunate ligament allow diagnosis of the lesion though, perhaps, in radial deviation, there is minor deformation of the hamate-triquetral-lunate interface, but this may be an effect of the projection. Only arthrography displays the triquetro-lunate ligamentous failure.

*Discussion.* Symptoms secondary to lesions between the lunate and triquetrum are more vague than those of the scapho-lunate ligament. Clinical examination certainly revealed pain in the perilunate region and ulnar compartment, but no functional disturbance was detectable. The patient was able to resume full-time work with no further trouble after ligamentoplasty. The re-establishment of functional anatomy normalized function, as was shown at follow-up 2 years later.

In this case the tracing of the ligamentous tear represents a mirror image of the scapho-lunate lesion discussed previously. Hence, the lesional mechanism must be the opposite to that of the previous cases, the pathology being entirely ulnar. The diagnosis of triquetro-lunate instability is difficult; the history arouses no suspicion, and radiology is of limited value. One would need to be able to measure the triquetro-lunate angle in the lateral film; however, because of superimpositions, this is usually impossible.

**De Quervain's Fracture-Dislocation**

The energy of the trauma will be absorbed by the various lesions, described below in a stepwise manner, until it is completely expended. We shall attempt to clarify the mechanism and treatment with several examples and on the basis of our anatomical knowledge.

As we have seen, the lesion may commence on the radial side (forced supination combined with hyperextension) or on the ulnar side (pronation and hyperextension).

*Sequence of Lesions*

*Radial onset; forced hyperextension and supination.*

1. This stage is facultative: fracture of the radial styloid (marginal fracture), or its equivalent, avulsion of the radial insertion of the distal V. In fact, the trauma may act directly on the scaphoid or scapho-lunate ligament by passing between the two V ligaments, without involving the radius.
2. Fracture of the scaphoid or rupture of the scapho-lunate ligament.
3. Dislocation of the loose structures binding the lunate and capitate (the rule when there is scapho-lunate dissociation) or fracture of the capitate (readily associated with the scaphoid fracture).
4. Tear of the triquetro-lunate ligament or fracture of the body of the triquetrum may take place.
5. Avulsion of the ulnar styloid or disruption of the ulnar portion of the proximal V (analogous to the events on the radial side).

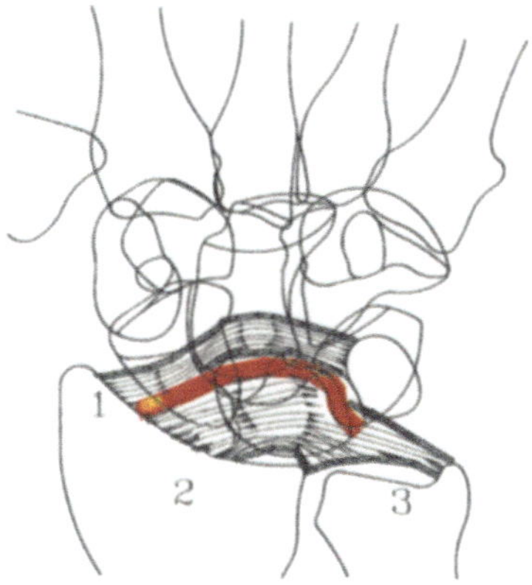


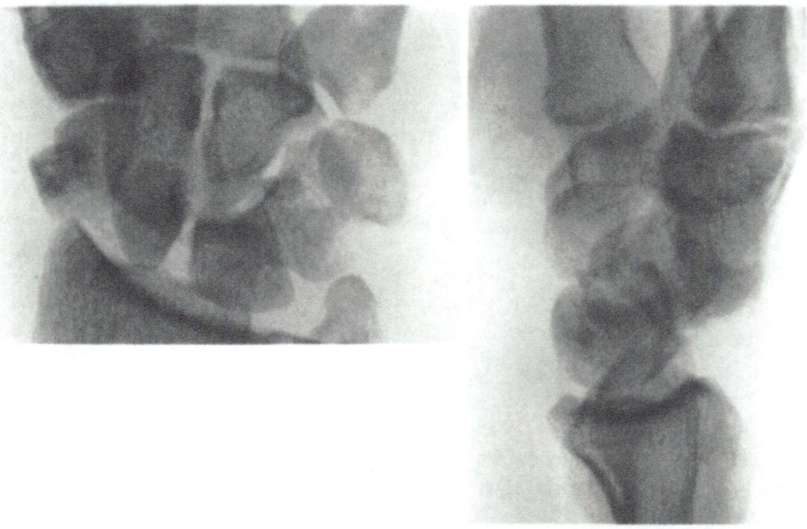

a

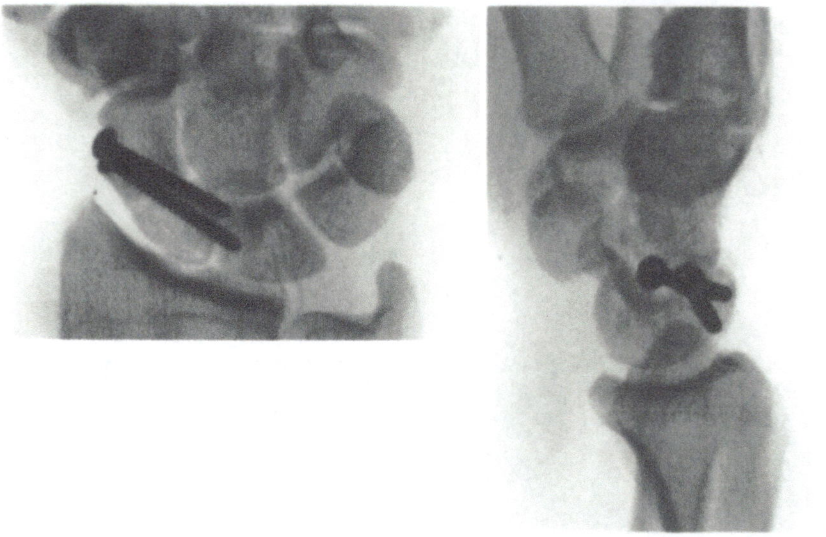

b

**Fig. III.9. a** De Quervain's fracture-dislocation with intact capitate but displaced fracture of the scaphoid, lunate in place without tilt; *diagram*, line of lesion.
*1* distal V
*2* proximal V
*3* ulno-carpal complex
**b** Postoperative views: the position of the lunate is perfect after reduction and osteosynthesis of the scaphoid

6. Progressive dislocation of the capitate in relation to the lunate. The distal V remains partly intact, though the deep attachments of the proximal V to the scaphoid must rupture if complete dislocation of the capitate is to occur. The superficial fibres joining the radius and capitate pass across the gap between the lunate and scaphoid or across the fractured scaphoid and remain intact; at the same time the deep fibres attaching the scaphoid to both the radius and capitate are ruptured. On the ulnar side, the capitate drags the triquetrum with it, the latter being freed from the lunate either by ligamentous tear or by fracture. The capitate ends up resting on the dorsal pole of the lunate (Fig. III.9a, b), which may be forced into a flexed position (Figs. III.10b and III.11b). The lunate pivots around the proximal V, to which it remains attached, and which acts as a hinge. It may even tilt through 180° and obstruct part of the carpal tunnel (Fig. III.12d) and may be responsible for acute compression of the median nerve.

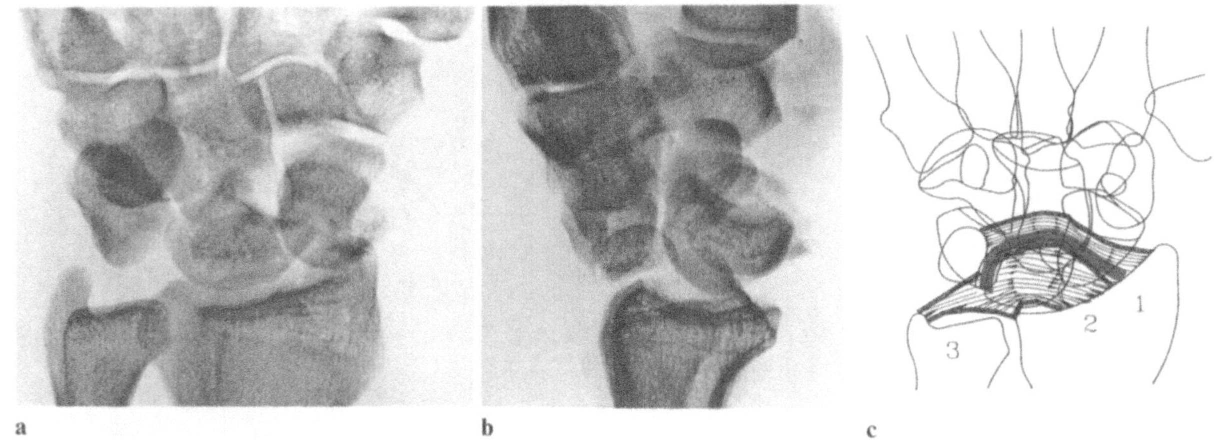


**Fig. III.10 a–c.** De Quervain's fracture-dislocation with fracture of the proximal pole of the capitate, rotated through 180°, fractured scaphoid and minor palmar lunate tilt.
*1* distal V
*2* proximal V
*3* ulnar complex

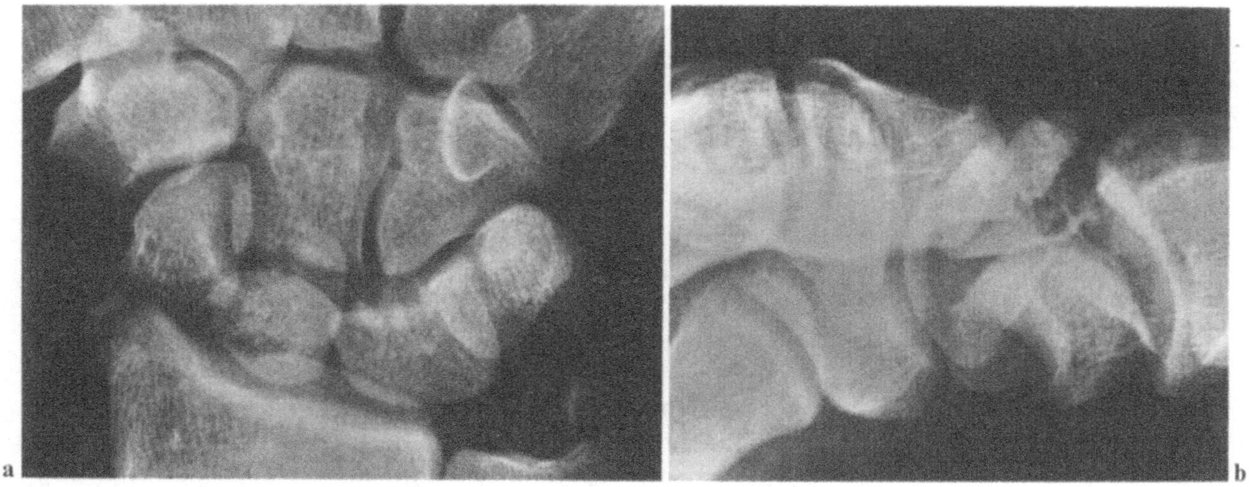


**Fig. III.11 a, b**

*Evaluation of lesions.* As a general rule the two V ligaments are preserved, the lesion being truly perilunate. On occasion the proximal radial attachments of the two Vs may be avulsed, with a consequent radio-scaphoid gap during ulnar deviation as shown in Fig. III.13.

The proof of integrity of the proximal V is given by the lateral film after reduction, where the lunate, as a rule, is in

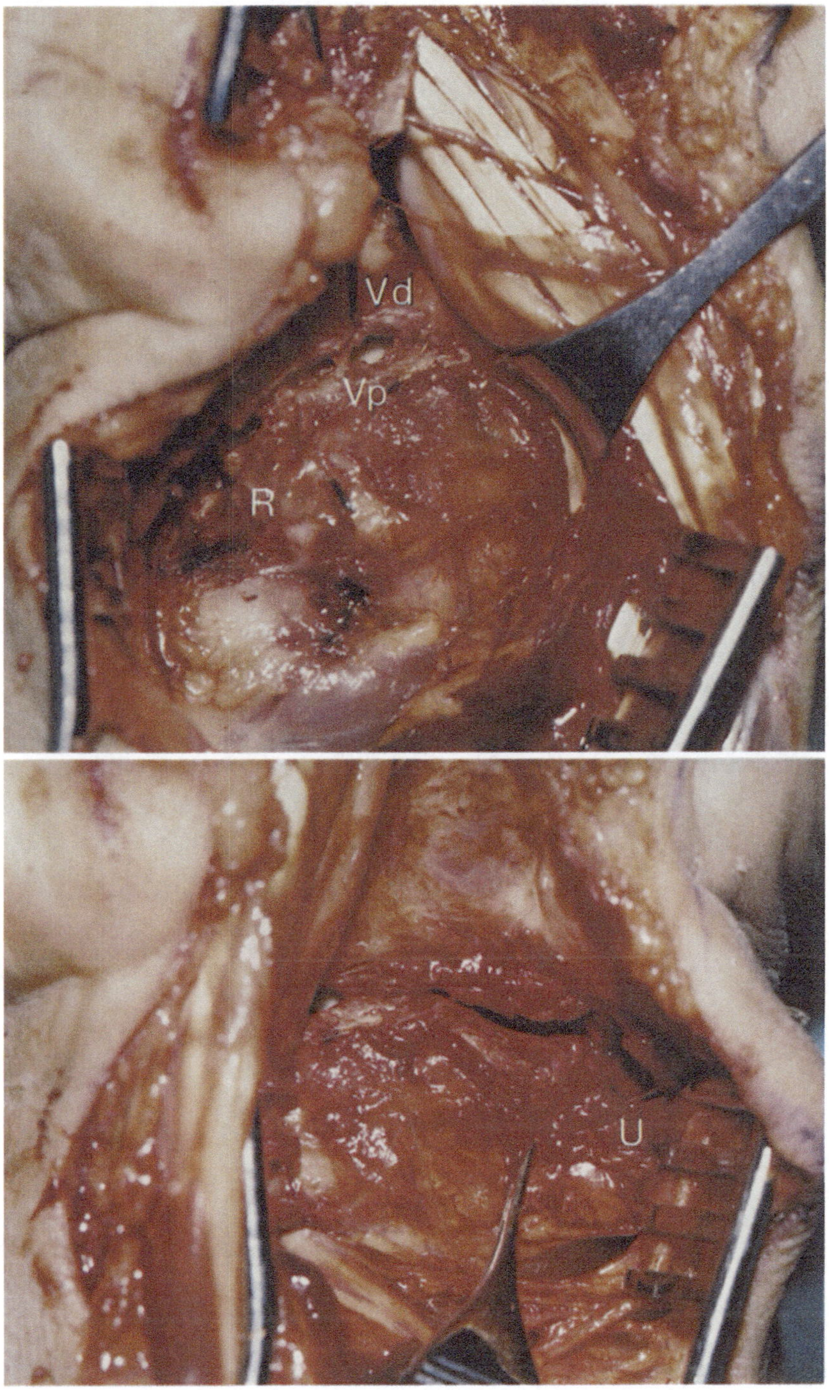


c

d

**Fig. III.11. a–d** De Quervain's fracture-dislocation. **a, b** Same lesion as in previous case but with more marked lunate tilt. **c, d** State of V ligaments after reduction: no lesion is visible.
*Vd* distal V
*Vp* proximal V

the normal position. This seems logical, since the line of injury passes between the two Vs. However:

- the integrity, i.e. the cohesion, of the proximal row is disrupted at two levels,
- the radio-scaphoid portion of the proximal V must be ruptured, a tear whose outcome is difficult to evaluate.

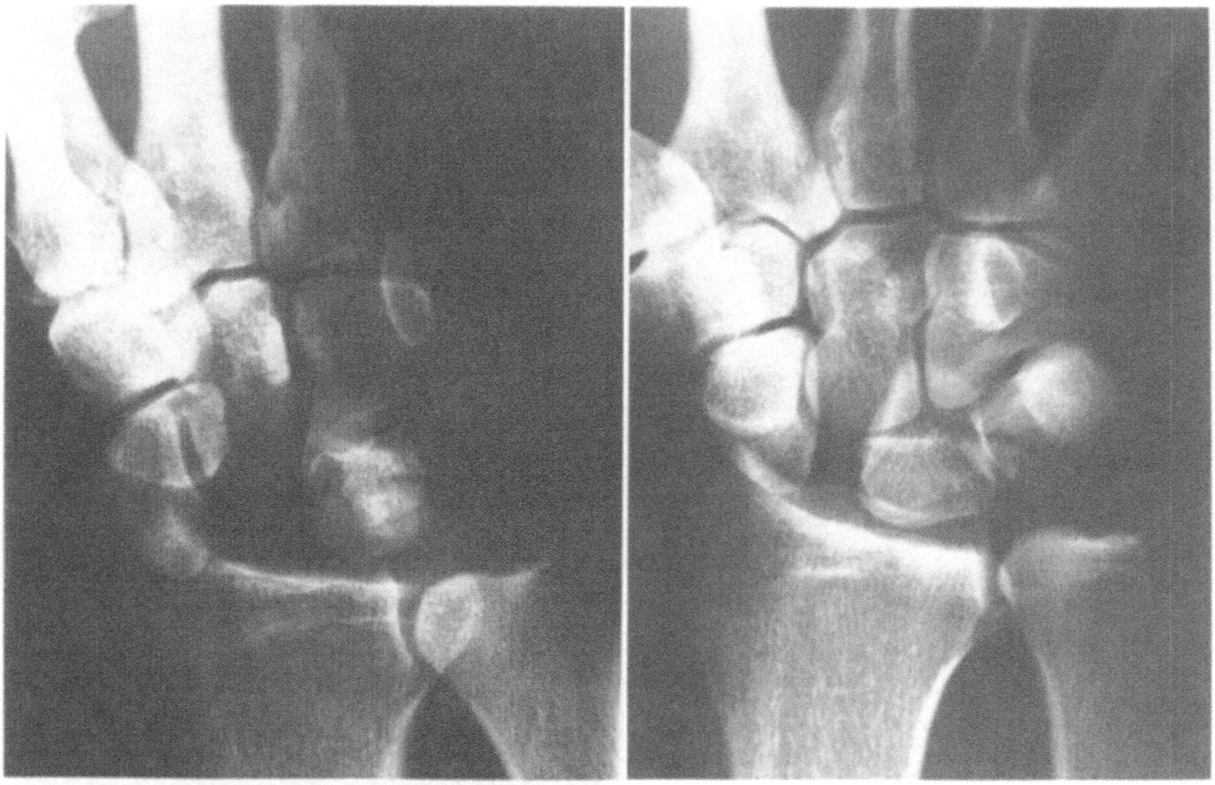

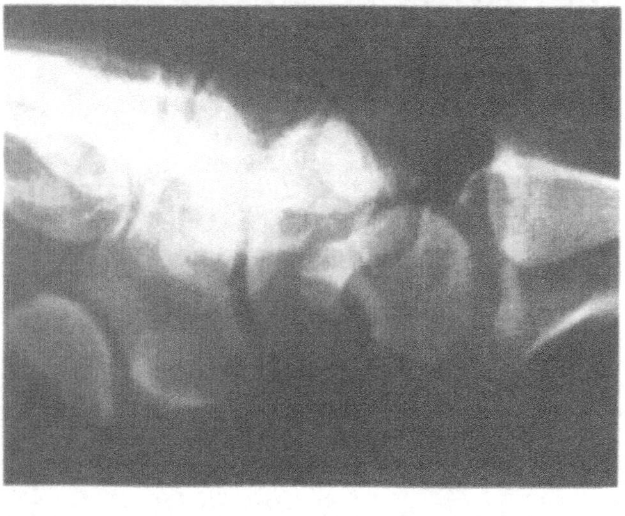

**Fig. III.12 a–e.** The radiological line of injury passes between the scaphoid and lunate. **d** Intra-operative view, palmar view: the torn ligaments of the lunate can be identified as a half-circle. **e** After reduction, the two V ligaments seem intact

*Discussion.* Only a perfect coaptation and an immobilisation for at least 6 weeks will allow healing of the torn ligaments. However, the proximal row is unstable by definition, and coaptation of the semi-circle of interosseous ligaments is particularly difficult to ensure. Therefore, it demands open reduction and stabilization with Kirschner wires. This surgical approach not only allows assessment of the lesions; it avoids the entrapment of the radio-capitate ligament between the two fragments of the scaphoid (Scharizer 1985). In the example of page 59 (Fig. II.13), despite conservative management, this complication did not occur. The perilunate dislocation was reduced by traction,

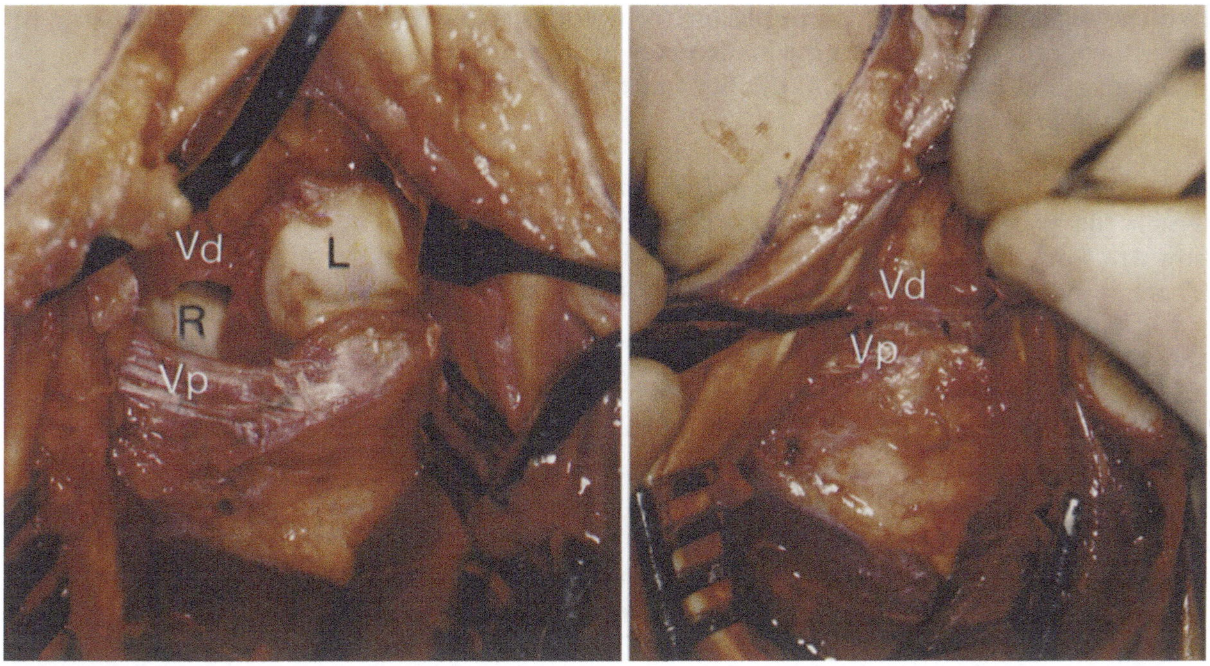

d e

Fig. III.12d, e

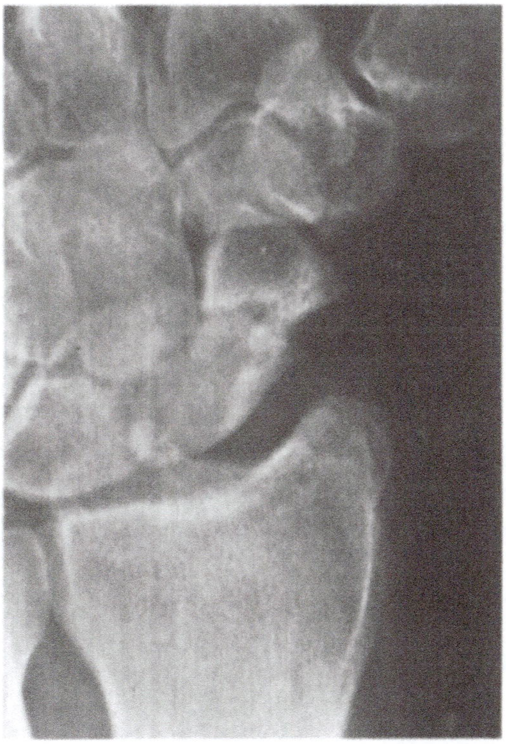

**Fig. III.13.** Subluxation of carpus secondary to avulsion of both V ligaments: status 6 months after De Quervain's fracture-dislocation treated by reduction and closed K-wiring and the reduction maintained in plaster for 6 weeks. However, the arthrogram demonstrates the inadequacy of the interosseous ligaments, and the functional disability underlines the dysfunction of the proximal row.

*Ulnar onset; forced hyperextension and pronation.*
When the two interosseous ligaments of the proximal carpal row are torn, the same ligamentous lesion as above is present. There is no need to describe this mirror sequence of events, since it is analogous to the order described above except that the lesion begins on the ulnar side, at the level of the ulnar styloid or between the lunate and triquetrum. It is impossible to tell whether the quality or the extent of the lesions are different.

## Conclusions

Conservative treatment makes it impossible to assess the extent of the lesions or to measure the quality of reduction. The aim of treatment of the dislocation, i.e. of De Quervain's fracture-dislocation, is to restore function. Only surgery will allow perfect coaptation of the fragments; and, for this, two approaches must be used: a dorsal and a palmar. These alone will permit exact assessment and complete, precise, surgical reconstruction. A fracture of the scaphoid can be advantageously pinned or stabilized by osteosynthesis, as in the example shown in Fig. III.9b. On the other hand, a fracture of the head of the capitate, which carries a risk of necrosis, can profitably be treated at the outset by arthrodesis of the central column or the whole carpal bones.

## References


Frykmann G (1967) Fracture of the distal radius including sequelae shoulder-hand-finger syndrome, disturbance in the distal radio-ulnar joint and impairment of nerve function. Acta Orthop Scand 108 [suppl]: 5–143

Mayfield JK, Johnson RP, Kilcoyne RK (1980) Carpal dislocation: Pathomechanics and progessive perilunar instability. J Hand Surg 5:226–241

Matti H (1936) Technik und Resultate meiner Pseudarthrosenoperation. Zentralbl Chir 63:1442–1453

Russe O (1952) Behandlungsergebnisse der Spongiosaauffüllung der Kahnbein-Pseudarthrosen. Z Orthop 81:466–473

Scharizer E (1985) Diskussionsbeitrag zum Thema: Anatomische Läsion bei der De Quervainsche Luxationsfraktur. Fruehjahrssymposium des Arbeitskreises für Handchirurgie der DGOT, Wengen: 31.3.–3.4.85

Weber ER (1980) Biomechanical implications of scaphoid waist fractures. Clin Orthop 149:83–89

Weber ER, Chao EY (1978) An experimental approach to the mechanism of scaphoid waist fracture. J Hand Surg 3:142–147

# B. Clinical Aspects

## 1. Instability of the Carpus and Pseudarthrosis of the Scaphoid

Linscheid et al., in 1972, suspected a diminished rate of union of both fractures and pseudarthroses of the scaphoid treated by Matti-Russe grafting in the presence of ligamentous instability. Brahin and Allieu (1984), 12 years later, asserted that only five of ten patients were cured by the Matti-Russe procedure in the presence of persistent malalignment of the lunate. Weber (1980) proposed a new classification of scaphoid fractures that was not based on the line of fracture, as with Trojan and Mourgues (1959), but on the displacement of the fragments, arguing that the more the fragments are displaced, the greater the ligamentous lesions, and the more difficult they are to treat.

Based on this information, we have reviewed and followed up 154 patients treated in our department for pseudarthrosis of the scaphoid in order to determine the factors influencing the rate of cure. Classically, osteosynthesis, a delay of over 1 year, a small-sized fragment, advanced age and instability are the factors that affect the chances of healing a pseudarthrosis. These factors have been reviewed and analysed by Nigst, among others, in the monograph *Fractures, Dislocations and Dissociations of the Carpal Bones* (1982) produced by a symposium on this subject held at Basel in June 1981.

### Case Material

The 154 patients reviewed represent 156 pseudarthroses of the carpal scaphoid, two cases being bilateral. The study extended from January 1961 to September 1984. The average follow-up from operation was 3.5 years, and at least 12 months had elapsed between the operation and the last check. Further, the X-rays needed to leave no doubt as to union; otherwise, the patients were reassessed with further films. Three cases were lost to follow-up; they have not been excluded from the study but have been considered failures. These three patients had all been treated by Matti-Russe grafting and while they certainly affect the statistics of cure for this operation, to exclude them would have reduced the objectivity of the statistics and might have suggested that we were trying to artificially improve the results of this procedure.

The ages range between 15 and 54 years with an average of 25 years. The graph in Fig. III.14 sets out the distribution according to age-group. The interval between fracture and operation for pseudarthrosis ranged from 4 months to 23 years, with an average of 2.7 years; in four cases the interval was unknown. We had 35 "small" fragments (i.e. the size is less than a quarter of the total length of the scaphoid) and 19 cases of arthrosis. We operated on 103 scaphoids primarily by the Matti-Russe

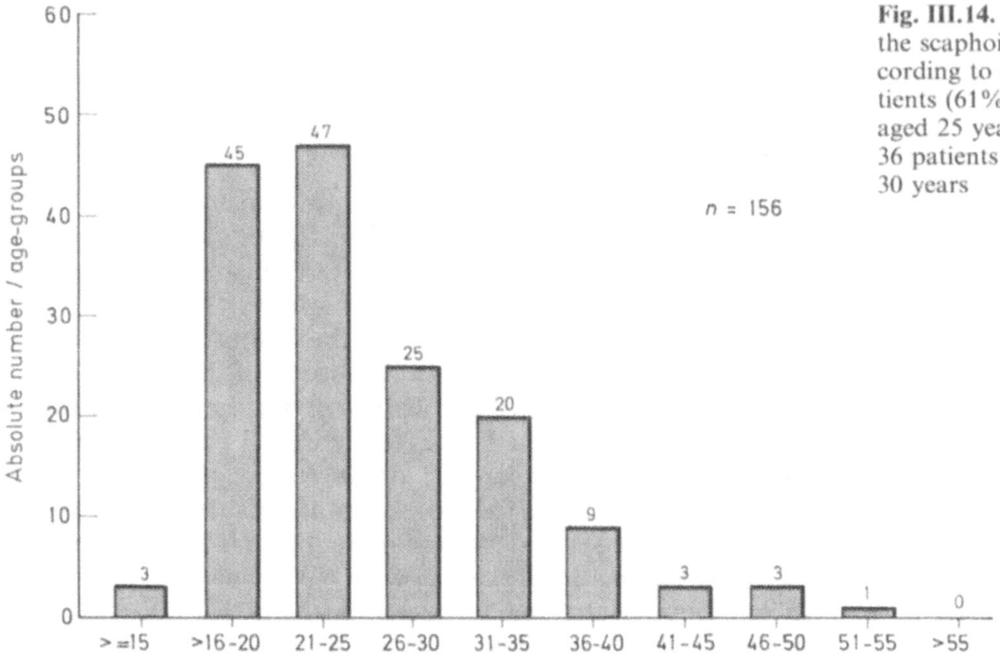


**Fig. III.14.** Pseudarthrosis of the scaphoid: distribution according to age-group; 95 patients (61% of the total) were aged 25 years or less and only 36 patients (23%) were over 30 years

technique, 23 by osteosynthesis and 30 by the "sandwich" technique. Finally, we had 26 cases of instability as defined by Linscheid (dorsiflexion of the lunate: 15° or more), of which 16 were operated by palmar grafting according to Matti-Russe. Tables III.1 and III.2 summarize the data.

### Type of Operation Related to Cure

Repeat operations were excluded; only cases having undergone no previous operative treatment have been analysed. We distinguish three types of operation: the Matti-Russe, the simple osteosynthesis (lag-screw) of the pseudarthrosis, and the "sandwich" technique: an interposed cortico-cancellous bone graft compressed by one or two lag-screws.

*Matti-Russe*

Among the 103 scaphoids operated by the Matti-Russe method, four techniques were distinguished:

1. The so-called simple Matti-Russe, i.e. with pegging of the graft but without supplementary measures (79 cases)
2. The Matti-Russe stabilized by Kirschner wires (17 cases)
3. The Matti-Russe supplemented by simple ligamentoplasty (two cases)
4. The Matti-Russe with ligamentoplasty and supplementary fixation by Kirschner wires (five cases)

Of these pseudarthroses, 85 were cured after the initial Matti-Russe operation, but three were unfortunately lost to follow-up. The cure-rate in this group, therefore, is 82.5% (85/103), with the missing patients considered as failures.

**Table III.1.** Pseudarthroses of the scaphoid

| | Number of patients | | Age | | | Interval | | | Fracture type | |
|---|---|---|---|---|---|---|---|---|---|---|
| | Total | % | Mean | Min. | Max. | Mean | Min. | Max. | Small fragments | Unstable |
| All scaphoids | 156 | | 25.4 | 15 | 54 | 2.7 | 0.25 | 23 (4 × inc) | 35 | 26 |
| MR (primary) | 103 | 66.03 | 25.7 | 15 | 54 | 3.2 | 0.25 | 23 (4 × inc) | 34 | 16 |
| OS (all) | 23 | 14.74 | 24.9 | 16 | 49 | 1.8 | 0.25 | 11 | 1 | 4 |
| Sandwich | 30 | 19.23 | 24.6 | 15 | 50 | 1.8 | 0.25 | 4 | 0 | 6 |
| MR (unstable) | 16 | 10.26 | 25.0 | 17 | 37 | 4.3 | 0.50 | 16 | 4 | |
| Instability (all) | 26 | 16.67 | 27.0 | 15 | 50 | 3.2 | 0.25 | 16 | 5 | |
| Arthrosis | 19 | 12.18 | 34.9 | 18 | 54 | 8.0 | 0.50 | 23 | 10 | |

Types of operation and cure-rates

| | N | Cured | % | Not cured | % |
|---|---|---|---|---|---|
| MR (all) | 103 | 85 | 82.5 | 18 | 17.5 |
| MR (no risks) | 53 | 45 | 84.9 | 8 | 15.1 |
| MR + arthrosis/ small fragment | 34 | 31 | 91.9 | 3 | 8.8 |
| OS (clinic) | 19 | 12 | 63.1 | 7 | 36.8 |
| Sandwich | 30 | 21 | 70.0 | 9 | 30.0 |

The results represent a group of 154 patients and 156 scaphoids. Of these patients, 135 were men (87.7%) and 19 were women (12.3%); MR, Matti-Russe operation; OS, osteosynthesis

**Table III.2.** Distribution of operations according to risk

| Operation | No risks | | | Arthrosis and/or small fragments | | | Instability | | |
|---|---|---|---|---|---|---|---|---|---|
| | Scaphoids | Primary cures | Cures | Scaphoids | Primary cures | Cures | Scaphoids | Primary cures | Cures |
| OS (clinic) | 15 | 9 | | | | | 4 | 3 | |
| Sandwich | 22 | 15 | | 2 | 1 | | 6 | 5 | |
| Secondary operation OS post-OS | | 1 | | | | | | | |
| Primary MR | | | | | | | | | |
| MR | 49 | 41 | | 22 | 20 | | 8 | 2 | |
| MR + K-wire | 4 | 4 | | 12 | 11 | | 1 | 1 | |
| MR + plasty | | | | | | | 2 | 2 | |
| MR + K-wire + plasty | | | | | | | 5 | 4 | |
| Secondary MR | | | | | | | | | |
| MR post-external OS | 4 | | 4 | | | | | | |
| MR post-internal OS | 1 | | 1 | | | | 1 | | 1 |
| MR post-sandwich | 7 | | 6 | 1 | | 1 | 1 | | 1 |
| MR post-OS + sandwich | 2 | | 2 | | | | | | |
| MR post-MR | 3 | | 1 | 2 | | 2 | 3 | | 3 |

*Osteosynthesis* (Fig. III.15)

Of the 23 scaphoids treated by primary osteosynthesis, 19 were operated at the outset in the clinic. We shall analyse only these 19 pseudarthroses treated in the department, as they represent a homogenous group in that only two surgeons were involved. This fact imparts some consistency to the analysis and allows valid conclusions as to method and risks. Only 12 of these pseudarthroses united after simple screwing, a success rate slightly below 64%. This is a figure markedly inferior to that of the Matti-Russe group. The advantage of the method lies in the short period of immobilization which, as a rule, does not exceed 15 days, the time for the skin wound to heal.

*The Sandwich*

For the 30 scaphoids treated by the sandwich method introduced by Segmüller (1973) over 10 years ago, 21 (70%) were cured by the operation. Again, immobilization in plaster did not exceed 15 days.

*Discussion.* The Matti-Russe method is a relatively reliable operation since it is not technically difficult and it produces a primary cure-rate of 83% across the board. This is more than can be said of osteosynthesis and the sandwich operation. These procedures, even if left to the experienced surgeon, have a cure-rate significantly lower than the Matti-Russe average with only 64% and 70% success, respectively (Fig. III.16).

**Analysis of Risk Factors**

*Success with the Matti-Russe Under Low-risk and High-risk Circumstances* (Table III.3)

Such an analysis can only be made for patients operated on using a single technique. As we have just seen the most reliable method is the Matti-Russe operation, and we have grouped the 103 patients so operated into three separate categories. The results appear as follows:

| | | | |
|---|---|---|---|
| 1. Instability (all forms): | 16 scaphoids; | 9 cures | (56.3%) |
| 2. Arthroses and/or small fragments: | 34 scaphoids; | 31 cures | (91.2%) |
| 3. "No risk": | 53 scaphoids; | 45 cures | (84.9%) |

*Discussion.* This initial comparative analysis makes it clear that the small fragment (Fig. III.17), whether alone or associated with arthrosis, is not a major risk factor. However, it is possible that this high cure-rate is related to the surgeon, these cases being handled by the more experienced. One must note the rather modest success in the group labelled as being without apparent major risks compared to the good results quoted in the literature. It embraces a series operated by a heterogenous group of surgeons, sometimes inexperienced, precisely because the risks ap-

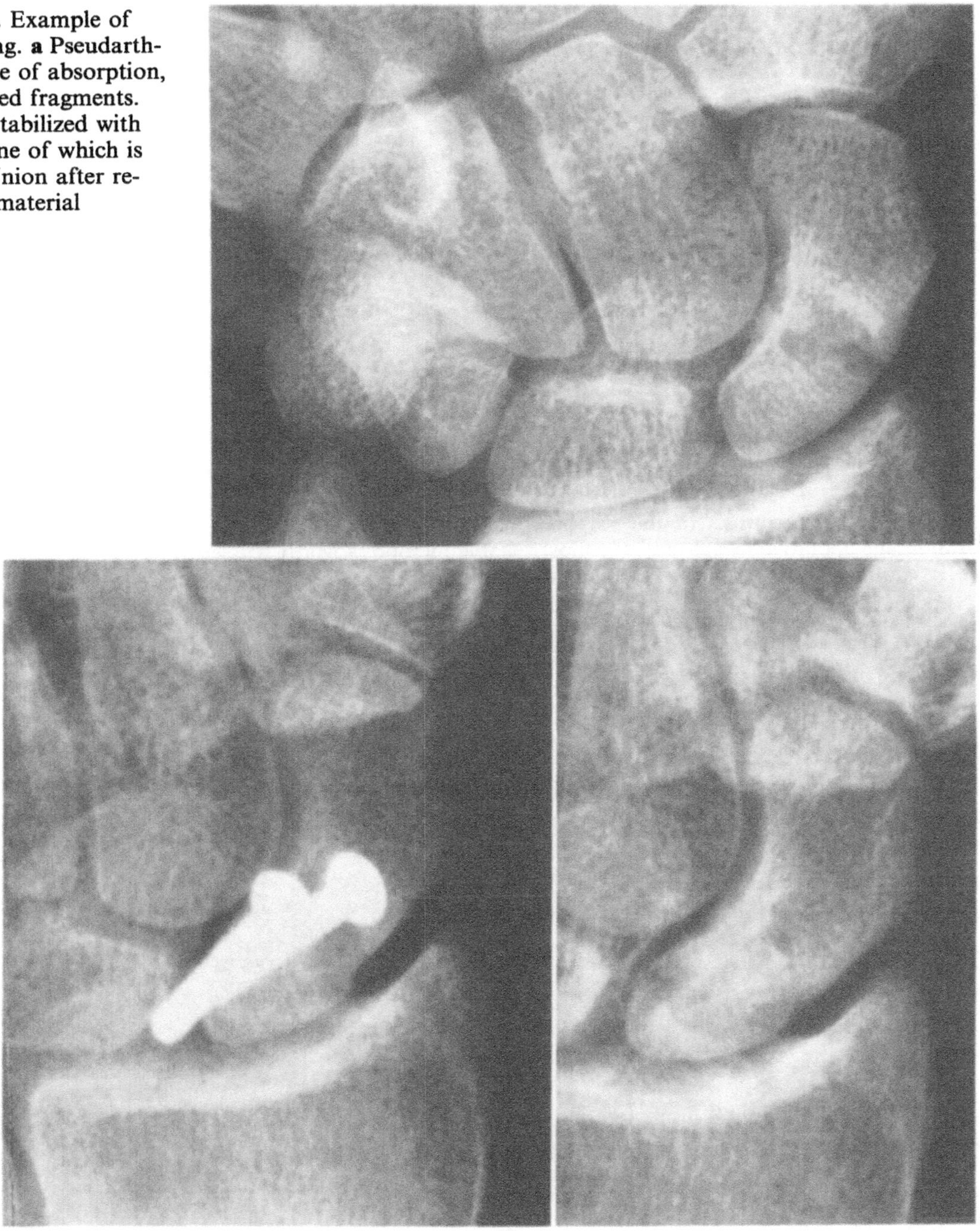

a

b

c

**Fig. III.15a–c.** Example of simple screwing. **a** Pseudarthrosis with zone of absorption, and undisplaced fragments. **b** Fragments stabilized with two screws (one of which is too long). **c** Union after removal of OS material

peared to be minor. On the other hand, this rate is also weighted by the three patients lost to follow-up. Therefore we can say that the Matti-Russe technique, in a group without obvious risks, gives a success rate of 85%, and we shall henceforth take this as the reference rate. The group with instability, whether isolated or combined with other lesions, gave the least favourable results: only 56% of operated scaphoids healed after the first operation. Figure III.18 illustrates the data of Table III.3 graphically.

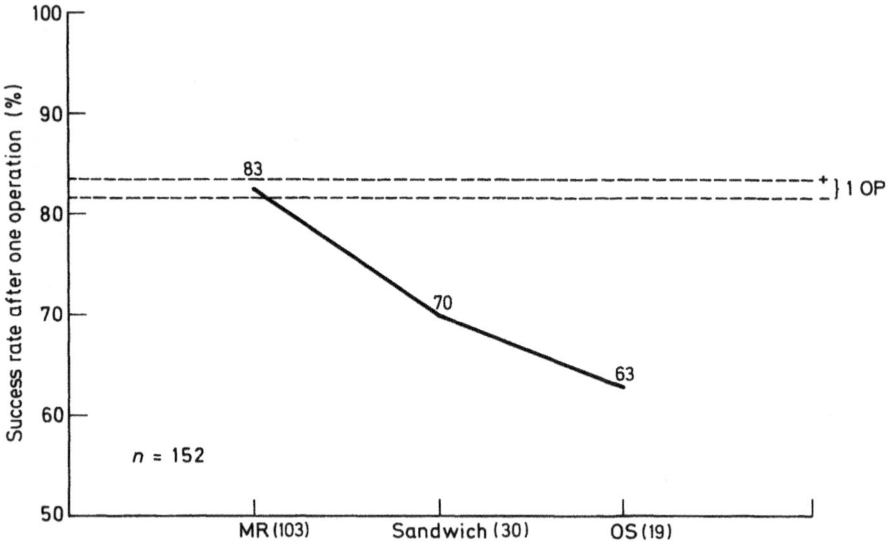


**Fig. III.16.** Pseudarthrosis of the scaphoid: comparison of success-rates of different operative techniques: the most reliable method is Matti-Russe (MR) grafting, with 83% cures after one operation

*Analysis of Cure-rate in Relation to Interval Between Fracture and Operation*

In 99 of our 103 cases the interval between fracture and operation could be precisely defined; in four cases it is unknown. This allows us to re-define three groups of patients:

- those operated up to 1 year after injury,
- those grafted after 1 year and up to 2 years,
- those treated after this interval.

The 16 unstable cases have been excluded since they have a cure-rate well below average, leaving a more homogenous group. Therefore these are 83 patients whom we have subdivided according to the criteria laid down. The results are collated in Table III.4.

Of the 39 patients operated in the 1st year, 34 were cured straight off, i.e. 87.2%. Nineteen patients were operated after 1 year but no later than 2 years after the fracture; 18 (95%)

**Table III.3.** Risk factors

| Risk | Total scaphoids | Cures | |
|---|---|---|---|
| | | (*n*) | (%) |
| None | 53 | 45 | 85 |
| Arthrosis and/or small fragments | 34 | 31 | 91 |
| Instability | 16 | 9 | 56 |
| Total | 103 | 85 | 82.5 |

**Fig. III.17. a** Pseudarthrosis and absorption cyst, with very small fragment. **b** Union at 20 months; bone remodelling is still in progress

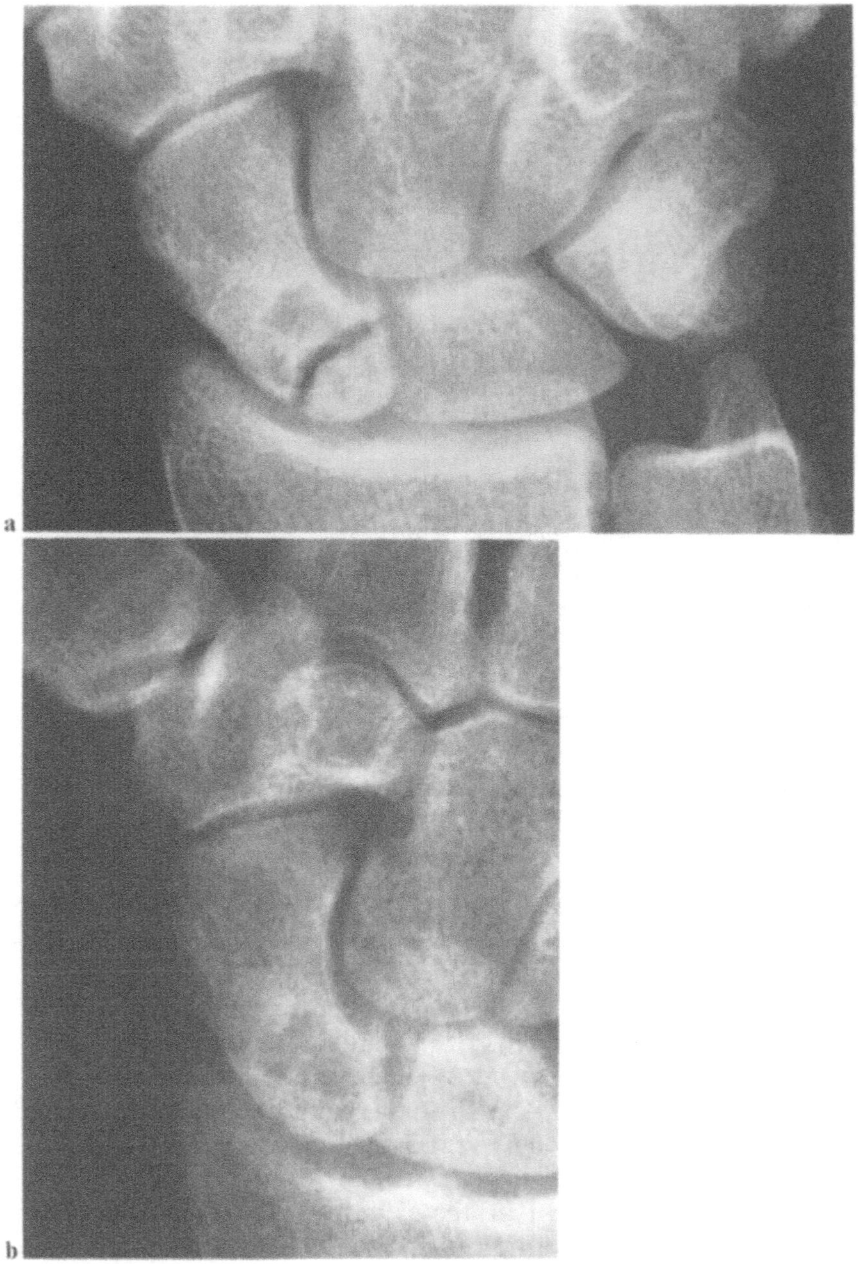

consolidated after the first operation. The remaining 25 patients were dealt with after 2 years and were successfully grafted in 20 cases (80% cures).

*Discussion.* For those patients operated after an interval of 2 years the cure-rate was slightly below average. Though this difference does not seem significant, it is worthwhile to emphasize that the average period between the time of fracture and the date of operation in the 11 patients in whom the first Matti-Russe procedure was a failure was 4.4 years. Thus it is legitimate

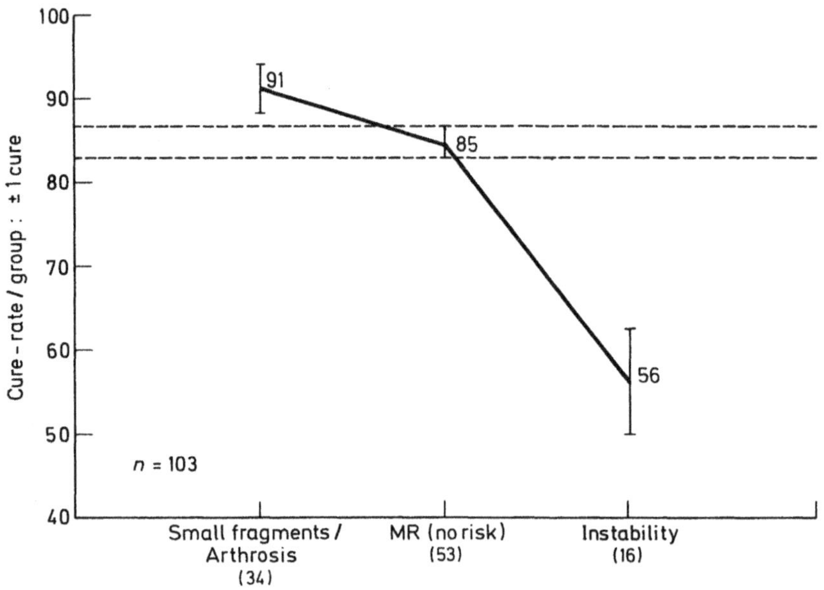


**Fig. III.18.** Graphical representation of data in Table III.3, the cure-rate in the unstable cases is very markedly inferior to the average

to state that prolonged delay lessens the chances of cure, but perhaps it takes longer than 5 years for this progressive secondary instability to affect the results of grafting.

*Analysis of Cure-rate in Relation to Age*

The unstable cases were directly excluded from this study, so that the analysis covers 87 patients subdivided into three categories:

1. Up to 25 years: 49 patients; direct cures: 43
2. Between 25 and 35 years: 30 patients; direct cures: 26
3. Over 35 years: 8 patients; direct cures: 7

The cure-rate was 87.7% in the first group, 86.6% in the second and 87.5% in the patients over 35 years of age (Fig. III.19).

*Discussion.* In the light of these figures, age as a risk factor seems insignificant, even though there were relatively few cases over 35 years.

**Table III.4.** Cure-rate related to interval between fracture and operation (unstable cases excluded)

| Interval | Operations | Cures | |
|---|---|---|---|
| | | (*n*) | (%) |
| 1 year or less | 39 | 34 | 87.2 |
| 1–2 years | 19 | 18 | 94.7 |
| Over 2 years | 25 | 20 | 80 |
| Total | 83 | 72 | 86.7 |

### Analysis of Matti-Russe Procedures with Kirschner Wire Fixation

We shall new examine the outcome of the cases stabilized by Kirschner wires. There are several indications, that may overlap, for the use of this technique:

1. There may be ligamentous instability with tilting of the lunate, and the surgeon can reduce this tilt by means of wires.
2. The surgeon may establish that the cortico-cancellous graft is not itself adequate to stabilize the fragments and that it is necessary to consolidate the construct.
3. In failed cases he may wish to supplement the graft in order to ensure maximum stabilization.
4. Finally, these problems may overlap.

Thirty scaphoids were stabilized by Kirschner wire (Table III.5). In 17 cases the first operation was supplemented by wiring, as the graft could not be held in place (proximal fragment too small or unstable); in five cases, supplementary stabilization was required for ligamentous instability and lunate tilting; the eight remaining cases were repeat operations after failed Matti-Russe or osteosynthesis procedures, in which the surgeon wished to ensure the maximum stability. It should be emphasized here that one of the 17 cases treated for bony instability also had ligamentous instability that was initially unrecognized.

*Discussion.* Supplementary wire stabilization appears to be an excellent technique, since 16 of the 17 Matti-Russe procedures so managed healed, i.e. 94%. The single failure was a case of ligamentous instability. Though treated primarily as such, failure

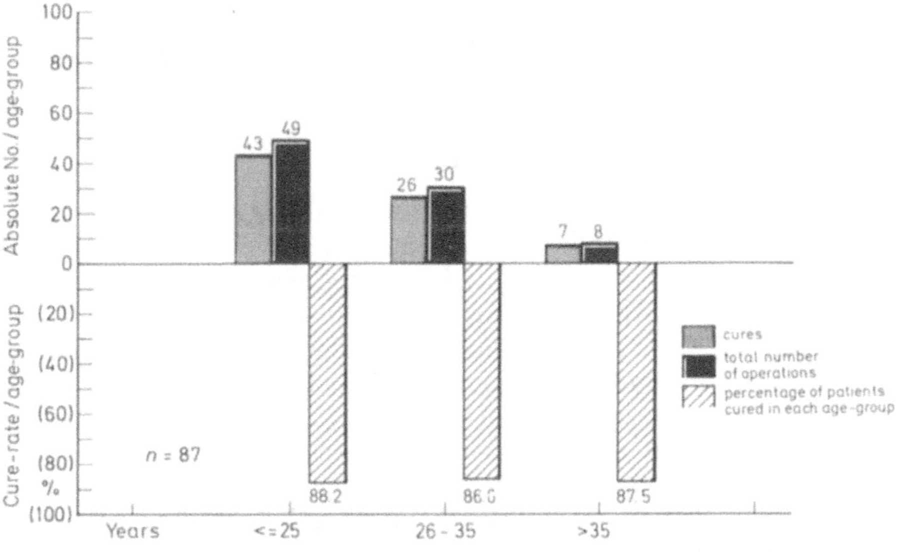


**Fig. III.19.** Cure related to age, excluding MR cases with instability: patient age does not appear to be an important risk factor

**Table III.5.** Matti-Russe and Kirschner wires

| Reason for use of wire | Operated | Cured | |
|---|---|---|---|
| | | ($n$) | (%) |
| Bony instability | 17 | 16 | 94 |
| Ligamentoplasty | 5 | 4 | |
| Repeat operation | 8 | 6 | |
| Total | 30 | 26 | 86 |

was probably a result of an error of technique associated with the difficulty of combining ligamentoplasty and cancellous grafting. For repeat operations the usefulness of supplementary stabilization is less evident, as we had two failures in the eight patients re-operated. Still, it is clear that in a case of this type many other factors play a role, for example, the type of previous operation and the approach employed (a dorsal approach disturbs the blood-supply of the scaphoid).

### Secondary Matti-Russe

Of the 25 scaphoids previously operated on without success, 22 healed with a second operation by the Matti-Russe technique (88% success).

*Discussion.* The risk of failure with re-operation is no greater than that of the first intervention. Therefore, there is no reason, because of initial failure, to abandon the Matti-Russe technique. Kleinert et al. (1985) have shown that resorting to Silastic implants does not modify the tendency of the carpus to collapse as described by Mack et al. (1984); Silastic is therefore of no use and possibly harmful, bearing in mind the risk of synovitis reported by Smith et al. (1985).

### The Problem of Statistical Evaluation

Are the different success rates of the various operations statistically significant? We shall endeavour to deal with this question here, not with the aim of irritating the reader with figures, but to try and clarify the difficulty of choosing adequate statistical tests and their interpretation. It should be appreciated that the comparison and evaluation of several tests or indices allows a more precise assessment of the situation. Unfortunately this approach is not the rule in many present-day medical/scientific studies. To mention a test and a percentage in passing, without defining exactly what they represent and how they have been calculated can be misleading and leads to misure of statistics. This is why different tests must be defined, discussed and analysed, with particular attention to their limitations.

We wish to substantiate two hypotheses: firstly, osteosynthesis (sandwich and/or simple screwing) gives a cure-rate significantly different from that of the Matti-Russe procedure; secondly, instability is an important prognostic factor and the cure-rate in stable cases is significantly different from that in unstable cases. This implies a modification of diagnostic and therapeutic attitudes.

The parameters analysed, the healing or non-healing of the fracture, are qualitative in the sense that these are data that can be stated but not measured. On the other hand, the choice of operation (such as the sandwich) is not related between patients, so that the samples analysed are independent of each other. The same applies to instability. In both cases we have independent and qualitative samples. Among the numerous tests or indices available, in our study four are capable of answering our questions:

1. the confidence interval,
2. the Phi coefficient,
3. the Chi-square test,
4. the Student's *t* test.

*Confidence Interval*

This allows definition of the limits of the possible fluctuations in sampling for a given risk of error. In fact, random sampling may produce any level of cure-rate; but even if all eventualities are possible, they are not all equally probable. A significant divergence between the observed and the true percentage is unlikely. The calculation of such an interval is determined by the following formula, assuming an error risk of 5%:

$$\mathrm{CI} = \mathrm{p} \pm 1.96 \cdot \sqrt{(\mathrm{p} \cdot \mathrm{q}/\mathrm{n})}$$

CI = confidence interval
p = % observed
q = 1 − p
n = number of subjects

Table III.6 sets out the data and gives the confidence intervals for all the groups studied. From a graph, we can ascertain that the cure-rates of the sandwich and osteosynthesis operations are outside the confidence interval of stable Matti-Russe procedures even for an error risk of 1%. The same is true for the unstable cases (Figs. III.20 and III.21).

In Fig. III.22 we have compared the confidence intervals for the Matti-Russe procedure in the stable and unstable situations. The number of the latter is small, so that the width of interval is greater. However, the resultant overlap is limited, leading one to suppose that these two groups are probably different. This overlap is greater when osteosynthesis is compared with the stable Matti-Russe procedures. To obtain a more precise idea of the true situation it is necessary to do further analysis, especially as the number of cases is limited. Strictly speaking,

**Table III.6.** Confidence intervals

| | n | g | p | q | CI | | a 5% | | a 1% | | np | nq |
|---|---|---|---|---|---|---|---|---|---|---|---|---|
| | | | (%) | (%) | 5% | 1% | Max. | Min. | Max. | Min. | | |
| **MR (all)** | **103** | **85** | **83%** | **17%** | **± 7.3%** | **± 9.6%** | **90%** | **75%** | **92%** | **73%** | **85** | **18** |
| **MR (stable)** | **87** | **76** | **87%** | **13%** | **± 7.0%** | **± 9.2%** | **94%** | **80%** | **97%** | **78%** | **76** | **11** |
| MR (unstable) | 16 | 9 | 56% | 44% | ±24.3% | ±31.9% | 81% | 32% | 88% | 24% | 9 | 7 |
| Sandwich | 30 | 21 | 70% | 30% | ±16.4% | ±21.6% | 86% | 54% | 92% | 48% | 21 | 9 |
| Screwing | 19 | 12 | 63% | 37% | ±21.7% | ±28.5% | 85% | 41% | 92% | 35% | 12 | 7 |
| **Sandwich + screws** | **49** | **33** | **67%** | **33%** | **±13.1%** | **±17.3%** | **80%** | **54%** | **84%** | **50%** | **33** | **16** |

Results based on the formula: $CI = p \pm a\sqrt{pq/n}$
p, cure-rate
n, number of scaphoids observed
g, number of scaphoids united after one operation
p, g/n
q, percentage of uncured patients: $(n-g)/n$
CI, confidence interval;
a, 1.960 for the 5% interval, 2.576 for the 1% interval
Conditions of validity: np or nq $\geq 10$

only the groups in bold type are statistically valid; the others do not meet the conditions of validity defined in Table III.6.

*Phi Coefficient*

This coefficient is particularly suited for evaluating two binomial samples. It provides information about the relationship between dichotomous groups. The more the coefficient approaches zero, the more marked is the disparity of the groups; on the other hand, a value of plus 1 or minus 1 indicates a virtually identical sample. This test satisfies the general formula set out in Table III.7.

*Chi-Square Test*

This permits determination of the disparity between two or more samples with a precise risk of error. When the samples are binomial and dichotomous, as in our case, this test must meet the following conditions to be valid: firstly, $ni * pi$ and $ni * qi$ must equal or exceed 10. Secondly, only one group may have a sample size below 5. Thirdly, no group may equal zero.

In our case, Phi squared multiplied by the number of cases observed $(n1 + n2)$ gives the value of Chi. The number of degrees of freedom is equal to 1 since we have a table of comparison with $2 \times 2$ parameters. The ad hoc tables contain the risk of error associated with the acceptance of the hypothesis of the disparity of the samples examined. Only two comparisons satisfy the conditions of validity of the test. These permit acceptance of our original hypotheses that the cure-rates are different. Though Schwartz and Lazar (1964) seem very tolerant as regards this test, certain statisticians, like Champion (1981), require that $n1 + n2$ should always exceed 25.

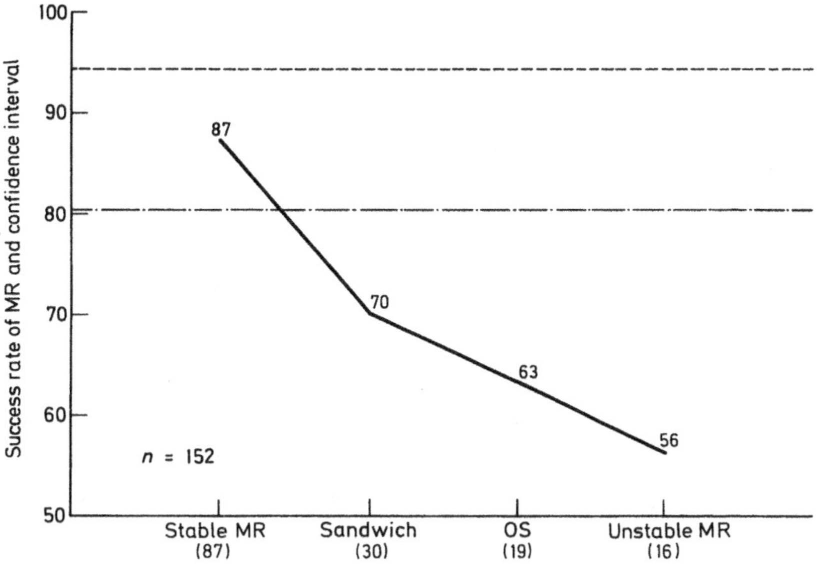


**Fig. III.20.** Confidence intervals of 5%

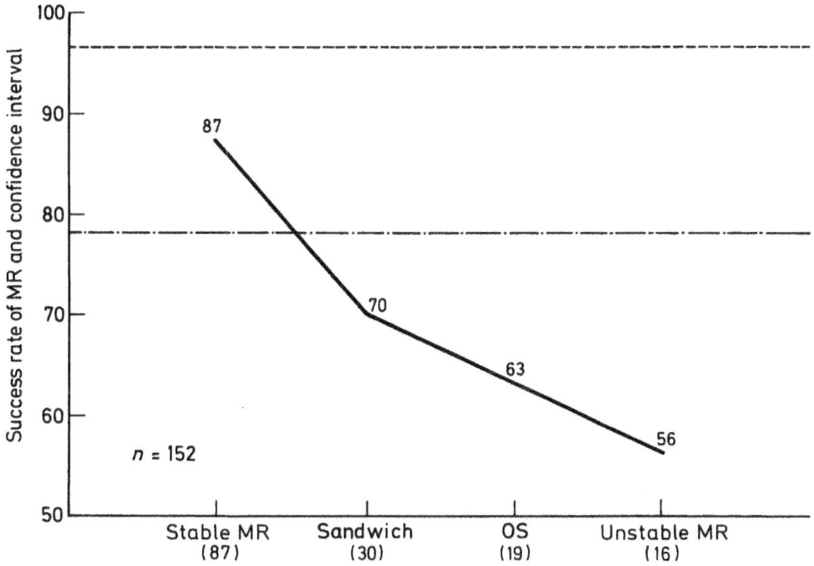


**Fig. III.21.** Confidence intervals of 1%

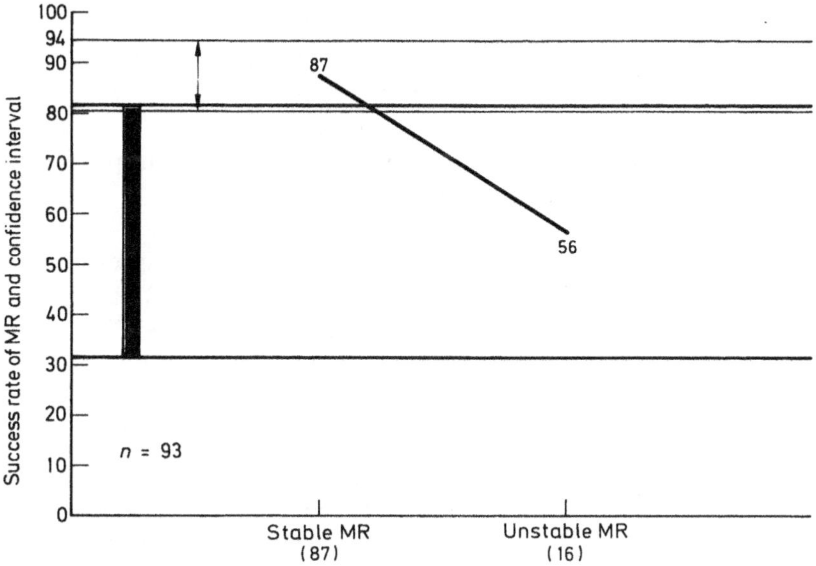


**Fig. III.22.** Comparison of 5% confidence intervals for stable and unstable MR procedures: the minimal overlap of the confidence intervals of the stable and unstable MR operation suggests that the two groups are statistically different

Table III.7. Phi coefficient and Chi-square test

| | n1 | n2 | k1 / n1p1 | k2 / n2p2 | n1−k1 / n1q1 | n2−k2 / n2q2 | Phi | Chi² |
|---|---|---|---|---|---|---|---|---|
| MR stable/MR unstable | 87 | 16 | 76 | 9 | 11 | 7 | −0.29 | 9.0 |
| MR stable/sandwich | 87 | 30 | 76 | 21 | 11 | 9 | −0.20 | 4.7 |
| MR stable/screwing | 87 | 19 | 76 | 12 | 11 | 7 | −0.24 | 6.5 |
| **MR stable/sandwich + screwing** | **87** | **49** | **76** | **33** | **11** | **16** | **−0.24** | **7.9** |
| **MR (all)/sandwich + screwing** | **103** | **49** | **85** | **33** | **18** | **16** | **−0.17** | **4.4** |
| MR unstable/sandwich + screwing | 16 | 49 | 9 | 33 | 7 | 16 | 0.10 | 0.6 |

$$\text{Phi} = \Phi = \frac{bc - ad}{\sqrt{(a+b)(c+d)(a+c)(b+d)}}$$

$a = k1 = n1 \cdot p1 \quad n1 = a + c$

$b = k2 = n2 \cdot p2 \quad n2 = b + d$

$c = n1 - k1 = n1 \cdot q1 \quad n = n1 + n2$

$d = n2 - k2 = n2 \cdot q2 \quad p1 = k1/n1$

$p2 = k2/n2$

$\text{Chi}^2 = \text{Phi}^2 \cdot (n1 + n2)$ or $X^2 = n\Phi^2$

Criteria of validity:
1. n1q1 and n1p1 $\geq 10$.
2. Only one size may be less than 5.
3. No sample may have the value 0.

The degree of freedom (table $2 \times 2$) is one. Thus, the test is significant with a 5% risk of error if Chi-square $\geq 3.841$

*Student's t Test*

This test is theoretically conceived for samples where the number of cases is less than 30. It therefore seems particularly well-suited to our situation. However, and this often fails to be recognized, there must be a normal distribution of the population. Now, the distribution of a binomial sample only satisfies this definition above 30 persons. However, if we use it as Kurtz suggests (1983), it does not add any fundamentally new factors to the previous conclusions, and confirms the values found by the earlier tests (Table III.8).

*Discussion: Limits and Problems of Statistical Analysis*

Unfortunately, the statistical analysis of the binomial and dichotomous samples cannot tell us what the results would be if the number of observations were multiplied by 10, since the Chi-square test does not satisfy the statistical definition in the strict sense when comparing stable and unstable Matti-Russe procedures. However, when the tests are so suggestive, it would be very questionable to continue with our present technique merely to produce convincing statistics!

*Unstable cases.* The very definition of instability is empirical; we have used the studies of Linscheid et al. (1972) to produce a definition. However, between the position called "normal" and the position called "unstable" there is a multitude of intermediate positions which are on a continuum of instability. Thus, the samples labelled "stable" certainly conceal a number of unstable cases whose role remains undefined. While our study takes no account of this "blurring", it nevertheless tends to demonstrate that the definition of instability given by Linscheid corre-

**Table III.8.** Student's *t* test

| | n1 | n2 | k1 / n1p1 | k2 / n2p2 | n1 − k1 / n1q1 | n2 − k2 / n2q2 | *t* | Degrees of freedom |
|---|---|---|---|---|---|---|---|---|
| MR stable/MR unstable | 87 | 16 | 76 | 9 | 11 | 7 | 3.0 | 101 |
| MR stable/sandwich | 87 | 30 | 76 | 21 | 11 | 9 | 2.2 | 115 |
| MR stable/screwing | 87 | 19 | 76 | 12 | 11 | 7 | 2.5 | 104 |
| **MR stable/sandwich + screw** | **87** | **49** | **76** | **33** | **11** | **16** | **2.8** | **134** |
| **MR (all)/sandwich + screw** | **103** | **49** | **85** | **33** | **18** | **16** | **2.1** | **150** |
| MR unstable/sandwich + screw | 16 | 49 | 9 | 33 | 7 | 16 | 0.8 | 63 |

$$t = \frac{p1 - p2}{\sqrt{pe \cdot qe\left(\frac{n1 + n2}{n1 \cdot n2}\right)}}$$

$pe = (k1 + k2)/(n1 + n2)$
Degrees of freedom $= n1 + n2 - 2$

The test is significant with a 5% risk of error if $t \geq 2.00$ and the number of degrees of freedom is above 60

sponds to a therapeutic threshold. As soon as the lunate tilt exceeds 15° ligamentoplasty is necessary in order to ensure cure, six of the seven unstable cases so treated having been primarily cured. This fact seems to confirm the importance of the ligamentous problem and its treatment. However, this "unstable" group is far from uniform; it also includes patients treated from the outset for their instability, which falsifies the objectivity of the study.

Moreover, this "unstable" group, despite its reduced population, still contains patients in whom the instability did not become manifest until after the operation – cases of latent instability in a manner of speaking. The intraoperative division of the radio-capitate ligament and of part of the radio-lunate ligament is probably related to this fact. Their reconstruction is imperative and routine in our department, but is it enough?

This account shows clearly how much prudence is required in interpreting the figures of statistical tables; it emphasizes how difficult it is, particularly in medicine, to be perfectly rigorous, especially in retrospective studies.

*Osteosyntheses (sandwich or simple screwing).* The factors influencing the results of these procedures are multiple: the exposure and its effects on vascularization, the size of the fragment, the axis of the fracture and of the screws, their number and anchorage, the compression obtained (either between the fragments or along the interposed graft), the quality of the bone, its resistance, the length of immobilization, the surgeon's experience and possible ligamentous problems. This list is almost longer than the list of cases treated by osteosynthesis, which indicates the difficulty of accepting the overall statistical verdict uncritically, although it is probably in large part true. It is difficult for the surgeon to master all of the above-mentioned problems. Despite everything, these techniques of osteosynthesis retain their indications; but they must be carefully weighed.

Thus, the statistical analysis of binomial and dichotomous samples remains of limited application; more so since the problem, once recognized, modifies the therapeutic approach and consequently the statistical data. While we may accept as valid the hypotheses we wished to demonstrate, statistical doubt persists. It should not be forgotten that the annual number of cases of pseudarthrosis of the scaphoid, which is doubtless on the increase, is small. In 21 years we have seen only 156 cases, an average of less than eight cases a year.

## Conclusions and Consequences

Two factors seem to influence the prognosis of the treatment of pseudarthrosis of the carpal scaphoid:

1. Osteosynthesis (sandwich or screwing)
2. Ligamentous instability

It is essential to stress here that, contrary to the general opinion, advanced age of the patient, the duration of the pseudarthrosis (up to a certain limit), size of the proximal fragment, arthrosis or even re-operation are not contra-indications to a Matti-Russe procedure. Now that instability occupies the foreground, it is important to recognize it. It is relatively common, since we encountered it 26 times in 156 scaphoid lesions (16%). Recognizing its existence can ensure a normal cure-rate! This is true for pseudarthrosis, but also for recent fractures of the scaphoid, as Weber (1980) has shown. All of this only reinforces our opinion that it is imperative to improve and standardize the radiological diagnosis.

## References


Brahin B, Allieu Y (1984) Les désaxations carpiennes d'adaptation. Ann Chir Main 3:357–363

Champion Dean J (1981) Basic statistics for social research. Macmillan, New York, pp 224–226

Kleinert JM, Stern PJ, Lister GD, Kleinhans RJ (1985) Complications of scaphoid silicone arthroplasty. J Bone Joint Surg [Am] 67:422–427

Kurtz NR (1983) Introduction to social statistics. International student edition. McGraw-Hill, New York

Linscheid RL, Dobyns JH, Boabout JW, Bryan RS (1972) Traumatic instability of the wrist: Diagnosis, classification and pathomechanics. J Bone Joint Surg [Am] 54:1612–1632

Mack GR, Bosse MJ, Gelberman RH, Yu E (1984) The natural history of scaphoid non-union. J Bone Joint Surg [Am] 66:504–509

Nigst H (1982) Pseudarthrosen des Scaphoids. In: Buck-Gramcko D, Nigst H (eds), Frakturen, Luxationen und Dissoziationen der Karpalknochen. Hippokrates, Stuttgart, pp 53–62

Schwartz D, Lazar P (1964) Eléments de statistique médicale et biologique. Editions Médicales Flammarion, Paris

Segmüller G (1973) Operative Stabilisierung am Handskelett. Huber, Bern, pp 99–104

Smith RJ, Atkinson RE, Jupiter JB (1985) Silicone synovitis of the wrist. J Hand Surg 10A:47–60
Trojan E, de Mourgues S (1959) Fractures et pseudarthroses du scaphoïde carpien. Etude thérapeutique. Rev Chir Orthop 45:614–677
Weber ER (1980) Biomechanical implications of scaphoid waist fractures. Clin Orthop 149:83–89

## 2. The Therapeutic Concept of Carpal Instability

### Ligamentoplasties and Partial Arthrodeses

The poor results of ligamentoplasties for post-traumatic wrist instability make the value of the procedure debatable (Palmer et al. 1978). The need to place the graft under correct tension to prevent its progressive failure makes the procedure unpredictable. However, we now know that ligamentoplasty may advantageously complement Matti-Russe grafting when scaphoid pseudarthrosis is associated with ligamentous instability (Fig. III.7, p. 74, and see p. 96 "unstable cases"). It is also justified between the lunate and triquetrum and is the treatment of choice for congenital laxity: over half of the patients in our series who benefited from a ligamentoplasty were less than 30 years of age (Table III.9). After age 30, partial arthrodesis is more valuable, allowing preservation of useful mobility while guaranteeing a lasting result. The average age of patients with partial arthrodesis reflects this approach.

Nowadays, partial arthrodeses are becoming increasingly fashionable, and yet no precise concept exists to guide the choice of the best possible fusion. We shall now set out our therapeutic principles, based on the observation of 41 partially arthrodesed wrists, our concept of stability (see p. 40) and our anatomical studies (see p. 16).

### Anatomical Review

There are three types of ligaments: "restraining" ligaments, "stabilizing" ligaments and "guiding" ligaments (see p. 39):

1. The "restraining" ligaments bind the bones of the distal row firmly together. As a result, they are virtually immobile in relation to one another. One may readily conclude that an arthrodesis between these bones will have practically no troublesome consequences.
2. The "stabilizing" ligaments are the proximal V and the interosseous ligaments joining the bones of the proximal row of the carpus. The proximal V controls the position and mobility of the lunate and, through it, that of the entire proximal row.
   The proximal interosseous ligaments, through the mobility they allow, make the proximal row a delicate and specialised anatomical unit.
3. The "guiding" ligaments, essentially the superficial fibres of

**Table III.9.** Case-series: partial arthrodeses, ligamentoplasties

| | | Partial arthrodeses | | Ligamentoplasties | Arthroplasties |
|---|---|---|---|---|---|
| No. of wrists | | 41 | | 15 | 5 |
| No. of men | | 26 | | 8 | 2 |
| No. of women | | 11 | | 6 | 3 |
| No. of patients | | 37 | | 14 | 5 |
| Mean age | | 46 years | | 19 years | – |
| Under 30 years | | 8 | | 9 | 1 |
| Over 30 years | | 33 | | 5 | 4 |
| *Aetiology:* | | | | | |
| Scaphoid pseudarthrosis | | 7 | | 0 | – |
| Traumatic instability | | 12 | | 10 | – |
| Congenital instability | | 0 | | 5 | – |
| Idiopathic arthrosis | | 11 | | 0 | 2 |
| Fracture-dislocation | | 3 | | 0 | – |
| Lunate necrosis | | 4 | | 0 | 3 |
| Polyarthritis (rheumatic) | | 3 | | 0 | – |
| Paralysis (Erb) | | 1 | | 0 | – |
| Total: | | 41 | | 15 | 5 |
| *Operations:* | | | | | |
| Arthrodeses: | SCL | 4 | Linscheid plasty | 8 | |
| | RL | 6 | RSL plasty | 3 | |
| | STT | 6 | RL plasty | 3 | |
| | LC | 9 | TH plasty | 1 | |
| | RSL | 10 | Simple resection | | 3 |
| | Other | 6 | Lunate prosthesis | | 2 |
| Total | | 41 | | 15 | |

Ligamentoplasties performed as part of a Matti-Russe operation are not included in this table. SCL, scaphoid-capitate-lunate; RL, radio-lunate; STT, scapho-trapezo-trapezoid; LC, lunate-capitate; RSL, radio-scapho-lunate; TH, triquetro-hamate

the distal V, keep the carpus centred by maintaining a constant distance between the radius and the head of the capitate.

To interfere with this delicate ligamentous system with an inadequate fusion may lead to painful and harmful functional limitations. The most adequate fusions can only be determined by a systematic analysis based on experience and an understanding of the anatomy and biomechanics.

## Systematic Analysis

*Proximal Row Arthrodesis*

The maximum interosseous mobility is between the scaphoid and the lunate, with much less motion between the lunate and triquetrum. The rocking of the scaphoid in flexion and extension is much more than that of the lunate. As Kauer (1980) has shown, this movement is possible thanks to the particular arrangement of the ligamentous fibres joining the two bones. Based on these, and the arguments below, fusion of the scaphoid and lunate would appear inadvisable.

1. In scapho-lunate dissociation, it is rare for the proximal V to be intact, resulting in the typical DISI position (Fig. III.23). Scapho-lunate fusion will not correct this ligamentous instability.
2. The scapho-lunate intersection supports the majority of the axial loads transmitted by the head of the capitate, which constantly tends to migrate between these two bones. Fusion in the presence of an unstable lunate will not correct the DISI and, indeed, may aggravate this instability. Radiologically, there will be a palmar subluxation of both bones (Fig. III.24). Thus, quasi-experimentally, the theory of Gilford et al. (1943) is insufficient.

On the other hand, fusion between the lunate and triquetrum, as proposed by Taleisnik (1984), seems more appropriate on the mechanical level. The triquetrum essentially undergoes only translation movements, the amplitude of which is comparable to those of the lunate, so that rotatory constraints seem of minor importance here. We have no experience with triquetro-lunate arthrodesis, partly because this lesion is rare, and partly because we prefer ligamentoplasty, which, at this site, seems to be justified. The constraints are relatively minor, and ligamentoplasty should re-establish the continuity of the proximal row and the control by the lunate. The procedure has predictable success. We may recall here the case of V.F., a manual labourer, cured by this procedure (p. 75).

*Conclusions.* An arthrodesis between the scaphoid and the lunate is undesirable, for mechanical and also pathophysiological reasons. This fusion is under extreme mechanical demands and takes no account of the pathology, namely the incompetence of the proximal V. Nor is it suitable for correction of the DISI. Thus, there exists no specific direct treatment for scapho-lunate dissociation, since it has been demonstrated (Palmer et al. 1978) that ligamentoplasty is not predictable in the radial compartment.

On the other hand, triquetro-lunate fusion is rational. However, we prefer ligamentoplasty; provided we can be assured that no other associated ligamentous lesions exist. The relatively minor mechanical stresses at this site allow this therapeutic approach.

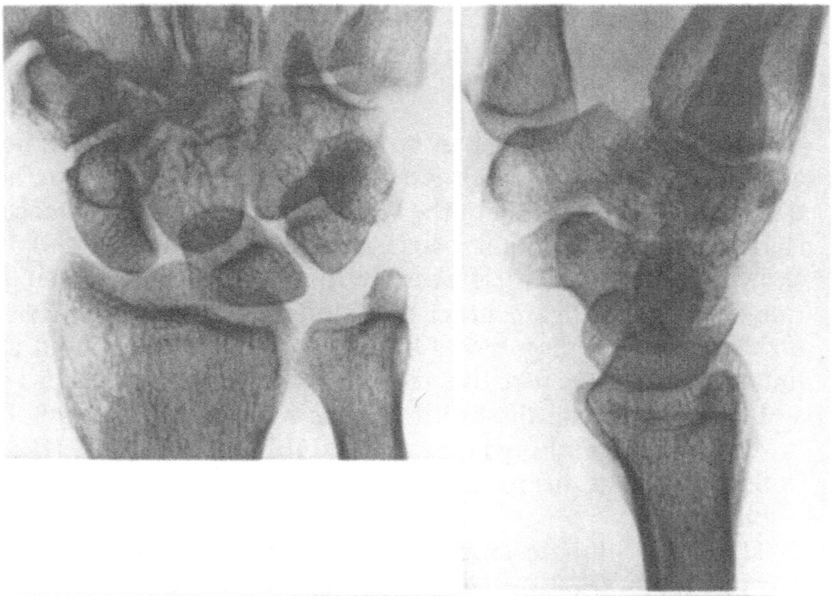

a

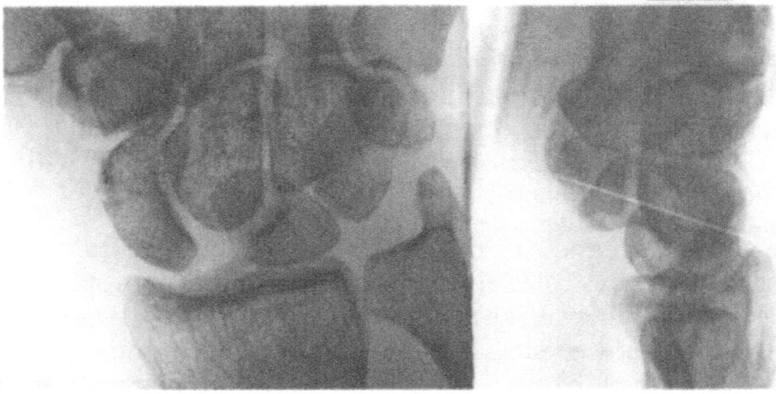

b

**Fig. III.23 a, b.** Scapho-lunate dissociation. **a** The lateral view taken without a guide does not define the exact extent of the lesions. **b** The guide brings out the subluxation of the lunate (DISI), the subluxation of the capitate and the abnormal scapho-lunate angle (90°)

*Proximal Row – Radius Arthrodesis*

Here three types of fusion may be envisaged:

- between the radius and the scaphoid (Fig. III.25),
- between the lunate and the radius (Fig. III.26),
- between these three bones.

*Radio-scaphoid arthrodesis.* This method blocks the most mobile bone of the proximal row. It does not interfere with the "guide" function of the distal V, since the immobile scaphoid contributes to maintaining a constant distance between the radius and the head of the capitate. The capitate remains fixed from then on, but, because its lateral movements are limited by the immobilized scaphoid, the resulting axial constraints on the lunate are minor. Though this arthrodesis is theoretically sound, it is difficult to effect in practice. The surfaces to be arthrodesed are small, the oblique axis of the scaphoid does not lend itself to a stable osteosynthesis, and, as a result, it is extremely difficult to neutralize the shearing forces. Finally, it is not easy to give the right orientation and adequate length to the radial compartment. Yet,

**Fig. III.24. a** Pre-operative ▷ films in flexion-extension; there is a marked permanent subluxation of the capitate, maximal DISI in dorsiflexion and absence of palmar flexion of lunate. **b** Scapho-lunate arthrodesis; the DISI has not been corrected, invalidating Gilford's thesis. The patient is not pain-free, though the pain is less

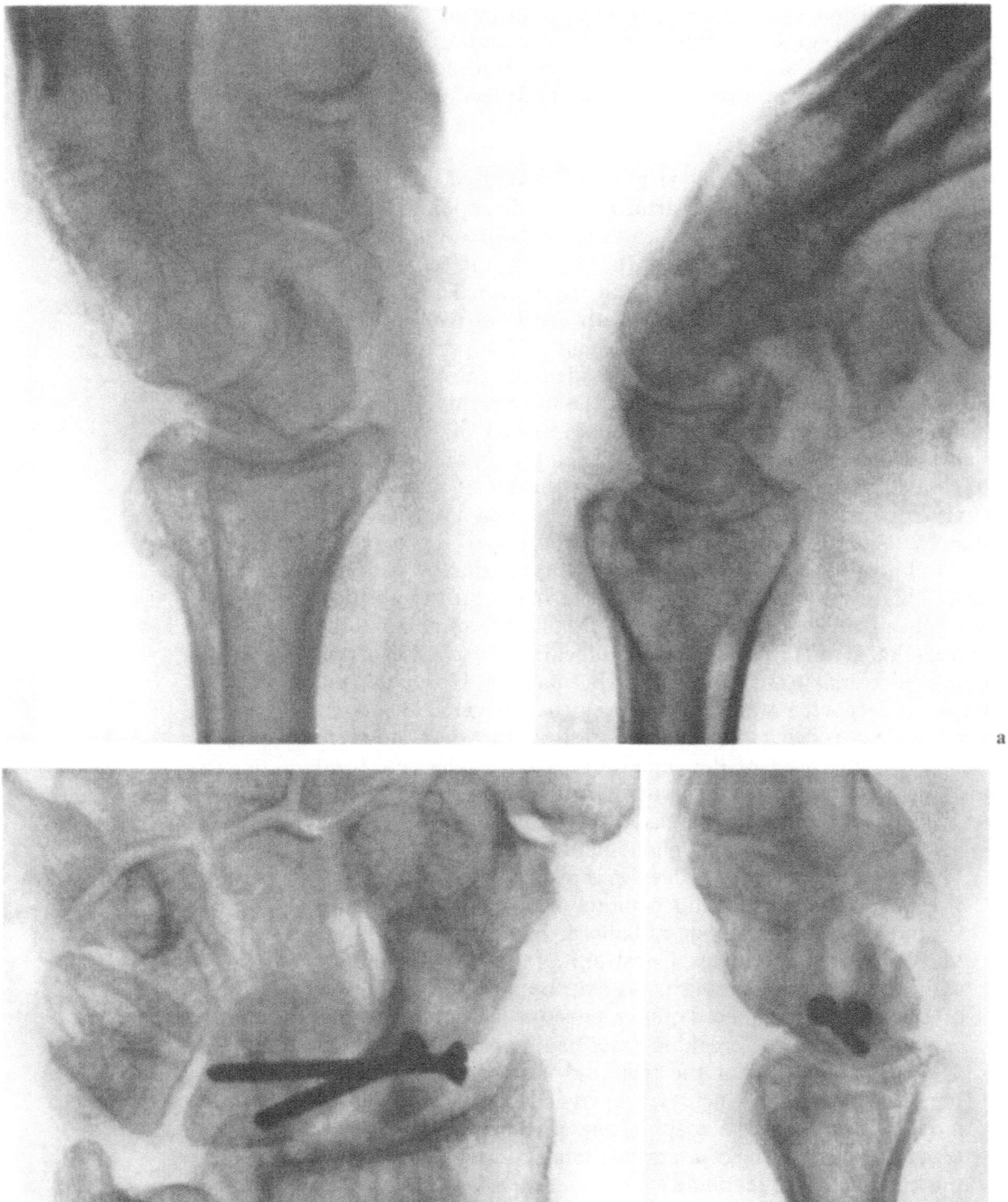

Fig. III.24 a, b

the re-establishment of this length is essential to normalization of the stresses on the other intracarpal articulations. After two fruitless attempts, we have abandoned this method in favour of radio-scapho-lunate fusion (Fig. III.29c) or reconstruction of the central column (Fig. III.32c).

*Radio-lunate arthrodesis*. This arthrodesis, proposed by Chamay et al. (1983) for rheumatoid arthritis, has disappointed us in post-traumatic cases. The three cases we operated on this basis had to be re-operated: the first after 3 years, the second after 9 months and the third as early as the 3rd month. The diagnosis in all three was lunate instability with DISI; in two cases the scapho-lunate ligament was functional. Postoperatively the symptoms in these three patients were identical: no pain at rest, but pain with any activity or during the movements of circumduction and abduction. They also complained of "creaking" – always painful – accompanied by an intracarpal "pressure" that was difficult to define but very unpleasant. It was striking in all three cases that these symptoms did not improve with time, but actually became worse.

In almost all traumatic cases, only the proximal V is damaged. The distal V, whose function is to maintain the position of the head of the capitate, remains intact. To immobilize the lunate (Fig. III.27) is equivalent to blocking the middle of the mobile proximal row and so disturb function. Normally, the lunate undergoes a translation movement (Kauer 1980) combined with a rocking movement during abduction-adduction. This allows the head of the capitate to keep a relatively fixed position in space, which is assured by the distal V. Once the lunate is fixed, this normal play is no longer possible, and during ulnar deviation the following phenomena occur:

1. The radial portion of the distal V is placed under tension.
2. Traction on the head of the capitate occurs, with a tendency for movement of this bone radially or laterally, in the direction of the resultant forces. Constraint of the capitate, hamate and triquetral articulations is present, because the distal part of the distal V is placed under tension. These constraints explain the pain and creaking described by patients.
3. The space reserved for the scaphoid is decreased, and this bone is subjected to increased axial load. It can no longer move normally. If the scapho-lunate attachments are ruptured, the head of the capitate also tends to infiltrate between the lunate and the scaphoid.
4. The phenomena described above appear only if the distal V is intact. This is not the case in rheumatoid arthritis, which probably accounts for the different results reported by Chamay. Indeed, three patients who underwent the same arthrodesis for carpal instability secondary to rheumatic ligamentous destruction have satisfactory and almost painless postoperative function.

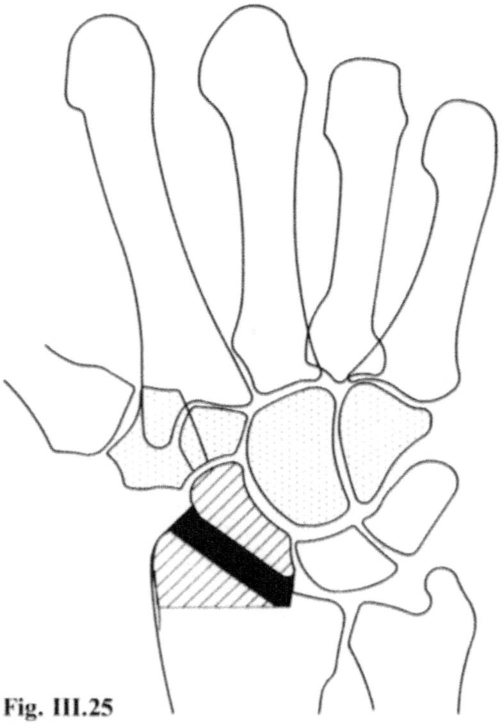

Fig. III.25

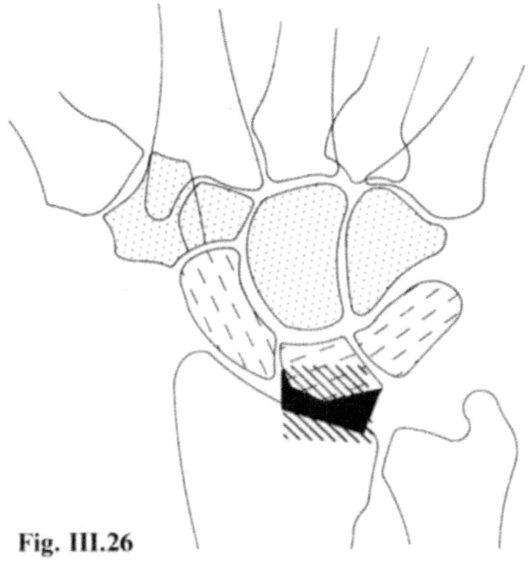

Fig. III.26

**Fig. III.25.** Radio-scaphoid arthrodesis; the small contact surface and oblique slope make fixation difficult. The operative indications are rare

**Fig. III.26.** Radio-lunate arthrodesis

*Conclusion.* Radio-lunate fusion is indicated for ligamentous destruction, which is the result of rheumatoid arthritis, where it prevents ulnar displacement of the carpus. As a corollary, it should not be contemplated in traumatic cases, in which the anatomy of the still healthy ligaments obstructs harmonious function of the adjacent bones.

*Radio-scapho-lunate arthrodesis.* Here the triquetrum remains the only free element. Stabilization of the scaphoid-lunate couple prevents any asynchonous ligament tension, since the major part of the two Vs is immobilized. The degree of residual mobility is minor, ranging from 10° to 30°, which is somewhat less than theoretical calculations would suggest (see examples: Figs. III.28 and III.29). The ten patients treated by this method are satisfied despite the handicap represented by the reduction of mobility.

*Discussion.* This arthrodesis may be contemplated in arthrosis of the radial compartment, whatever the cause. However, we generally prefer, if possible, to perform a fusion between the distal and proximal rows. This preserves the movement of the wrist better, which after all is the aim of a partial rather than a total arthrodesis.

### *Proximal Row-Distal Row Arthrodesis*

*Scaphoid-trapezium (with or without trapezoid; STT) arthrodesis.* This has been advocated by Watson (1980). He advises it in the treatment of scapho-trapezo-trapezoid arthrosis, rotatory

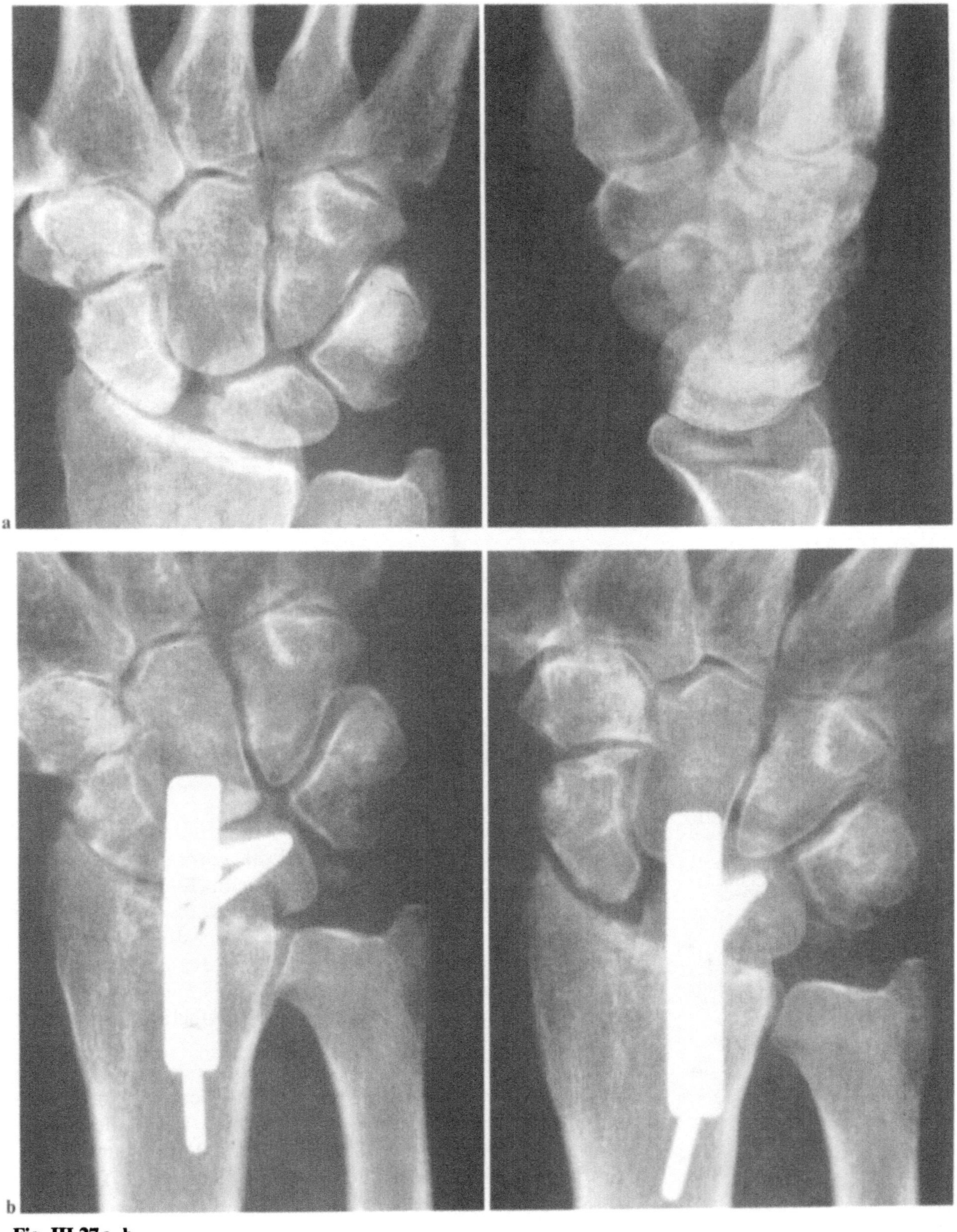

**Fig. III.27 a, b**

Fig. III.27 a–c. Radio-lunate arthrodesis. a Pre-operative films show scapho-lunate dissociation and DISI. b Post-operative films in radial and ulnar deviation show blockage of the keystone of the proximal row, persistence of scapho-lunate dissociation, possible interposition of the head of the capitate between the lunate and the scaphoid and abnormal load on the scaphoid. c Schematic representation of abnormal load; these, and the pain, are increased in the presence of an intact distal V ligament

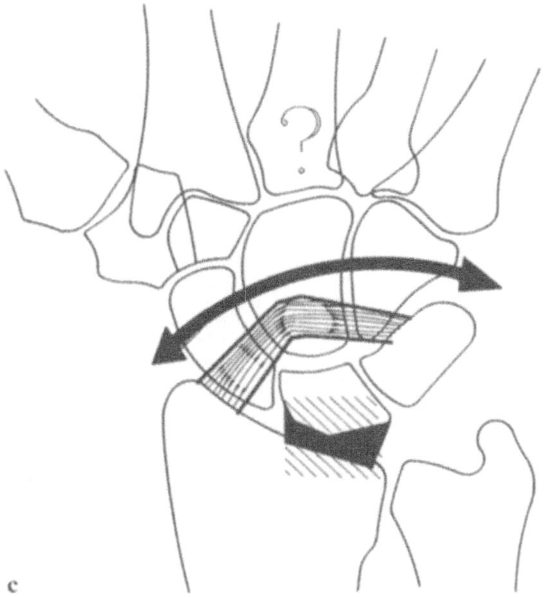

c

instability of the scaphoid and Kienböck's disease (Watson et al. 1985). To date, we have arthrodesed six cases according to Watson's principles, but with different operative techniques (see Fig. III.30). For us, the indications are almost exclusively limited to arthrosis. The proposal to use the method in Kienböck's disease is attractive, but it remains to be shown that the pressures acting on the lunate are reduced to the same extent by this method as by shortening the radius, or lengthening of the ulna. However, it takes over 15 years to determine the long-term outcome of a procedure in the wrist joint. Lengthening of the ulna loads the ulnar compartment of the carpus; fixation of the scaphoid overloads the radial side; perhaps a combination of these two methods would add their respective advantages.

There is still controversy regarding the role of this operation in scapho-lunate dissociation. We know that this instability is often combined with a lesion of the proximal V, and a resultant palmar subluxation of the lunate, which installs itself in DISI. The horizontal position of the scaphoid produced by its fixation to the trapezium and trapezoid makes this bone one with the distal row of the carpus. The lunate can no longer function normally and forces are transmitted more through the scaphoid. The DISI is partly reduced, since axial forces are channelled through the scaphoid, and the diastasis disappears. Only experience and time will allow us to judge the long-term value of this operation in this type of lesion. In our opinion, the major problem is determination of the position for the scaphoid. If it is too horizontal, degenerative changes may result from excessive pressure on the radial compartment; if too vertical, it will only partly limit the consequences of the collapse. Of the 13 cases published by Watson, only four had rotatory instability.

The preservation of some residual mobility represents the major advantage of this technique. In certain cases, Watson sug-

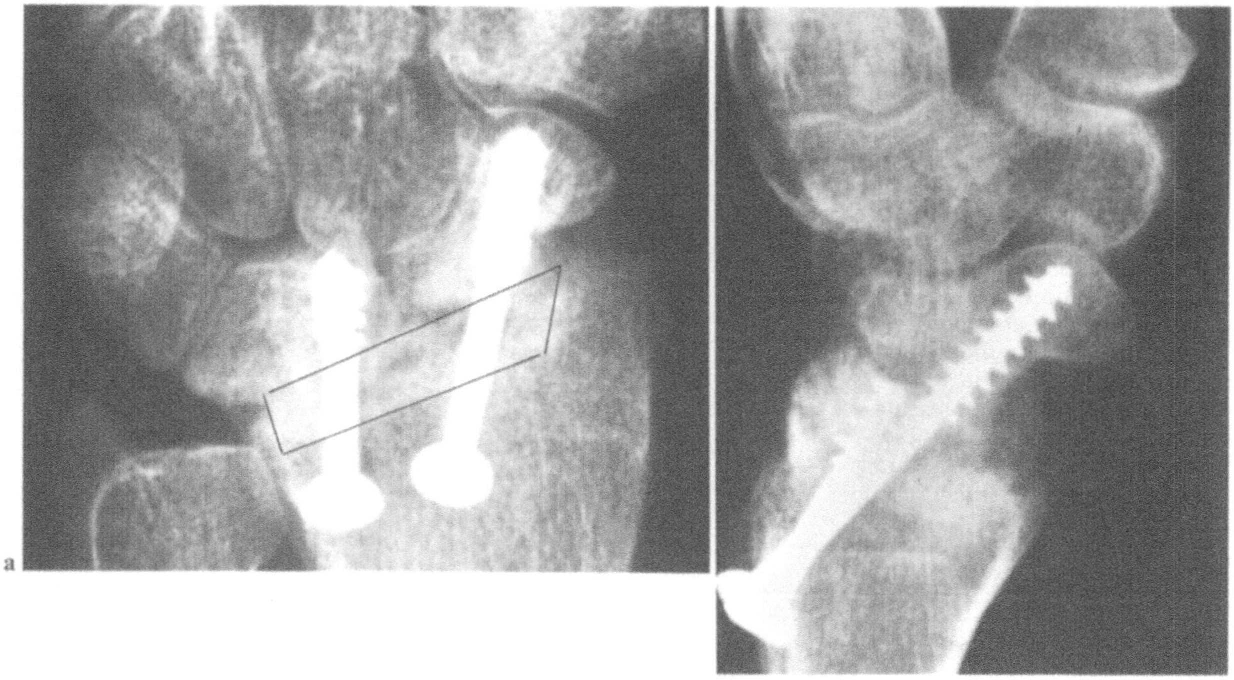

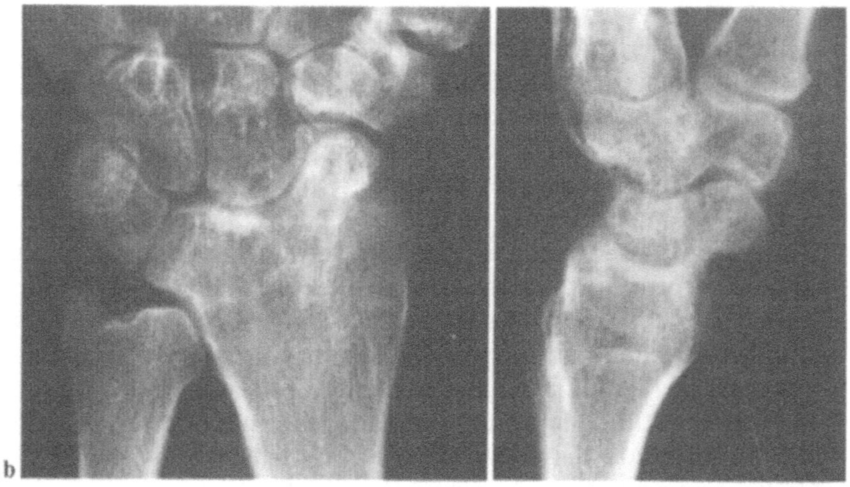

**Fig. III.28 a, b.** Radio-scapholunate arthrodesis. **a** Technique of screwing and grafting: the washer guarantees interfragmentary compression; the axis of the scaphoid is very vertical, the ideal of 45° being very difficult to achieve; the area *outlined* on the film defines placement of the graft. **b** After removal of the osteosynthesis material there is no pain and 30° residual flexion-extension

gests combining it with a Silastic lunate prosthesis. The concept is excellent, and we too have used such a combination. But the major problem remains wear of the prosthetic material which has poor resistance to shear. In the example shown in Fig. III.31, 3 months after implantation, the deterioration of the subluxated prosthesis is evidence of the problem. The prosthesis only acts as a spacer; it cannot compensate for loss of the support from missing bone. At the functional and anatomical levels, the constraints imposed on the distal V by the forced immobility of the scaphoid seem to be compensated for by the residual mobility of the proximal row; which can absorb, without obvious difficulty, the flexion and extension necessary to maintain the position of the head of the capitate.

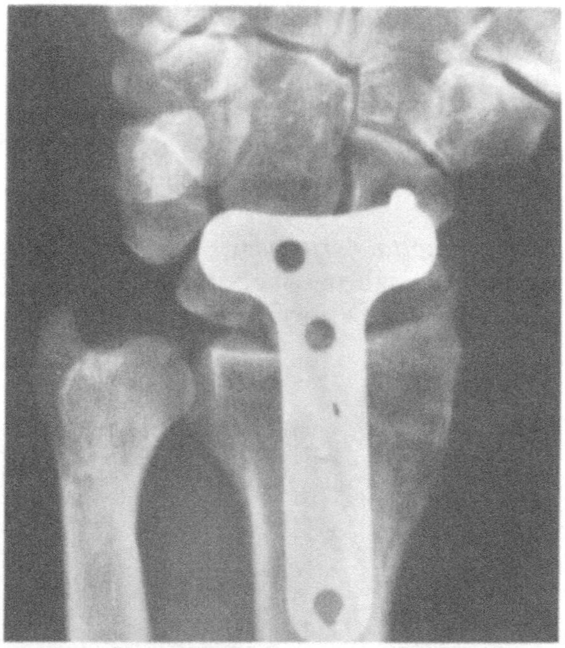

a

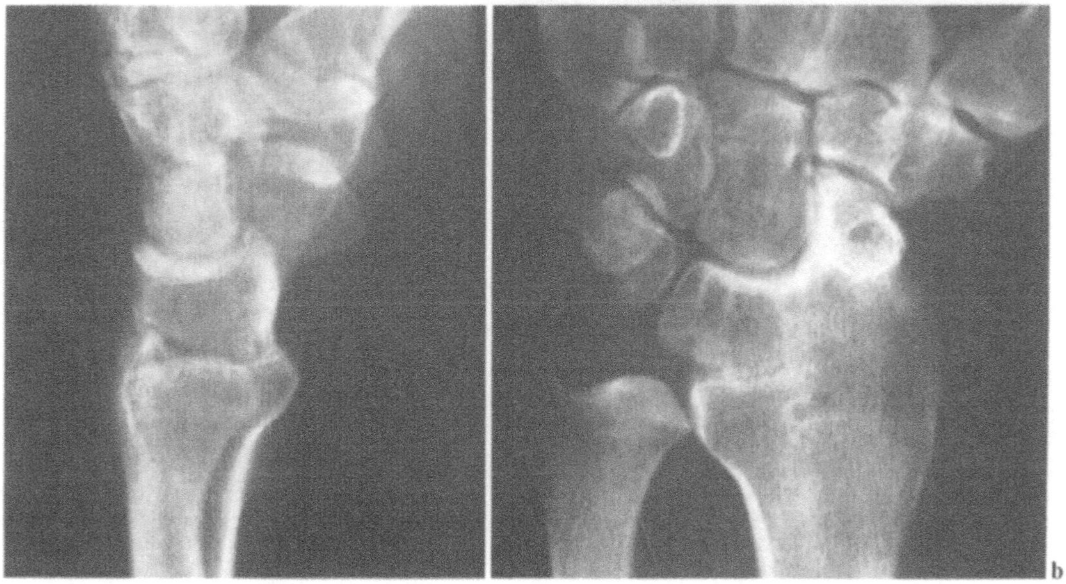

b

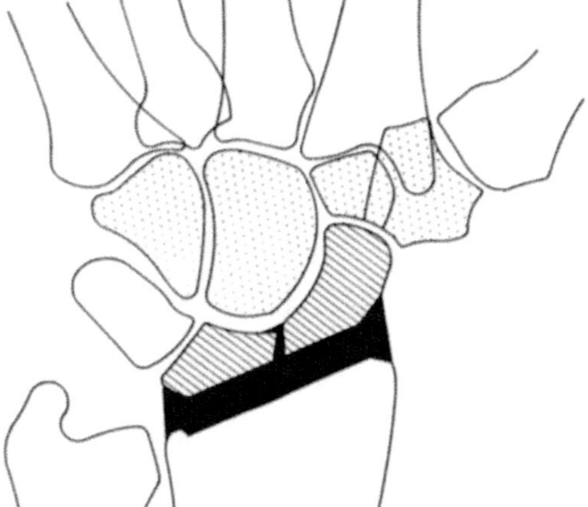

c

**Fig. III.29 a–c.** Radio-scapho-lunate arthrodesis. **a** Neutralization plate with cortico-cancellous bone graft, a considerable amount of metal. **b** After removal of the metal, the radiographic appearance is the same as in Fig. III.28 b. **c** Diagram of operation: graft bed in *black*. The aim is to decompress the ulnar compartment

*Discussion.* The best indication for this technique is scapho-trapezo-trapezoid arthrosis. Some doubt exists regarding its role in Kienböck's disease and scapho-lunate dissociation. However, the excellent residual mobility and the relative simplicity of the operation are significant advantages provided the radial compartment is free from arthrosis.

*Scapho-capitate arthrodesis.* This exceptional fusion is equivalent to an STT arthrodesis, but is technically more difficult to carry out. We have performed it once, 10 years after resection of the

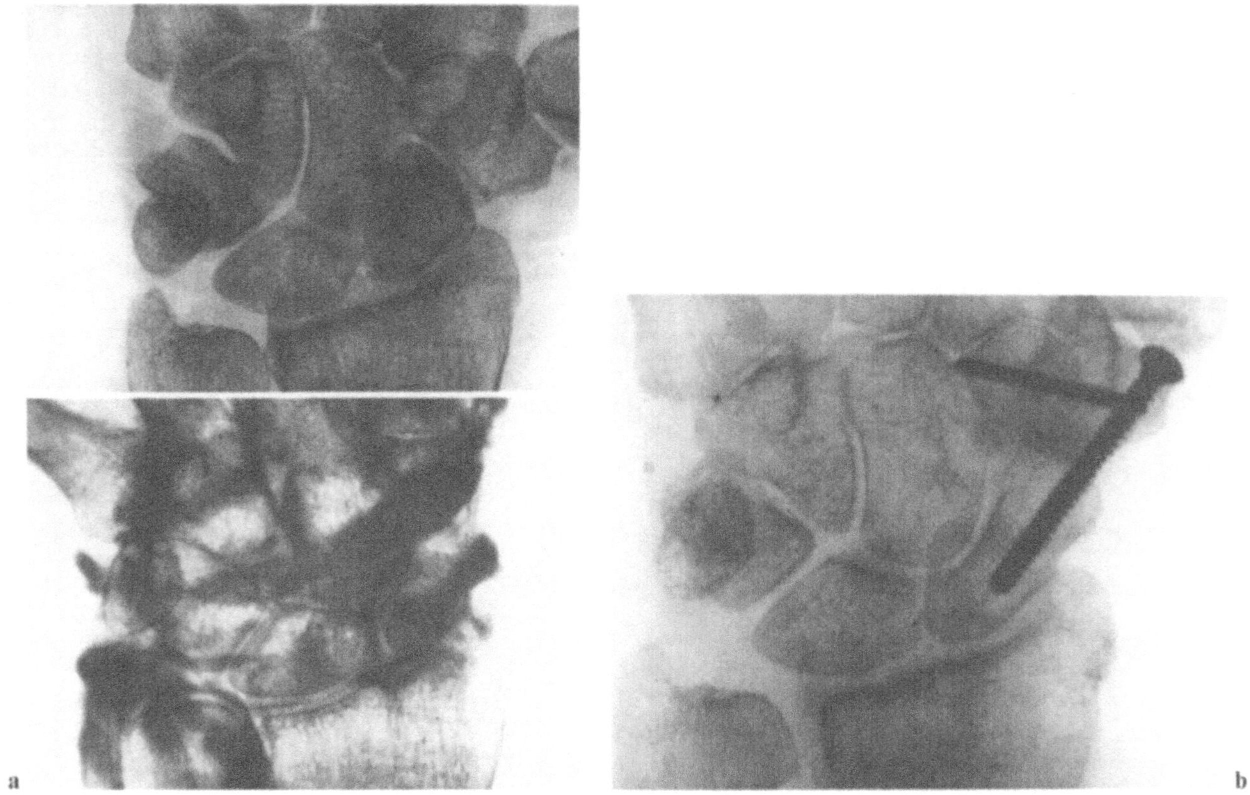

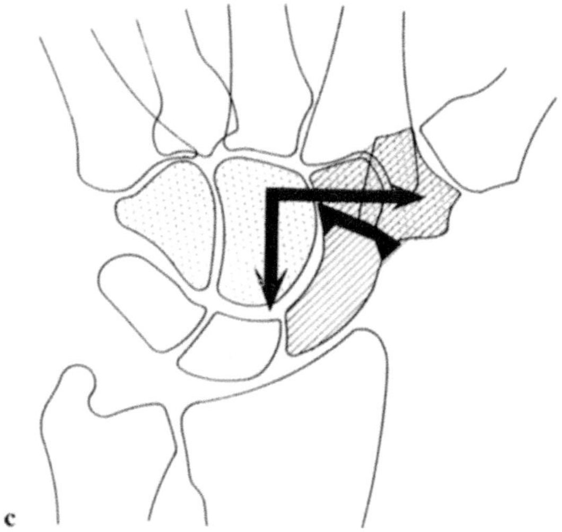

**Fig. III.30 a–c.** Scapho-trapezo-trapezoid (STT) arthrodesis. **a** Scapho-lunate instability and ligamentous rupture are demonstrated in the arthrogram. **b** This technique requires a lag-screw between the trapezium and the scaphoid, and trapezo-trapezoidal stabilization by pin. **c** Radial block (*arrows*) created by means of the distal interosseous ligaments is probably equivalent to scapho-capitate arthrodesis

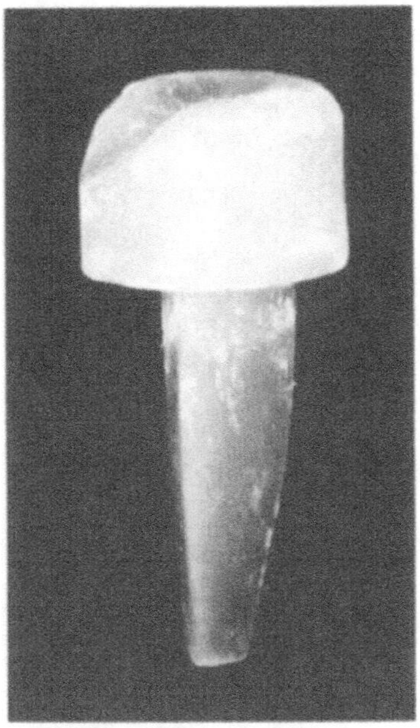

**Fig. III.31.** Condition of a prosthesis 3 months after implantation, showing extreme wear associated with subluxation. The Silastic has no resistance to friction and no supportive function; it acts only as a spacer

lunate for severe avascular necrosis. This scapho-capitate fusion was combined with a lunate prosthesis, the patient, a mechanic, was able to return to work.

*Capitate-lunate arthrodesis* (see Figs. III.32 and III.33). This is the carpal arthrodesis we perform most often in our department. We have carried out 13 fusions of this type and so far none has had to be re-operated. Fusion of the central column of the carpus does not disturb free ligamentous play (the same argument as for STT fusion) but leaves the patient with good mobility. It is possible even with advanced collapse of the carpus and can also be combined with a total or partial prosthesis of the scaphoid. Two examples demonstrate this, one with a pseudarthrosis going back for over 20 years and advanced collapse (Fig. III.32) and the other with a prosthesis and resection of the radial styloid (Fig. III.33). Pain relief is generally achieved after 6 months.

The problem of stabilization is not yet completely solved. The plate used by us (a AO 2.7 mm T-plate) abuts against the radial socket with consequent discomfort, some limitation of function and synovial irritation. This discomfort disturbs early rehabilitation but disappears once the osteosynthesis material is removed.

*Discussion.* It is interesting to note that the 20-year-old pseudarthrosis of the scaphoid has destroyed the radial compartment and the capitate-lunate articulation but has, as is usual, spared the radio-lunate joint. This is why we favour arthrodesis of the central column; it eliminates the pain while conserving the mobility required for the actions of everyday life. It can also be combined with a scaphoid prosthesis but this alternative remains the exception, experience having shown that even a partly arthrotic scaphoid can function well once the central column is reconstructed. In any case, we are very cautious in the use of prostheses, their future being so uncertain.

*Triquetro-hamate arthrodesis.* Theoretically, this arthrodesis should not disturb the function of the distal V. However, the indications for this type of fusion are limited. For us, if intracarpal ligamentoplasty still has a place, it is precisely for these ulnar intracarpal instabilities, where the mechanical constraints are of less importance than on the radial side.

*Global intercarpal arthrodesis (including Graner's operation).* The indications for this are few. The indication of choice is a severe injury, such as a De Quervain's fracture-dislocation with avulsion of the proximal pole of the capitate, since the fused carpus seems well supported (see p. 5). We do not recommend the operation of Graner et al. (1966), advocated for severe lunate osteomalacia; it is difficult and, for vascular reasons, is often associated with necrosis of the proximal pole of the osteotomized

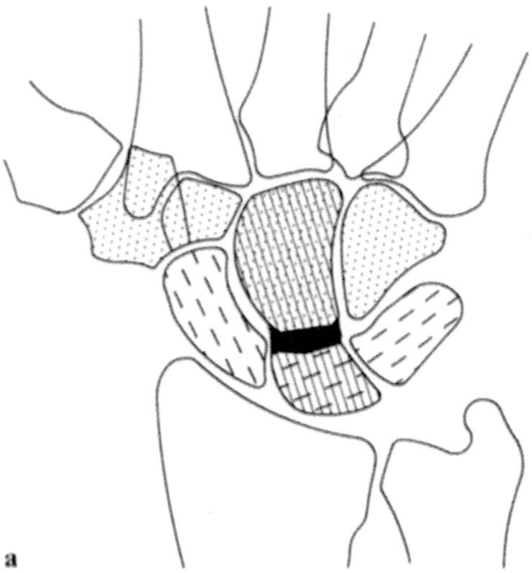

a

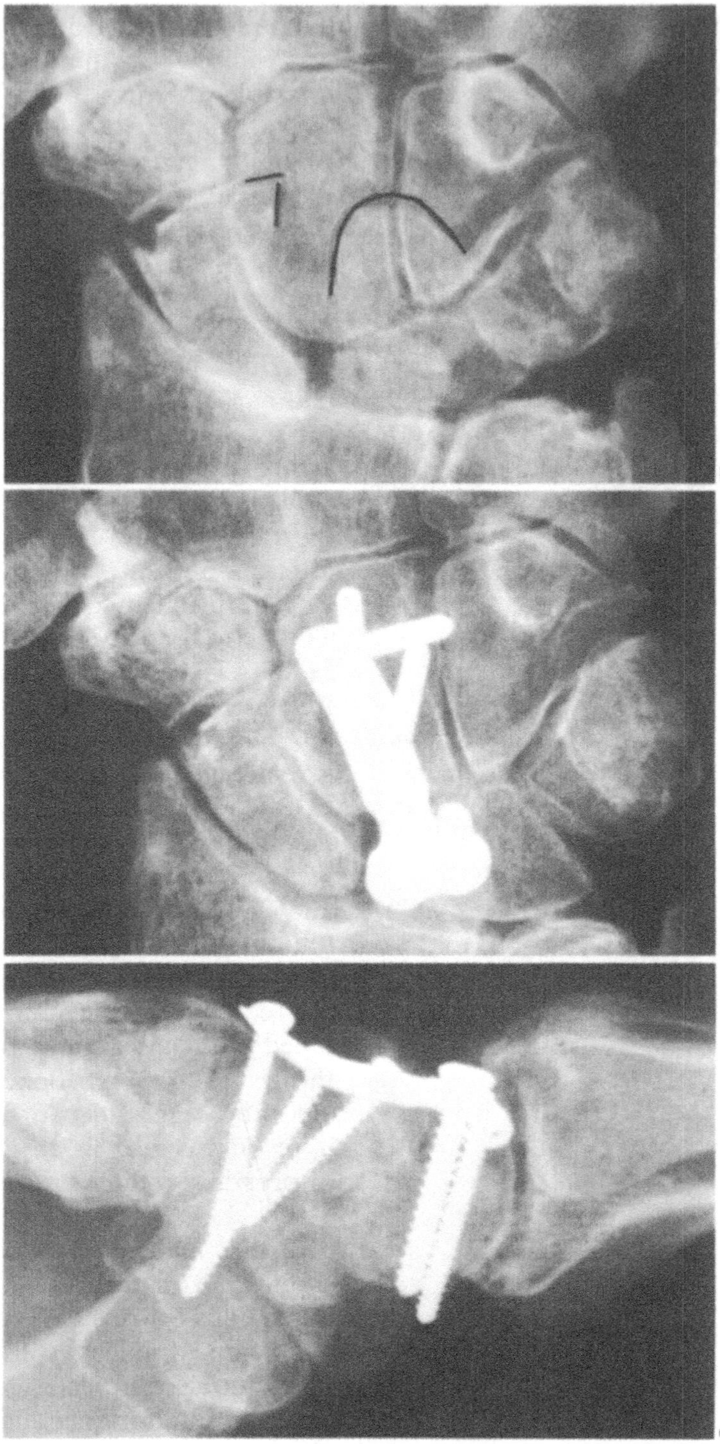

b

c¹

c²

**Fig. III.32 a–c.** Capitate-lunate arthrodesis. **a** *Diagram:* creation of two rotatory columns based on Taleisnik's thesis of the reconstruction of a central column. **b** Massive collapse, scapholunate dissociation. **c** Reconstruction of a central column (PA and lateral views)

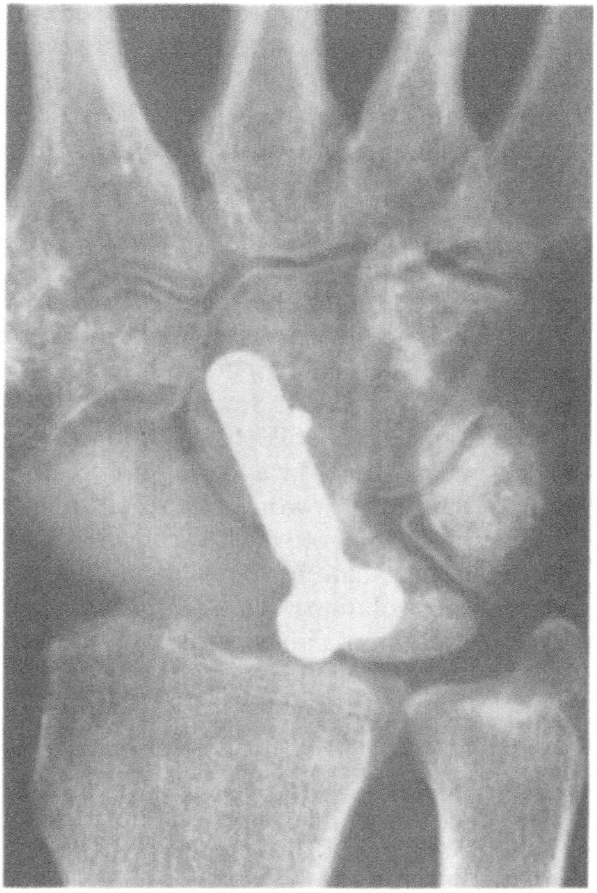

**Fig. III.33.** Reconstruction of the central column with replacement of the scaphoid by a Silastic prosthesis which has no function. *NB:* the resection of the styloid may damage the distal V, risking ulnar subluxation of the carpus

capitate. If shortening of the radius is no longer possible, we feel that a tri-scaphoid arthrodesis or a fusion between the scaphoid, lunate and radius is preferable. The choice depends on the degree of collapse of the lunate and the state of the radial compartment.

**Discussion**

The aim of partial arthrodesis is to preserve the best possible function while abolishing the pain. From this clinical review we may draw the following general principles:

1. Arthrodeses between the proximal and distal rows of the carpus preserve mobility better than arthrodeses between the radius and the proximal row and carry virtually no risk of impaired ligamentous function.
2. Arthrodesis between the scaphoid and the lunate is not sound mechanically and functionally.
3. Arthrodesis between the lunate and radius must remain the exception.

4. Ligamentoplasty may replace arthrodesis in the ulnar compartment, where the stresses are less severe than on the radial side.
5. Pre-operative assessment must be strict: (a) to localize the arthrosis and ligamentous inadequacy; (b) to analyse the tilt; (c) to assess collapse and shift.

## Conclusions

Partial arthrodesis of the carpus should not be contemplated unless the surgeon feels capable of ridding the patient of pain: (a) by restoring carpal height, with reconstruction of the central column or an equivalent procedure; (b) by preserving what ligamentous function is still present and/or compensating for that which is defective; (c) by avoiding the creation, through his operation, of new stresses which can result in iatrogenic symptoms.

It is plain that only with knowledge of the biomechanics and functional anatomy can the surgeon decide when to apply such delicate solutions. Total arthrodesis of the wrist may still be the procedure of choice, especially for patients who do heavy work.

## References


Chamay A, Della Santa D, Vilaseva A (1983) L'arthrodèse radio-lunaire facteur de stabilité du poignet rhumatoïde. Ann Chir Main 2:5–17

Gilford WW, Bolton RH, Lambrinudi C (1943) The mechanism of the wrist joint with special reference to fractures of the scaphoid. Guy's Hosp Rep 92:52–59

Graner O, Lopes EI, Carvalho BC, Atlas S (1966) Arthrodesis of the carpal bones in the treatment of Kienböck's disease, painful ununited fractures of the navicular and lunate bones with avascular necrosis, and old fracture-dislocations of carpal bones. J Bone Joint Surg [Am] 48:767–774

Kauer JMG (1980) Functional anatomy of the wrist. Clin Orthop 149:9–20

Palmer AK, Dobyns JH, Linscheid RL (1978) Management of post traumatic instability of the wrist secondary to ligament rupture. J Hand Surg 6:507–532

Taleisnik J (1984) Triquetrohamate and triquetrolunate instabilities (medial carpal instability). Ann Chir Main 3:331–343

Watson HK (1980) Limited wrist arthrodesis I. The triscaphoid joint. J Hand Surg 5:320–327

Watson HK, Ryu J, DiBella A (1985) An approach to Kienböck's disease: triscaphoid arthrodesis. J Hand Surg 10A:179–187

CHAPTER IV

# Fractures of the Distal Radius

## A. The Specific Problem

This is considered a routine, frequent fracture, reputedly easy to treat, since the treatment is generally left to the assistant. In fact, this fracture is not well understood, and the therapeutic criteria are vague. This is because:

- an analytical morphological basis is lacking;
- conservative treatment appears to give good results;
- malunion seems to be well tolerated;
- the population affected, often elderly and female, does not arouse interest.

In practice, despite numerous studies (Castaing 1964; Chamay 1977; Chamay et al. 1983; Clancey 1984; Cooney et al. 1979), no-one acknowledges the problems of malunion, since no relationship has ever been demonstrated between the severity of the malunion and the patient's discomfort (Fourrier et al. 1981). We now propose to study:

1. The population involved in this type of injury
2. The consequences of malunion in an apparently apathetic population – the elderly
3. The possibilities of conservative management
4. The practical implications of a classification developed with therapeutic aims
5. The basis of rational treatment

### Distribution of Radial Fractures According to Age and Sex

During the 3-year period from the start of 1980 to the end of 1982, the St Gallen orthopaedic clinic treated 653 fractures of the distal radius. Of these patients, 200 were aged 30 or under, 102 were between 31 and 51, while the remaining 351 were aged 51 or over. From Figs. IV.1 and IV.2, three interesting facts emerge:

1. Below the age of 30 years this fracture affects mainly men (69%).
2. Between 30 and 51 years, men and women are affected equally.
3. After the 51st year, women are predominantly affected (86.6%).

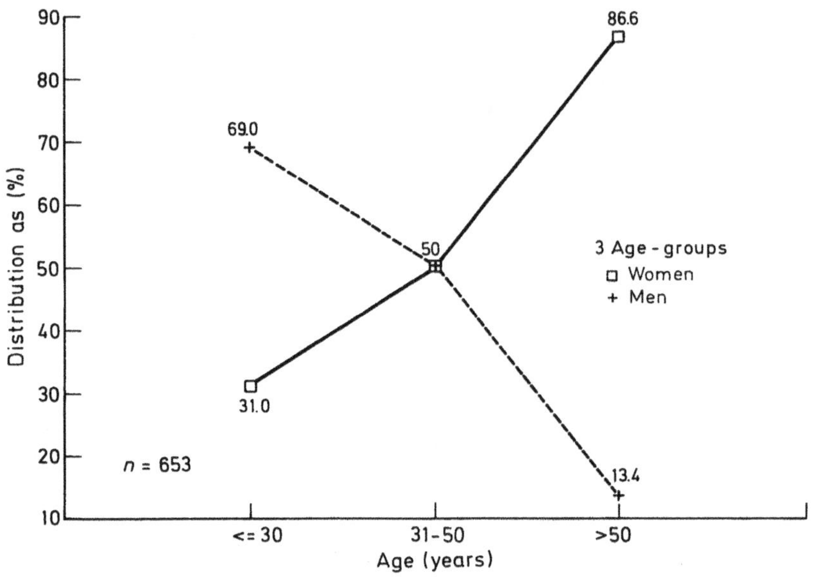


**Fig. IV.1.** Distribution of fractures of the lower radius according to age and sex (1980–1982): men are mainly affected before the age of 30 years, and women after the age of 50 years

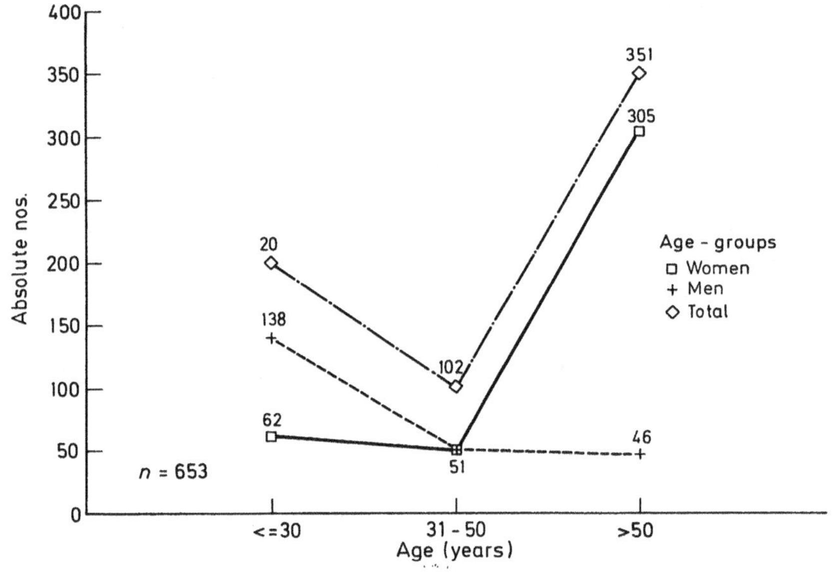


**Fig. IV.2.** Distribution in terms of absolute numbers; the increased incidence of this fracture among women over 50 years of age is characteristic

## Current Treatment of Fracture of the Radius

During these 3 years only 54 of the 653 fractures were operated on, i.e. 8.3%; an external fixator was used 41 times and osteosynthesis was performed 13 times. If we consider the 41 patients managed by external fixator (Fig. IV.3), we note that:

- men were treated 25 times and women 16 times,
- it was employed only 13 times in patients over 50,
- it was employed in the under-50 women only seven times, and in the over-50 women only nine times.

Put into percentages, these figures reflect a casual attitude about the outcome, especially in women. Indeed, of the 305 women over 50 years only nine were given the benefit of external fixation; 2.6% of the population concerned. For those under 50 years the rate was more favourable, since seven out of 113 (6.2%)

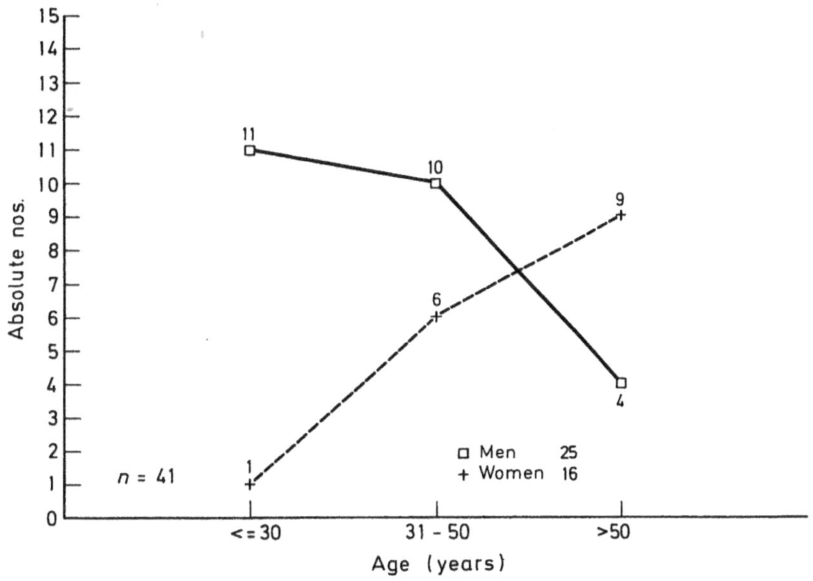


**Fig. IV.3.** Treatment by external fixation (1980–1982)

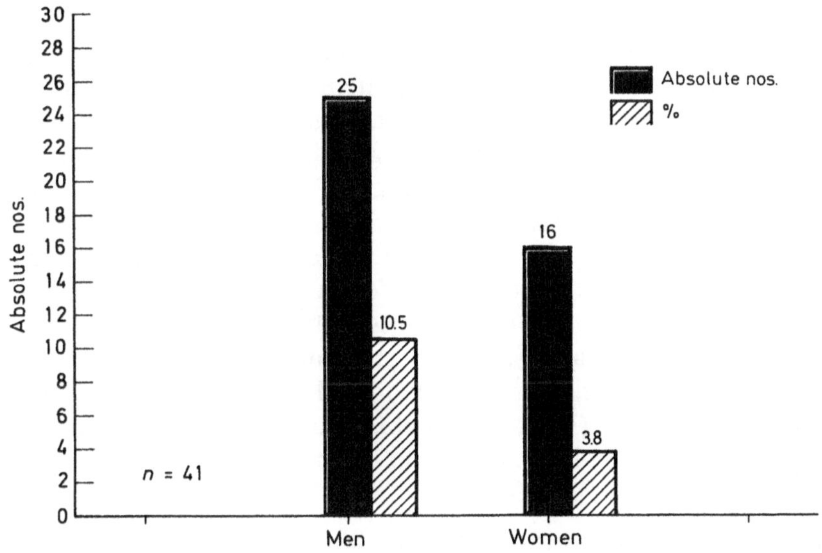


**Fig. IV.4.** Fractures of distal radius 1980–1982; men are more readily treated by external fixation than women are

were so treated. The men were more spoiled: for the under-50s there were 21 fixators for 290 fractures (11%) and four out of 47 for the over-50s (8.5%). Overall, 10.5% of the men were treated by external fixator compared with only 3.8% of the women (Fig. IV.4). Were the women not as well treated? Our next task is to look at the results of present treatment. Does it assure as good results as the optimists would have us believe?

## Tolerance of Malunion

The clinical, radiological and subjective analysis of 43 fractures, selected at random, allows us to address this question. The patients, all aged 60 years or over, should be generally tolerant of malunion. The primary treatment had been conservative in every case, without recourse to Kirschner wires, external fixator or osteosynthesis. The group included 39 patients: five men and

34 women. The proportion of men (5/39; 12.8%) is similar to our 3-year findings for this age group: 46 men among a total of 351 fractures (13.3%). The average age of the group was 71.7 years (60–88). The interval between fracture and follow-up was always greater than 1 year, with a maximum of 24 months and an average of 13.6 months.

### Analysis of Results

The results are summarized in Table IV.1. We grouped our patients into five subjective classes and four radiological groups. We then sought to establish a "structure-pain" relationship and a "function-pain" relationship.

### Subjective Results

Table IV.2 summarizes the subjective classes, defined according to the patient's symptoms, and shows their distribution. The percentage of perfect results is small: 20.9%. Even regarding "moderate discomfort" as a favourable result gives only 50% good results! Class III represents patients complaining of inability to perform stressful activities (e.g. being unable to lift a saucepan full of water or a shopping-bag). Though not often considered serious, this is very disabling to some patients. Perhaps this group has acceptable results from certain points of view, but they can hardly be classed as "good". Still, if these class III cases are added to the two previous classes, we find only 70% tolerable results after conservative management. This means that 30% have bad results: about one patient in three. Our figures are quite comparable to those of Castaing (1964) with 433 fractures (right-hand column of table). Are we to conclude that 20 years later we are no further advanced?

### Relationship Between Reduction and Symptoms

The structural findings from an analysis of the radiographs allow us to define four radiological groups (Table IV.3). Three possible deformations have been allowed for: the distal radius may tilt in the frontal and/or sagittal planes, and/or exhibit shortening. Consequently, the radiograph may show either undisplaced fractures or fractures with one, two or three deformities. Radiological group 0 corresponds to almost perfect anatomical reduction (allowing $\pm 2$ mm of shortening and $\pm 5°$ of tilt in either of the two planes of space). Radiological group 1 is characterized by an isolated deformity (tilt in only one plane or shortening only). A tilt plus shortening, or a combined tilt in two planes, defines radiological group 2. Finally, a combination of all three factors defines group 3. Analysis of Table IV.4, in which we have sought correlations between the radiological and subjective groups, is difficult because the number of cases in each group is small. However, we are immediately struck by the fact that there are only two anatomical reductions. This allows a preliminary conclusion: plaster immobilization in the elderly is ineffective. As the number of fractures in group 0 is too small, groups 0 and 1 have been analysed together, thus accounting for 17 fractures spread over five classes. The findings in Table IV.4 lead us to the following conclusions:

1. Most of the good radiological results, i.e. 11, correspond to subjective classes I and II, and only six to classes III and IV. No favourable radiograph was found in class V.
2. The greater the anatomical deformation, the smaller the number of good subjective results obtained.
3. Of the four mediocre subjective results, despite satisfactory anatomical reduction, one was secondary to reflex sympathetic dystrophy, one presented a caput ulna syndrome, and in the other two there had not been perfect structural restoration.
4. Subjective classes I and II were marked by a higher rate of radiologically satisfactory results (Fig. IV.5): 55%. In classes III–V the rate was less than 30%. This illustrates the relationship between quality of anatomical reduction and quality of life. But, is this statistically significant? Detailed statistical analysis of the results will be carried out, in an effort to demonstrate that it is.

### Relationship Between Mobility and Symptoms

The measurements of mobility in degrees are reported in Table IV.5, and are expressed by the differences between the so-called normal function of the sound side and that of the injured side. In cases of bilateral fracture, the difference is calculated in relation to the mean for "normal" mobility in the group examined. From this detailed table of values we can construct a graph comparing the average losses of mobility for each individual type of movement, as well as the global losses for our five subjective classes. The differences in mobility between subjective classes are not very marked, except for class V, for which they are very definite. The difference is also apparent if the classification is simplified by comparing only two groups of patients, satisfied and unsatisfied (Fig. IV.6).

### Statistical Analysis of Results

Such an analysis must be precise and clear. The reader must be able to check the various stages constantly, particularly the tests employed to verify the results. This approach applied along with various checks is the only way to counter the well-known adage: "With statistics, one can prove anything!". The significance of $P$ depends not only on the choice of test, but also on how the data are ordered. Kurtz's book, *Introduction to Social Statistics* (1983), may prove very helpful to the reader. To our knowledge, no statistical demonstration has been made to prove that a relationship exists between the quality of the anatomical result and the satisfaction of the patient. On the con-

**Table IV.1.** Fractures of the distal radius in the third age-group (over 51 years). $n=39$ (5 men, 34 women), average age 71 years

| | Age | Hand | | Pronation | | Supination | | Flexion | | Extension | | Radial deviation | | Ulnar deviation | |
|---|---|---|---|---|---|---|---|---|---|---|---|---|---|---|---|
| | | R | L | Ref. | Fract. | Ref. | Fract. | Ref. | Fract. | Ref. | Fract. | Ref. | Fract. | Ref. | Fract. |
| A.I. | 74 | | × | 90 | 0 | 90 | 0 | 65 | −10 | 55 | 5 | 20 | 10 | 50 | −20 |
| B.A. | 72 | | × | 90 | 0 | 80 | −10 | 65 | −20 | 45 | −15 | 50 | −30 | 40 | −10 |
| B.A. | 81 | | × | 90 | 0 | 90 | 0 | 90 | −20 | 65 | − 5 | 25 | 10 | 45 | −10 |
| B.L. | 79 | | × | 80 | 0 | 90 | −10 | 60 | −30 | 60 | 30 | 30 | −10 | 35 | − 5 |
| B.M. | 62 | | × | 88 | 0 | 87 | 0 | 64 | 0 | 61 | 0 | 32 | 0 | 40 | 0 |
| B.M. | 62 | × | | 88 | 0 | 87 | 0 | 64 | 0 | 61 | 0 | 32 | 0 | 40 | 0 |
| D.A. | 71 | | × | 80 | 0 | 80 | 0 | 60 | −10 | 60 | 0 | 35 | −15 | 40 | 0 |
| E.F. | 65 | × | | 90 | 0 | 90 | 0 | 80 | 0 | 70 | −10 | 50 | −10 | 40 | −10 |
| E.M. | 65 | | × | 88 | 0 | 87 | 0 | 64 | 0 | 61 | 0 | 32 | 0 | 40 | 0 |
| E.M. | 65 | × | | 88 | −10 | 87 | −20 | 64 | −15 | 61 | −20 | 32 | −20 | 40 | −10 |
| F.A. | 64 | | × | 88 | −10 | 87 | 0 | 64 | −10 | 61 | −15 | 32 | 0 | 40 | 0 |
| F.A. | 64 | × | | 88 | 0 | 87 | 0 | 64 | 20 | 61 | 0 | 32 | 0 | 40 | 0 |
| F.K. | 76 | × | | 90 | 0 | 90 | 0 | 70 | −15 | 65 | −10 | 40 | 0 | 40 | 0 |
| F.F. | 97 | | × | 90 | 0 | 90 | 0 | 65 | −20 | 45 | −30 | 15 | − 5 | 40 | −10 |
| F.M. | 72 | | × | 90 | 0 | 80 | 10 | 55 | −15 | 50 | − 5 | 35 | −10 | 50 | −20 |
| G.C. | 61 | | × | 80 | 0 | 80 | 0 | 60 | −15 | 70 | −10 | 30 | − 5 | 50 | −20 |
| G.E. | 65 | | × | 90 | 0 | 90 | −10 | 65 | −20 | 70 | −10 | 35 | − 5 | 40 | − 5 |
| G.I. | 67 | | × | 90 | 0 | 70 | 0 | 60 | −10 | 55 | 0 | 30 | −10 | 40 | − 5 |
| G.L. | 60 | × | | 88 | 0 | 87 | 0 | 64 | 0 | 61 | 0 | 32 | 0 | 40 | 0 |
| G.L. | 60 | | × | 88 | 0 | 87 | 0 | 64 | 0 | 61 | 0 | 32 | 0 | 40 | 0 |
| H.M. | 62 | × | | 90 | 0 | 90 | 0 | 65 | −15 | 70 | 20 | 30 | 0 | 40 | −10 |
| H.M. | 78 | | × | 90 | 0 | 90 | 0 | 55 | − 5 | 50 | − 5 | 30 | 0 | 30 | 0 |
| M.M. | 88 | × | | 90 | −10 | 90 | −20 | 55 | −25 | 55 | − 5 | 40 | −25 | 40 | −10 |
| H.O.♂ | 75 | | × | 90 | 0 | 90 | 0 | 55 | −15 | 50 | −10 | 30 | −15 | 40 | − 5 |
| H.W.♂ | 72 | × | | 80 | 0 | 90 | −20 | 40 | 0 | 55 | 0 | 25 | − 5 | 30 | 0 |
| K.E. | 65 | | × | 90 | 0 | 90 | 0 | 80 | −20 | 70 | −10 | 40 | 5 | 40 | − 5 |
| K.H.♂ | 68 | × | | 90 | 0 | 90 | 0 | 85 | −10 | 70 | −25 | 35 | 0 | 40 | −10 |
| L.G. | 65 | | × | 90 | −30 | 90 | −10 | 60 | −25 | 70 | 0 | 40 | − 5 | 45 | −15 |
| M.B. | 83 | | × | 90 | 0 | 90 | 0 | 60 | −10 | 50 | 0 | 30 | 0 | 40 | −10 |
| M.E. | 74 | | × | 90 | 0 | 90 | 0 | 70 | −40 | 70 | −15 | 35 | −10 | 40 | −10 |
| M.F. | 72 | | × | 90 | 0 | 90 | 0 | 50 | 0 | 60 | − 5 | 20 | 10 | 30 | 10 |
| M.I. | 81 | | × | 90 | 0 | 80 | 0 | 40 | −10 | 50 | −15 | 25 | 0 | 35 | 0 |
| M.M. | 60 | | × | 85 | 0 | 85 | 0 | 60 | 0 | 70 | −10 | 25 | 5 | 25 | 10 |
| R.I. | 70 | × | | 90 | 0 | 90 | 0 | 70 | −20 | 65 | − 5 | 25 | − 5 | 40 | −10 |
| R.M. | 80 | × | | 90 | −10 | 90 | −20 | 60 | −15 | 80 | −30 | 40 | −15 | 40 | −15 |
| S.C. | 65 | | × | 90 | 0 | 90 | 0 | 85 | −15 | 75 | −15 | 25 | −20 | 45 | −30 |
| S.H.♂ | 69 | | × | 90 | 0 | 90 | 0 | 70 | −10 | 60 | −10 | 20 | 0 | 45 | 0 |
| S.I.♂ | 71 | | × | 90 | −45 | 90 | −45 | 50 | −20 | 50 | −20 | 30 | −10 | 40 | −10 |
| T.E. | 69 | | × | 90 | 0 | 90 | −10 | 70 | −25 | 50 | −10 | 40 | 0 | 30 | −15 |
| W.A. | 70 | | × | 80 | 0 | 80 | 0 | 70 | −15 | 60 | −30 | 45 | −25 | 35 | − 5 |
| W.A. | 79 | × | | 90 | −30 | 90 | −10 | 70 | −40 | 50 | 0 | 30 | −10 | 40 | −10 |
| W.E. | 62 | | × | 90 | 0 | 90 | 0 | 70 | −15 | 65 | −20 | 25 | 0 | 45 | 0 |
| W.L. | 62 | | × | 80 | 0 | 80 | 0 | 60 | 0 | 50 | 0 | 30 | 0 | 40 | − 5 |

| Radiology Tilt in PA and sagittal planes (degrees) | | Shortening (mm) | X-ray groups: Radiology | | | | Clinical group: Subjective class | | | | | Remarks, Other pathology |
|---|---|---|---|---|---|---|---|---|---|---|---|---|
| | | | 0 | 1 | 2 | 3 | I | II | III | IV | V | |
| 14 | 0 | 2.00 | | × | | | × | | | | | Post-operative RSD, but minor |
| 0 | 18 | 3.50 | | | × | | | | × | | | |
| 2 | 2 | 3.50 | | × | | | × | | | | | |
| 2 | 46 | 4.00 | | | × | | | × | | | | Painful shoulder |
| 0 | 12 | 4.50 | | | × | | | × | | | | Distal ulnar instability |
| 0 | 8 | 2.00 | | × | | | | × | | | | |
| 3 | 10 | 0.00 | | × | | | × | | | | | |
| 0 | 34 | 0.00 | | × | | | | | | × | | |
| 10 | 5 | 3.00 | | | × | | | | × | | | |
| 0 | 20 | 5.50 | | | × | | | | | | × | Ulnar head syndrome |
| 0 | 10 | 0.00 | | × | | | × | | | | | |
| 0 | 40 | 6.00 | | | × | | | | × | | | Radial epicondylitis |
| 0 | 0 | 0.00 | × | | | | | | | × | | Stiffness related to RSD |
| 35 | 24 | 16.00 | | | | × | | | × | | | |
| 11 | 32 | 2.00 | | | × | | × | | | | | |
| 0 | 16 | 0.00 | | × | | | | | × | | | Ulnar head syndrome |
| 0 | 46 | 3.00 | | | × | | | × | | | | |
| 0 | 44 | 1.00 | | × | | | | | × | | | |
| 0 | 18 | 3.00 | | | × | | | × | | | | Carpal tunnel syndrome |
| 0 | 10 | 3.00 | | | × | | | | × | | | Ulnar head syndrome |
| 5 | 34 | 3.50 | | | × | | × | | | | | |
| 2 | 20 | 3.00 | | | × | | | × | | | | Bilateral carpal tunnel syndrome, inability to lift saucepans or do housework |
| 10 | 34 | 6.50 | | | | × | | | × | | | |
| 0 | 15 | 3.50 | | | × | | | | × | | | |
| 4 | 10 | 4.00 | | | × | | | | × | | | |
| 7 | 23 | 0.00 | | | × | | | × | | | | Left-handed woman |
| 13 | 0 | 4.00 | | | × | | | × | | | | |
| 4 | 24 | 6.00 | | | × | | | | | × | | Carpal tunnel syndrome |
| 17 | 22 | 5.50 | | | | × | | | | × | | Intra-articular fracture |
| 4 | 14 | 3.00 | | | × | | | | | | × | RSD finger-palm distance 3.5 cm |
| 0 | 20 | 1.00 | | × | | | | | | × | | |
| 0 | 8 | 0.00 | | × | | | × | | | | | Painful shoulder, subcapital fracture |
| 0 | 21 | 0.00 | | × | | | | × | | | | |
| 3 | 6 | 1.00 | | × | | | × | | | | | |
| 17 | 10 | 3.00 | | | | × | | | | | × | RSD |
| 25 | 10 | 2.50 | | | | × | | | × | | | |
| 5 | 0 | 3.00 | | × | | | | × | | | | |
| 10 | 4 | 5.50 | | | × | | | | | | × | Polyarthritis |
| 2 | 16 | 0.50 | | × | | | | | | × | | Ulnar head syndrome |
| 5 | 23 | 1.00 | | × | | | | × | | | | |
| 10 | 45 | 3.00 | | | × | | | × | | | | |
| 9 | 4 | 3.00 | | | × | | | | | × | | Left-handed woman |
| 0 | 4 | 0.00 | × | | | | × | | | | | |

RSD, reflex sympathetic dystrophy

**Table IV.2.** Subjective classes

| Class | | *n* | Castaing |
|---|---|---|---|
| I | Perfect results, no disability | 9 (20.9%) | 21.2% |
| II | Satisfactory, moderate disability | 11 (25.6%) | 24.9% |
| III | Fair, major disability | 12 (27.9%) | 25.6% |
| IV | Poor, no movement | 7 (16.3%) | 18.9% |
| V | Bad, activity very much reduced | 4 (9.3%) | 9.4% |
| | Total: | 43 (100%) | |

This distribution is the same as that reported by Castaing (1964) in 433 fractures in patients of all ages; *n*, number of patients

**Table IV.3.** Radiological groups

| Group | | *n* |
|---|---|---|
| 0 | No deformity | 2 (4.7%) |
| 1 | One deformity | 15 (34.9%) |
| 2 | Two deformities | 20 (46.5%) |
| 3 | Three deformities | 6 (13.9%) |
| | Total: | 43 (100%) |

**Table IV.4.** Distribution of radiological groups by subjective class

| Radiological group | Subjective class | | | | | |
|---|---|---|---|---|---|---|
| | I Perfect | II Satis. | III Fair | IV Poor | V Bad | Total |
| 0 | 1 | 0 | 0 | 1 | 0 | 2 |
| 1 | 6 | 4 | 2 | 3 | 0 | 15 |
| 2 | 2 | 7 | 6 | 2 | 3 | 20 |
| 3 | 0 | 0 | 4 | 1 | 1 | 6 |
| Total | 9 | 11 | 12 | 7 | 4 | 43 |

**Table IV.5.** Subjective class related to mobility

| | Pronation | Supination | Flexion | Extension | Deviation | | Total |
|---|---|---|---|---|---|---|---|
| | | | | | Radial | Ulnar | |
| I. Perfect | − 1.1 | 1.1 | −12.2 | − 2.2 | − 1.1 | − 8.3 | − 23.8 |
| II. Satisfactory | 0.0 | − 1.8 | −10.0 | − 6.4 | − 2.7 | − 1.8 | − 22.7 |
| III. Fair | − 3.3 | − 5.0 | −15.0 | − 7.1 | −10.4 | − 8.3 | − 49.2 |
| IV. Poor | − 4.3 | − 2.9 | −12.9 | − 7.9 | − 0.7 | − 5.7 | − 34.3 |
| V. Bad | −16.3 | −21.3 | −22.5 | −21.3 | −13.8 | −11.3 | −106.3 |

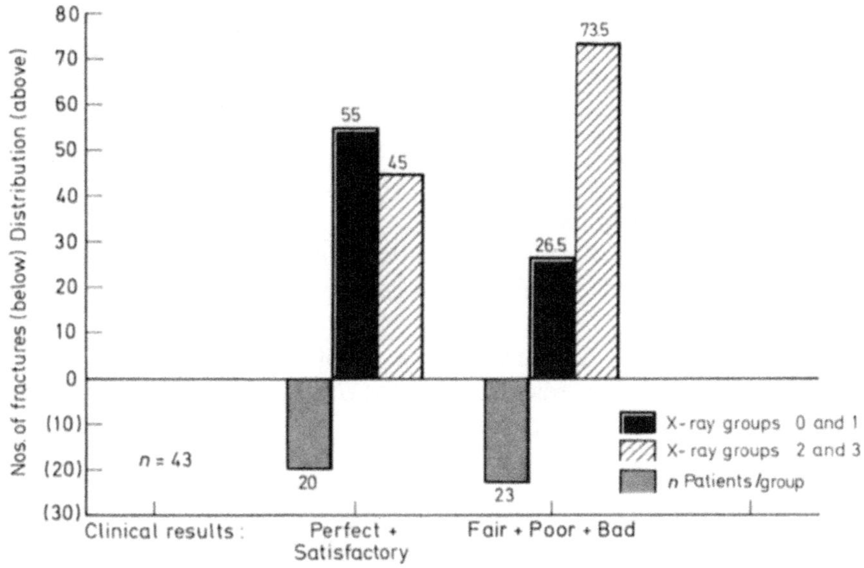


**Fig. IV.5.** Comparison of clinical and radiological results; there are more satisfactory results in the radiological groups with the least deformity

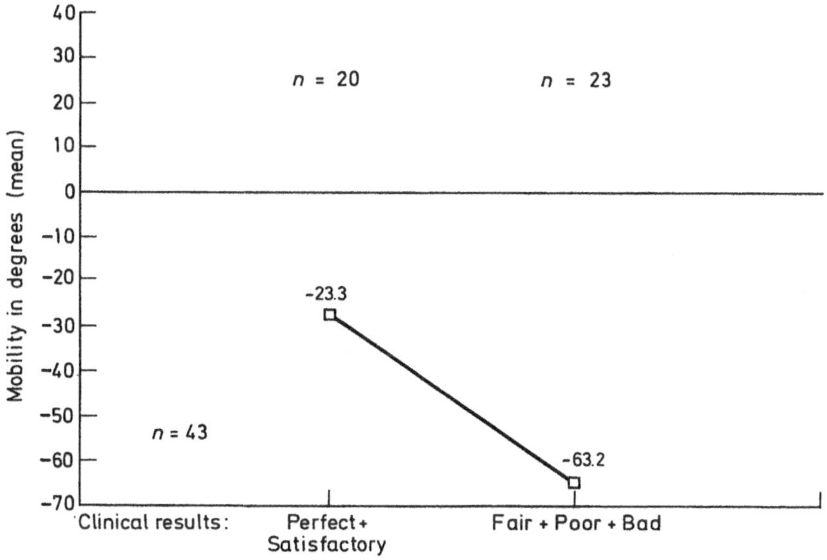


**Fig. IV.6.** Relationship between class of result and global mobility; satisfactory result seems to go together with mobility

trary, exceptions are always quoted to prove the benign nature of malunion. Fourrier et al. (1981) failed in this approach, thus reinforcing the opinion of the sceptics, and confirming that tolerance increases with age.

*Aims of Statistical Analysis*

Our goal is:
- to determine whether a relationship exists between structure and symptoms,
- to discover the factors influencing or disturbing this relationship,
- to determine the role of age,
- to define the most adequate treatment.

Our initial hypothesis will be the usual one: namely, that there is no correlation between the radiological or anatomical result obtained and the subjective result, the patient's comfort.

*Method*

We shall proceed in two stages:
- the first consists of seeking an index that allows determination of the degree of correlation between structural and clinical status,
- the second is to determine the risk of error associated with the acceptance or rejection of the initial hypothesis in the light of the degree of correlation.

*Choice of Tests*

The variables to be analysed are ordinal, since they are ordered as functions of precise criteria; they are mutually dependent, since the subjective result is compared with the radiological image, which reflects the morphology. Morphology is the independent criterion on the basis of which the quality of the subjective result is judged.

The statistical index *gamma* is the index best suited to analysis of this type of problem because it measures the association between ranks. It corresponds to the formula:

$$gamma = \frac{n \text{ agreements} - n \text{ inversions}}{n \text{ agreements} + n \text{ inversions}} = \frac{\text{fa} - \text{fi}}{\text{fa} + \text{fi}}$$

Agreements occur when the rank of the dependent variable agrees with that of the independent, for instance a patient of radiological group 2 and clinical category III in relation to a patient of radiological group 3 and clinical category IV. Inversion refers to the contrary case, i.e. a patient of group 1 and class III in relation to a patient of group 3 and class I. The number of agreements is indicated by fa, the number of inversions by fi. The methodology is well described in Kurtz's book (1981) and will not be discussed further.

For the data in Table IV.6, this index is 0.43 with 343 agreements and 137 inversions, i.e. 480 pairs compared, from a total of 903 possible pairs. This positive result suggests that a correlation exists between the quality of the anatomical result and the quality of life. This contradicts our working hypothesis. We now need to calculate the risks of error associated with rejection of our hypothesis. The formula:

$$Z = \gamma \sqrt{\frac{\text{fa} + \text{fi}}{n\,(1 - \gamma^2)}}$$

answers our question.

**Table IV.6.** The *gamma* index and its statistical significance. The *gamma* index measures the correlations between two ordinal variables, the order of the observations being defined by the independent variable, in our case radiology, from 0 to 3. The value of *gamma* ranges from +1.00 (perfect correlation) to −1.00 (inverse correlation). Zero signifies disorder.

$$\gamma = \frac{\text{fa} - \text{fi}}{\text{fa} + \text{fi}}$$

where fa = $n$ agreements and fi = $n$ inversions

For Table IV.4.

| Radiological group | Subjective class | | | | | |
|---|---|---|---|---|---|---|
| | I Perf. | II Satis. | III Fair | IV Poor | V Bad | Total |
| 0 | 1 | 0 | 0 | 1 | 0 | 2 |
| 1 | 6 | 4 | 2 | 3 | 0 | 15 |
| 2 | 2 | 7 | 6 | 2 | 3 | 20 |
| 3 | 0 | 0 | 4 | 1 | 1 | 6 |
| Total | 9 | 11 | 12 | 7 | 4 | 43 |

fa = 343 and fi = 137 imply a *gamma* of 0.429.

The test of significance of *gamma* is $Z$. $Z$ makes it possible to determine whether the calculated *gamma* coefficient is really significant. It is applicable only if $n \geq 10$.

$$Z = \gamma \sqrt{\frac{\text{fa} + \text{fi}}{n(1 - \gamma^2)}} = 1.58$$

The significance of $Z$ is found in the standard distribution table. Our hypothesis implies a one-tailed test.

The conditions are valid if $n \geq 10$. The results are significant at 5% if $Z \geq 1.64$ (one-tailed test).

In this case, $Z$ equals 1.58. The tables allow us to find the value of the risk *alpha* or *P*. Here, this risk is 0.057 or 5.7% for a one-tailed test. We are at the limit of significance. Are we consequently to admit that it is statistically impossible to reject the initial hypothesis solely on the basis of an *alpha* risk of 5% taken as a limiting value?

### *The Problem of Associated Pathology*

Fractures of the radius may be associated with reflex sympathetic dystrophy (RSD), carpal tunnel syndrome, epicondylitis or shoulder pain. We define these as associated pathology and have added to the list the "ulnar head" syndrome. This is often evidence of an invisible ligamentous lesion that may occur despite perfect anatomic reduction and therefore qualifies as an associated lesion.

**Table IV.7.** *Gamma* index of patients divided into categories: satisfied and unsatisfied

| | Satisfied | Unsatisfied | Total |
|---|---|---|---|
| Group 0 | 1 | 1 | 2 |
| Group 1 | 10 | 5 | 15 |
| Group 2 | 9 | 11 | 20 |
| Group 3 | 0 | 6 | 6 |
| Total | 20 | 23 | 43 |

This analysis includes 246 agreements, 64 inversions, 310 pairs out of 904 possible pairs; *gamma* = 0.587. The corresponding $Z = 1.92$, therefore $P = 0.024$ (one-tailed curve)

*The Pain Threshold*

The *gamma* test is very sensitive and covers all the factors influencing the results. These factors are extremely numerous, starting with the pain threshold.

In dividing our patients into five classes, we distinguish the degree of dissatisfaction – eminently variable from one subject to another – influenced by associated pathology or local pain not related to the X-ray film. To eliminate this over-elaborate differentiation, we now distinguish two categories of patients: the satisfied and the unsatisfied, without any fine tuning. This yields four pairs of figures (Table IV.7).

The *gamma* index rises to 0.58. The possible correlation seems statistically proved, since the $Z$ corresponding to this value, i.e. 1.92, represents a $P$ of 2.4%. Thus, the initial hypothesis can be rejected. Once the gradation of dissatisfaction is suppressed, the correlation, so often denied, can be demonstrated statistically!

*Reflex Sympathetic Dystrophy (RSD)*

RSD can have severe functional sequelae and cripple the hand. Its incidence appears particularly high in our series (4/43 or 9.3%). It varies enormously according to the author quoted: Castaing found 17% in 433 fractures and Meine (reported by Coquoz, 1982) only 4.2% in 549 cases. It is probably a matter of definition but despite this, whatever the definition chosen, the frequency of this complication still seems unduly high.

To convince ourselves, we reviewed all the cases of dystrophy occurring in patients operated in the department (including traumatic cases) between 1st July 1984 and 30th April 1985: 15 out of 974 patients, i.e. 1.5%. Is this rate significantly different from that observed in patients suffering from a distal radius fracture?

**Table IV.8 a–c.** The Chi-square test: proof of the independence of two qualitative variables; in our case: table of contingency 2 × 2, number of degrees of freedom = 1, the values are nominal (occurrence versus non-occurrence of RSD). To test the hypothesis that the incidence of RSD is the same in the different samples compared, the following conditions were applied: the sample size should be such that no scale categories have zero observations; no more than 20% should have less than 5; it is always a two-tailed test. With the number of degrees of freedom = 1, the test is significant at:

1. 5% if it is equal or superior to 3.85
2. 2% if it is equal or superior to 5.42
3. 1% if it is equal or superior to 6.64
4. 1‰ if it is equal or superior to 10.83

$Chi^2 = (Oi - Ei)/Ei$
Oi, observed sample totals
Ei, calculated sample totals

**a** Comparison of incidence of RSD in the sample of operated patients (974) within Meine's "radius" sample of 549 post-fracture patients

| | Operated in clinic | Meine's radius |
|---|---|---|
| No. with RSD | 15 | 23 |
| No. without RSD | 959 | 526 |
| Total | 974 | 549 |

$Chi^2 = 10.13$
*Conclusion:* the incidence of RSD differs significantly ($P \simeq 1\%$) between the two samples; its probability is greater in Meine's patients.

**b** Comparison of incidence of RSD in our sample of 43 post-fracture cases with that in our sample of 974 operated cases

| | Our post-fractures | Operated cases |
|---|---|---|
| No. with RSD | 4 | 15 |
| No. without RSD | 39 | 959 |
| Total | 43 | 974 |

$Chi^2 = 13.53$
*Conclusion:* the incidence of RSD differs significantly ($P < 1‰$) between these two samples.

**c** Comparison of incidence of RSD in our sample of 43 patients after radial fractures with that in Meine's sample of 549 patients after radial fractures

| | Our cases | Meine's cases |
|---|---|---|
| No. with RSD | 4 | 23 |
| No. without RSD | 39 | 526 |
| Total | 43 | 549 |

$Chi^2 = 2.39$
*Conclusion:* the incidence of RSD does not differ significantly between these two samples

**Table IV.9 a, b.**

**a** Analysis of all classes: $n = 39$ (excluding patients with RSD)

| | Class | | | | | Total |
|---|---|---|---|---|---|---|
| | I | II | III | IV | V | |
| Group 0 | 1 | 0 | 0 | 0 | 0 | 1 |
| Group 1 | 5 | 4 | 2 | 3 | 0 | 14 |
| Group 2 | 2 | 7 | 6 | 2 | 2 | 19 |
| Group 3 | 0 | 0 | 4 | 1 | 0 | 5 |
| Total | 8 | 11 | 12 | 6 | 2 | 39 |

*Gamma* = 0.453
268 agreements
101 inversions
741 possible pairs
$Z = 1.52$ and $P = 0.064$ (limit of significance below that of the complete sample)

**b** Division into two categories: satisfied and unsatisfied

| | Satisfied | Unsatisfied | Total |
|---|---|---|---|
| Group 0 | 1 | 0 | 1 |
| Group 1 | 9 | 5 | 14 |
| Group 2 | 9 | 10 | 19 |
| Group 3 | 0 | 5 | 5 |
| Total | 19 | 20 | 39 |

200 agreements
45 inversions
245 pairs out of 741 possible pairs
*Gamma* = 0.633; corresponding $Z = 2.00$, therefore $P = 0.023$ (one-tailed curve, statistically significant)

To answer this question we carried out a Chi-square test. We had samples independent of one another, i.e. binomial; hence, we could compare the percentages observed by a contingency table of $2 \times 2$. The conditions of validity of the test and the Chi-square formula are set out in Table IV.8, together with the results. It is to be noted that the incidence of RSD in the control population, i.e. the 974 operated cases in the department, is significantly lower than for each of the post-fracture samples studied (Meine's 549 cases and our 43 cases) and with a *P* of about 1‰. As well, there is no significant statistical difference between the incidence of RSD observed by ourselves and by Meine.

If RSD is more frequent after fracture of the radius, it is probable that it disturbs the relationship between structure and quality of life. To verify this hypothesis we withdrew the four cases of RSD from the comparative table and repeated the

**Table IV.10 a, b.**
**a** Analysis of all classes: $n=33$ (excluding 10 patients with RSD and other pain syndromes)

| | Class | | | | | Total |
|---|---|---|---|---|---|---|
| | I | II | III | IV | V | |
| Group 0 | 1 | 0 | 0 | 0 | 0 | 1 |
| Group 1 | 4 | 4 | 2 | 3 | 0 | 13 |
| Group 2 | 2 | 4 | 5 | 1 | 2 | 14 |
| Group 3 | 0 | 0 | 4 | 1 | 0 | 5 |
| Total | 7 | 8 | 11 | 5 | 2 | 33 |

*Gamma* = 0.423
195 agreements
79 inversions
528 possible pairs
$Z=1.32$ and $P=0.093$ (limit of significance below that of the complete sample)

**b** Division into two categories: satisfied and unsatisfied

| | Satisfied | Unsatisfied | Total |
|---|---|---|---|
| Group 0 | 1 | 0 | 1 |
| Group 1 | 8 | 5 | 13 |
| Group 2 | 6 | 8 | 14 |
| Group 3 | 0 | 5 | 5 |
| Total | 15 | 18 | 33 |

152 agreements
30 inversions
182 pairs out of 520 possible pairs
*Gamma* = 0.670; corresponding $Z=2.02$, therefore $P=0.021$ (one-tailed curve, statistically significant)

*gamma* analysis. Table IV.9 summarizes the findings; the results are interesting.

- *Gamma* for the complete table of the remaining 39 patients shows an index of correlation that is better, but the $Z$ is diminished because the number of observations is fewer.
- *Gamma* for the simplified table (only two groups) fulfills our expectations: both *gamma* and $Z$ increase in parallel, but so moderately that the role of RSD in affecting the final outcome is doubtful.

### *Associated Conditions*

It is clear that, to gain a better grasp of the relationship between structure and discomfort, it is necessary to eliminate all focal painful points, i.e. not only RSD but also pain syndromes in the upper extremity. This is why we have discarded from our table the ten patients suffering from painful conditions unrelated

**Table IV.11 a, b.**
**a** Analysis of all classes: $n=28$ (only patients with no particular complaint)

| | Class | | | | | Total |
|---|---|---|---|---|---|---|
| | I | II | III | IV | V | |
| Group 0 | 1 | 0 | 0 | 0 | 0 | 1 |
| Group 1 | 4 | 4 | 1 | 2 | 0 | 11 |
| Group 2 | 2 | 3 | 4 | 1 | 1 | 11 |
| Group 3 | 0 | 0 | 4 | 1 | 0 | 5 |
| Total | 7 | 7 | 9 | 4 | 1 | 28 |

*gamma* = 0.527
155 agreements
48 inversions, 203 pairs out of 378 possible pairs
$Z=1.64$ and $P=0.0505$ (limit of significance virtually reached)

**b** Division into two categories: satisfied and unsatisfied

| | Satisfied | Unsatisfied | Total |
|---|---|---|---|
| Group 0 | 1 | 0 | 1 |
| Group 1 | 8 | 3 | 11 |
| Group 2 | 5 | 6 | 11 |
| Group 3 | 0 | 5 | 5 |
| Total | 14 | 14 | 28 |

127 agreements
15 inversions
142 pairs out of 378 possible pairs
*gamma* = 0.789; corresponding $Z=2.87$, therefore $P=0.002$ (one-tailed curve, statistically very significant, correlation incontestable)

to the wrist and repeated our calculations. On the other hand, the ulnar head syndrome remains included in the analysis (Table IV.10).

With the five-column table, the *gamma* index is 0.423 and the corresponding $Z$, 1.32. With two columns we obtain a *gamma* of 0.670 and a $Z$ of 2.02. The correlation again exists, provided we suppress the nuances and retain only two classes. Is this bound to be the case?

To settle this question, we have excluded from the analysis all persons presenting with any upper extremity complaints, including the ulnar head syndrome. Only 28 persons remain who meet these criteria.

The results in Table IV.11 are very interesting. For the total of all classes, *gamma* equals 0.527 and $Z$ is 1.64, so that the 5% limit of significance is virtually attained. For the simplified table, the correlation seems certain since $P$ equals 2‰ for a *gamma* value of 0.789.

## Conclusions

This statistical analysis demonstrates several important points that have not been clearly defined before:

1. There is a relationship between the quality of the anatomical result and patient satisfaction, but this relationship is not linear; the pain threshold differs for each patient, hence the intensity of complaints in patients with other painful conditions in the upper extremity. This makes analysis particularly difficult.
2. The absence of a linear relationship explains the contradictory current opinions. Once the criteria for assessing the results are modified in the direction of greater tolerance, the correlations become blurred. Nothing is more subjective than the patient's assessment; nevertheless, we were surprised to find that our study, with only 43 cases, gave subjective results superimposable on those of Castaing (Table IV.12).

**Table IV.12.** Subjective results of Castaing ($n=433$) compared with our own study ($n=43$)

| | Class | | | |
|---|---|---|---|---|
| | I | II | III | IV and V |
| Castaing | 21.2 | 24.9 | 25.6 | 28.3 |
| St Gallen | 21.0 | 25.5 | 28.0 | 25.5 |

This study did not permit assessment of the influence of the different degrees of osseous tilt. We feel that protrusion of the ulna plays an important role, though the correlation is not significant. In this context, we regret that Castaing's analysis did not employ strict statistical methods; the comparison of results would have been easier.

3. The fracture is not better tolerated with age. Our results are identical to those of Castaing who had a younger patient population.
4. Only anatomical reduction will predictably give a satisfactory clinical result. Therefore, by definition, this must be the aim of treatment.

## Discussion

In the light of our analysis it is clear that anatomical reduction, and only anatomical reduction, offers the best chance for a good result. This well-known orthopaedic axiom is thus verified for fractures of the distal radius also.

To discern the cause of certain failures, one would have to assess only the anatomically perfect results. Now, these are the exception. For that to become the rule, a better understanding of the fracture, its physiology and morphology are needed. This should be the basis of a classification oriented towards treatment. In the light of our clinical results we propose a rational basis for treatment of fracture of the distal radius, exploiting the possibilities of both conservative and surgical treatment, and particularly of the external fixator.

## B. Morphology and Classification of Fractures of the Distal Radius in Relation to the Quality of the Bone: Therapeutic Implications

The usual classifications, complex and elaborate, have often been purely descriptive, or sometimes derived from experimental studies (Frykmann 1967). None to our knowledge is primarily therapeutically oriented. That is why we now propose a classification based on the morphology of the fractures in relation to the age of the patients, and therefore to the quality of the bone.

### Anatomy

As with every long bone, the distal radius includes:
- the epiphysis; a block extending from the radio-carpal joint to the diaphyseal-metaphyseal junctional zone,
- the metaphysis; or zone for growth in length, between the epiphysis and the diaphysis, virtually absent in the adult,
- the diaphysis; the middle section which encloses the medullary canal surrounded by a cortex of thick compact bone.

### Physiology

In women, the mineral content of the bone attains its maximum at around 35 years of age, after which it diminishes by 10% per decade (Karjalainen and Alhava 1977; Mazess and Cameron 1973; Moore et al. 1975). In men the physiology is quite different: the loss of mineral salts from bone is negligible up to age 55 and then occurs at a rate of 4.4% per decade, less than half the rate for women. The diagrammatic representation of these data (Fig. IV.7) perfectly illustrates the problem: at 75 years of age the mineralization of a man's bone is comparable to that of a woman of 45 years. The woman of 75 years has lost 35% of her mineral salt content. Hence it is understandable that, under comparable conditions, a fall does not have the same consequences for both sexes. In women the greatly demineralized bone undergoes telescoping, while in men the fracture is still comparable to that of a youth. Therefore, a morphological analysis of the fracture must be the key element of a practical classification.

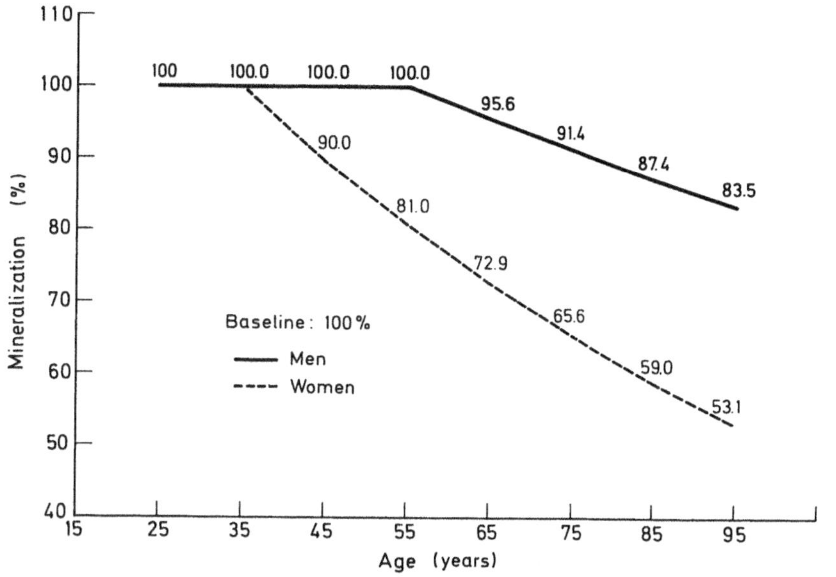


**Fig. IV.7.** Demineralization of the skeleton in relation to age and sex; mineralization of the male skeleton at age 75 years is equal to that in women of 45 years. Mineralization is expressed as a percentage. From Karjalainen and Alhava (1977), Mazess and Cameron (1973), Moore et al. (1975)

## Morphology

Since the bony texture changes with age, there is a distinction between the normally mineralized immature bone, normally mineralized adult bone and bone undergoing demineralization.

### *Normally Mineralized Immature Bone*

This type of bone is vulnerable in the metaphyseal zone; the epiphyseal part usually remains intact. It is possible to have an undisplaced linear fracture or impaction, i.e. a meshing of the distal spongiosa, so that the bone density increases at the site of the fracture. This gives the typical image of the torus or buckle fracture. There is no loss of bone substance (Fig. IV.8).

### *Normally Mineralized Adult Bone*

This bone generally shatters, but the bony volume is preserved. However, the fragmentation of the metaphyseal zone has the same consequences as a loss of substance in terms of stability, and therefore of treatment. The distal epiphyseal block, if it is intact, is unstable on the diaphysis (Fig. IV.9b).

### *Bone Undergoing Demineralization*

This is the rule in women after 50 years (by this age there is already a loss in mineral content of 15%), and sometimes from the age of 40 years, whereas it is exceptional in men, even after the age of 60 years. The fracture shows telescoping, the bone

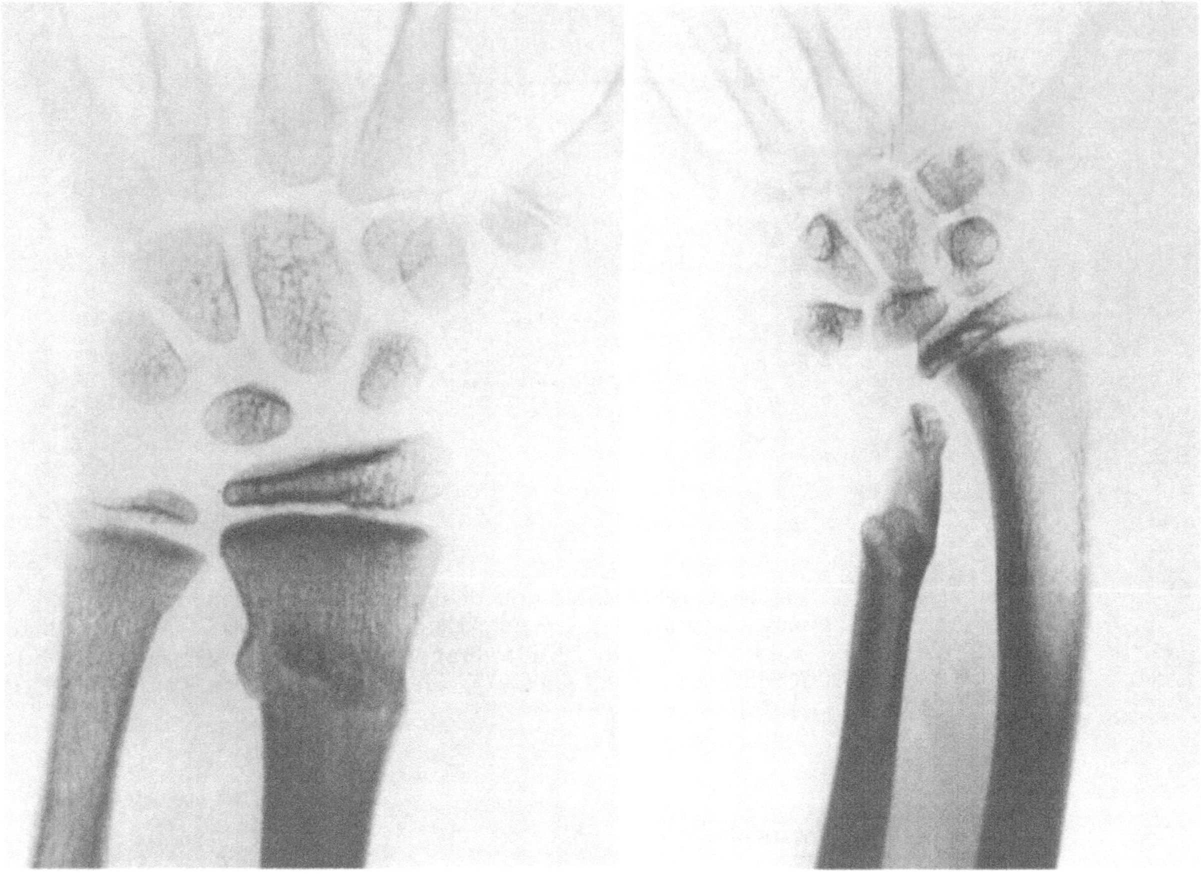
a b

**Fig. IV.8a, b.** Typical torus fracture. The fracture line does not pass through the joint but through the ulnar growth-plate, resulting in partial arrest of growth with malalignment of the radius and carpus. Treatment consists of repeated sessions of ulnar elongation (as with the external fixator)

trabeculae being crushed against each other, so that a reduction of bone volume ensues. This produces a loss of substance that is more or less marked depending on the violence of the impact. The telescoping absorbs energy, thus usually preserving the epiphyseal zone: this is the classical form of the fracture described by Colles and by Pouteau (Fig. IV.10).

*Note.* Involvement of the epiphyseal zone signifies an intra-articular fracture, a sub-classification possible for the three categories mentioned above. Very rare in immature bone and rare in bone undergoing demineralization, it is relatively common in the adult. In this case the fragmentation may affect the entire articulation or only part, then constituting the Barton type of marginal fracture.

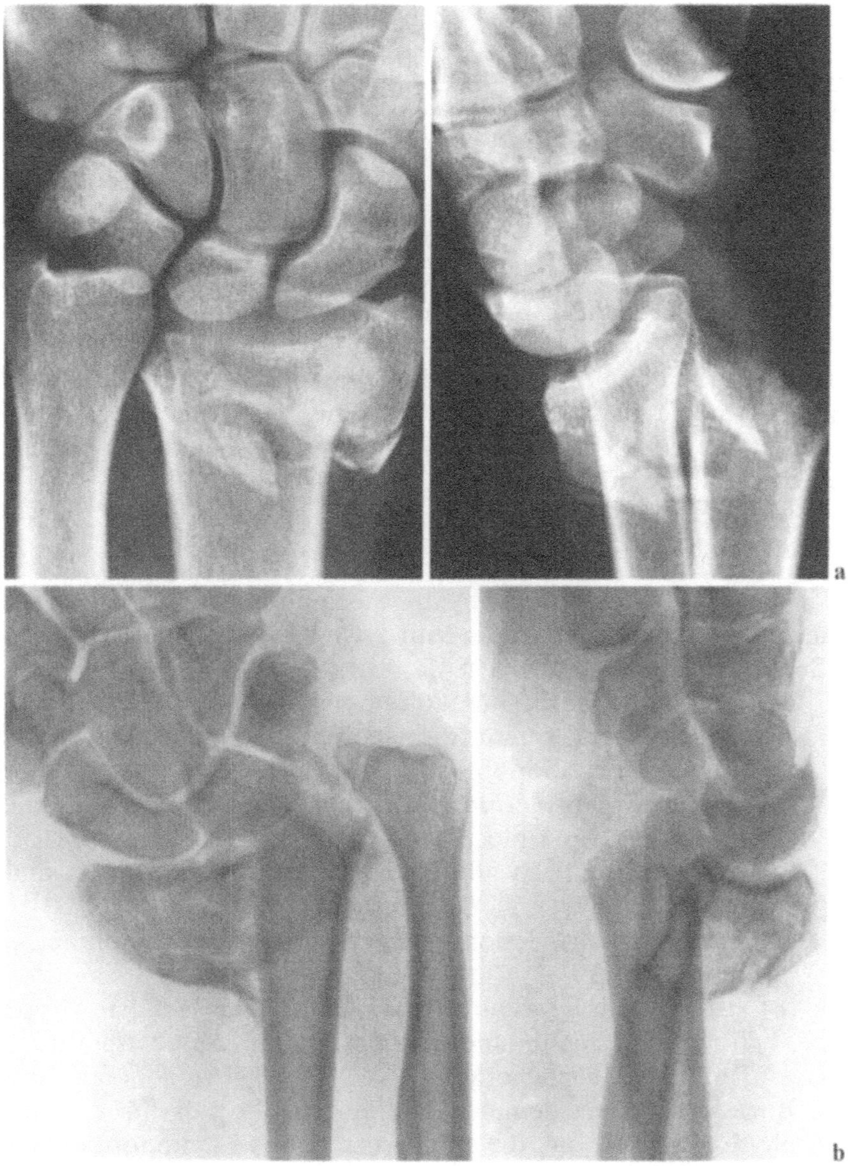


**Fig. IV.9 a, b.** Fracture with shattering, either of the metaphyseal zone only (**a**) or including the epiphysis (**b**); this produces an unstable and/ or a deformable epiphysis

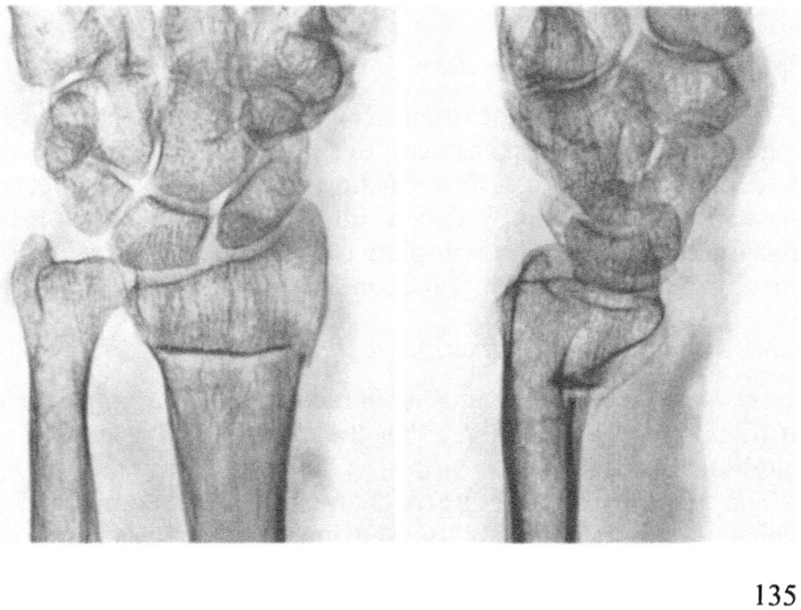

**Fig. IV.10.** Typical fracture of osteoporotic bone, with virtually no fracture line. The *dense line* is due to the cortex being driven into the spongiosa. Note: this fracture is stable, disimpaction creates an unstable situation which requires cancellous bone grafting

## Pathomechanics

The form of the fracture depends not only on the texture of the bone but also on the way the force is applied to the bone (Mayfield et al. 1980). For example, a fall on the hyperextended hand produces tension on the palmar aspect of the distal radius while the dorsal aspect is subjected to great compression. The zone under tension exhibits a sharp fracture line, and that subjected to compression undergoes impaction, fragmentation or telescoping depending on the degree of mineralization of the bone. In all three cases this amounts to a loss of substance. Between the zone of pressure and the zone of tension there is an intermediate zone, difficult to define, where shearing forces are active. Table IV.13 summarizes the physiological and pathomechanical factors.

## Classification of Fractures and Relation to Treatment

This has been established by us on anatomical, physiological and mechanical foundations with a view to planning treatment (Sennwald and Segmüller 1984):

1. Normally mineralized immature bone presents either:
   (a) a metaphyseal fracture: the epiphysis remains as a single fragment or "monoblock"
   (b) an epiphyseal fracture: with a linear fracture dividing the epiphysis: "split block" (marginal or Aitken fracture)
2. Normally mineralized adult bone (men up to 60 years and women under 40 years) may present:
   (a) a metaphyseal lesion: the epiphysis remains intact – "monoblock"
   (b) an epiphyseal fracture with either a simple Barton type fracture – "split block" – or a comminuted fracture – "multifragment block"
3. Bone undergoing demineralization usually presents a metaphyseal fracture, i.e. the epiphysis remains a "monoblock".

These data are summarized in Table IV.14.

### *Fracture of the Immature Bone, Normally Mineralized*

If the epiphysis is intact (monoblock), even if complicated by angulation or wide displacement, this presents no major difficulties, and consolidates after reduction and 3 weeks of effective plaster immobilization. When one finds an additional intra-articular fracture line, the growth-plate is involved and the reduction must be perfect, i.e. open reduction is required.

### *Adult Bone, Normally Mineralized*

In the absence of disease, this is characterized by varying degrees of fragmentation involving either the metaphyseal region or the epiphyseal zone.

– The metaphyseal fracture is characterized by comminution, which often implies instability. The dimensions of this zone rare-

**Table IV.13.** Pathomechanics of distal fractures of the forearm

| | |
|---|---|
| Quality of bone | Growing skeleton<br>Normally mineralized adult skeleton<br>Skeleton undergoing demineralization |
| Mode of action of forces | Compression<br>Traction<br>Shearing (mixed) |

**Table IV.14.** Morphology of distal fractures of the forearm

| Quality of bone | Site | Typology |
|---|---|---|
| Normally mineral-ized, immature | Metaphyseal<br>Epiphyseal | Epiphysis = "monoblock"<br>Epiphysis = "split block" (Aitken or marginal fracture) |
| Normally mineralized adult bone:<br>men $<$ 60<br>women $<$ 40 | Metaphyseal<br>Epiphyseal | Epiphysis = "split block"<br>Epiphysis = "monoblock"<br>– simple = marginal or Barton fracture = split block<br>– comminuted = "multifragmented block" |
| Bone undergoing demineralization<br>men $\geq$ 60<br>women $\geq$ 40 | Metaphyseal | Epiphysis = "monoblock" (telescoping) |

ly permit effective plaster immobilization (Fig. IV.11), and in general stable osteosynthesis is the method of choice. Progress in the field of external fixation makes this an option, but only in experienced hands. Though it obviates the need for a surgical approach to the wrist, its insertion remains difficult, and calls for precise anatomical knowledge of nerve and tendon pathways. When the distal segment is massive, the fixator can be applied without crossing the radio-carpal joint (Fig. IV.12), an important advantage in rehabilitation. The dorsal ligaments of the wrist, given their poor development and oblique course, do not constitute an anatomical structure adequate to reduce and maintain separated fragments. They should be called upon for assistance by longitudinal traction only if it is absolutely necessary, as in comminuted fractures.

– The complex epiphyseal fracture (neither split nor comminuted) often imposes a combination of several methods of treatment: for example, reduction of the articular fracture by screw or Kirschner wire, then, as a second stage, maintenance of the whole by stable osteosynthesis or external fixator.

The marginal fracture forms part of this group, and can be elegantly treated with a buttress plate placed on the dorsal, radial or palmar aspect, according to the fracture type.

Table IV.15. Classification by mode of treatment

| Type | Quality of bone | Treatment |
|---|---|---|
| Single epiphyseal fragment or monoblock (extra-articular) | Child | Plaster and/or reduction |
| | Adult, no defect: minor impaction, RU index < 3 mm, minor fragmentation and tilting < 8° | Plaster and/or reduction |
| | Adult, with defect: marked impaction, RU index > 3 mm, marked fragmentation | Ext. fix. ± OS[a] OS ± ext.fix.[a] |
| Fragmented epiphysis, no monoblock (intra-articular) | Marginal, child (Aitken: split block) | OS |
| | Marginal, adult (split block: radial, ulnar, palmar or dorsal) | OS |
| | Comminuted (or multifragmented block) | Ext. fix.[b] or OS[b] |

RU, radio-ulnar index; ext. fix., external fixation; OS, osteosynthesis

[a] Homogenous or autogenous cancellous graft in fracture gap
[b] Reduction and joint remodelling by means of cancellous graft

Fig. IV.11 a, b. Reduction of fracture shown in Fig. IV.9a. This is satisfactory as regards restoration of length, but there is residual tilt in both planes and shortening, with chronic pain ▷

– The comminuted epiphyseal fracture (multifragment) occurs in young men involved in high-energy accidents (as in moto-cross activities); it is characterized by extreme comminution of the centre or margins of the joint (Fig. IV.13).
– With central involvement, only an external fixator crossing the joint offers an acceptable solution. However, the comminution, the devitalization of the fragments and the difficulty of obtaining perfect reduction (some fragments may not reduce) may necessitate cancellous bone grafting, in the style used for reduction of depressed tibial plateau fractures. This allows remodelling of the radio-carpal joint, while preventing the carpus from becoming embedded in the radial epiphysis.
– For marginal joint involvement, a buttress plate combined with autogenous or homogenous cancellous grafting offers the best solution. The use, even temporarily, of the external fixator will avoid difficult manipulations, which can injure the soft tissues, especially the median nerve.

### *Adult Bone Undergoing Demineralization*

Because the fracture is impacted, with loss of bone substance, reduction with disimpaction of the fragments creates an unstable situation. For this reason, reduction should be avoided unless the impaction exceeds 3 mm, there is greater than 8° of dorsal angulation or greater than 8° of radial angulation. Under these conditions, we have found that, with conservative management,

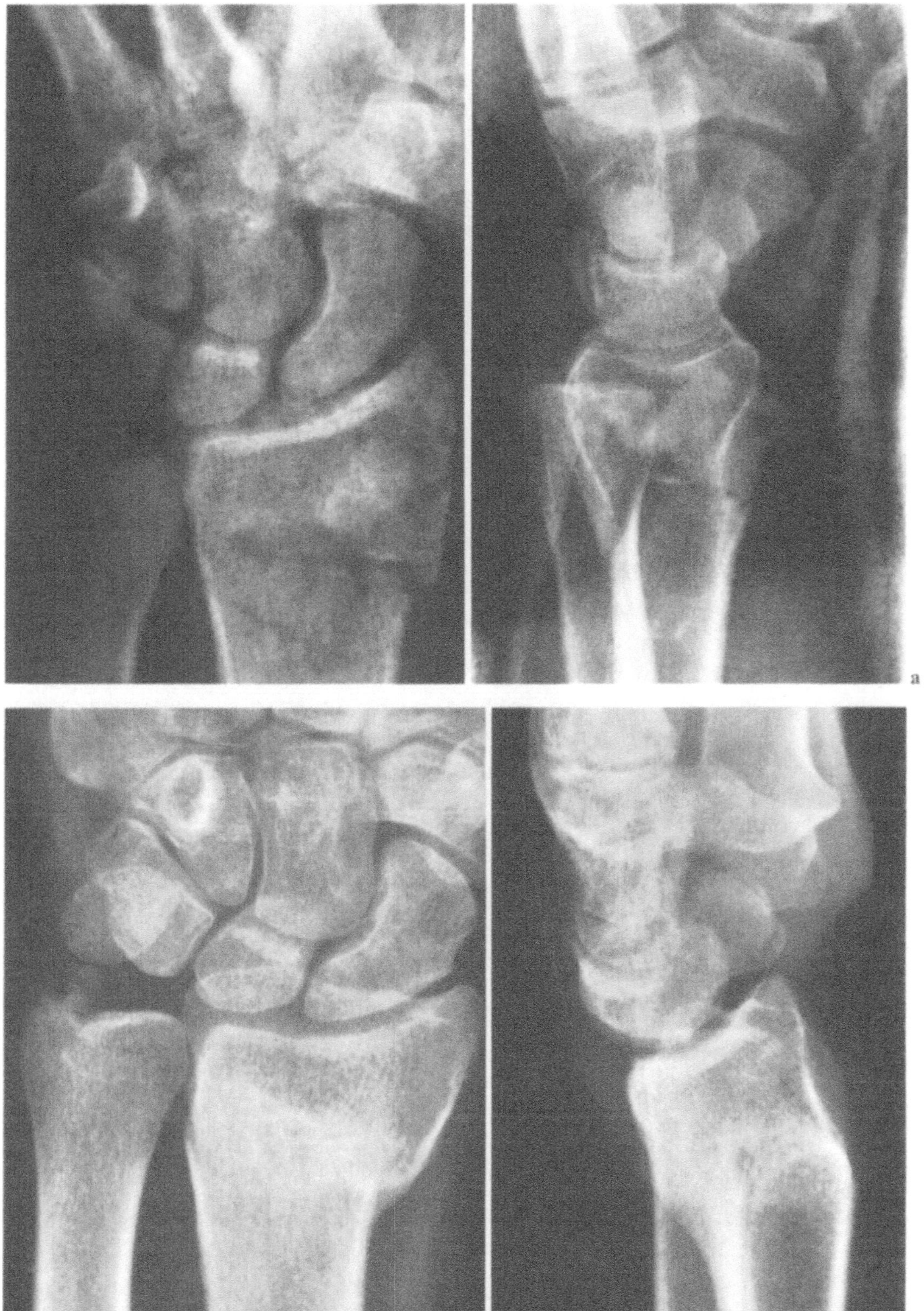


Fig. IV.11 a, b

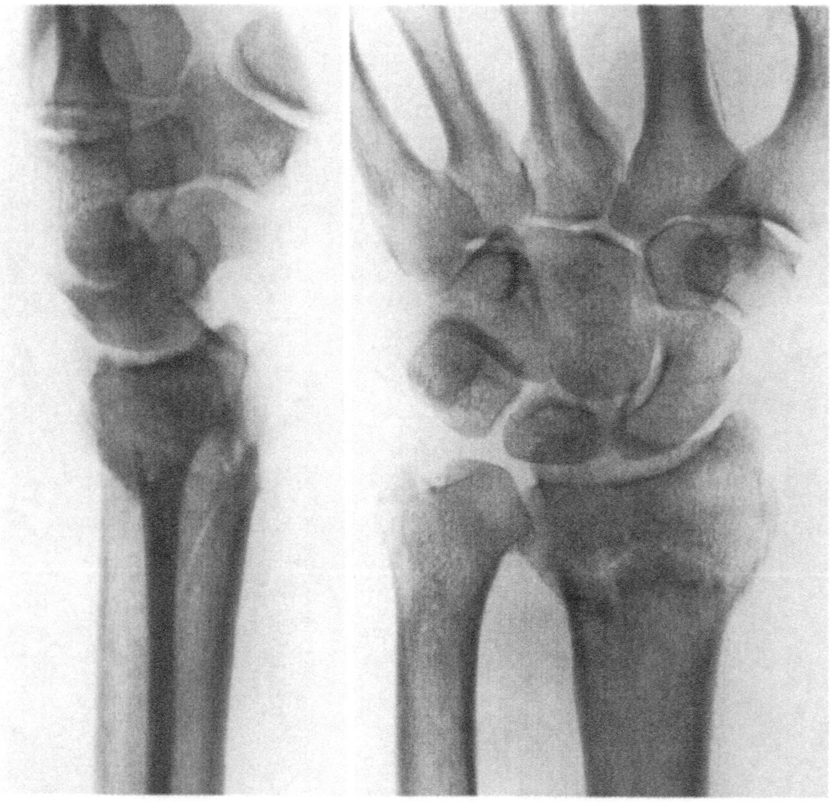

a

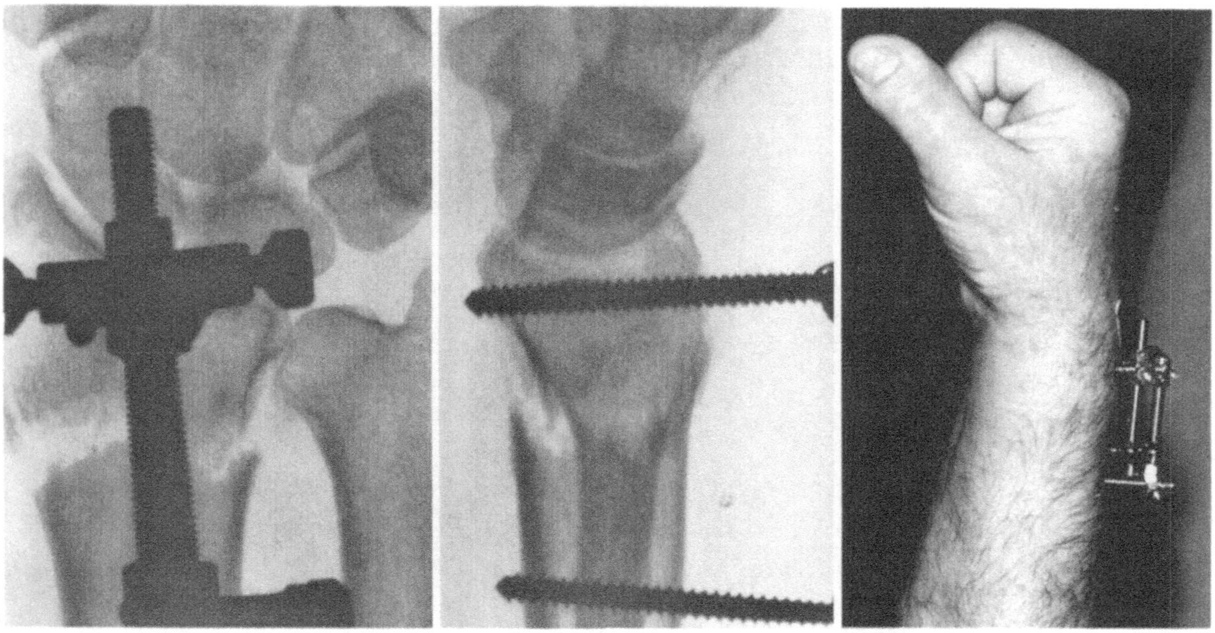

b

**Fig. IV.12 a, b.** Monoblock fracture comparable to Fig. IV.9 a: a method of stabilization by external fixation, using 3.5 mm AO cortical screws; two placed distally fix the transverse bar, while the two proximal ones fix the longitudinal bar. The final construct has minimal bulk

**Fig. IV.13a–c.** Comminuted epiphyseal fracture, reduction by external fixator without cancellous graft, removal of material after 6 weeks and secondary deformity; this demonstrates that the fixator must stay in place for at least 8 weeks. Alternatively, for faster recovery, cancellous grafting can be done, with the possible added advantage of joint remodelling

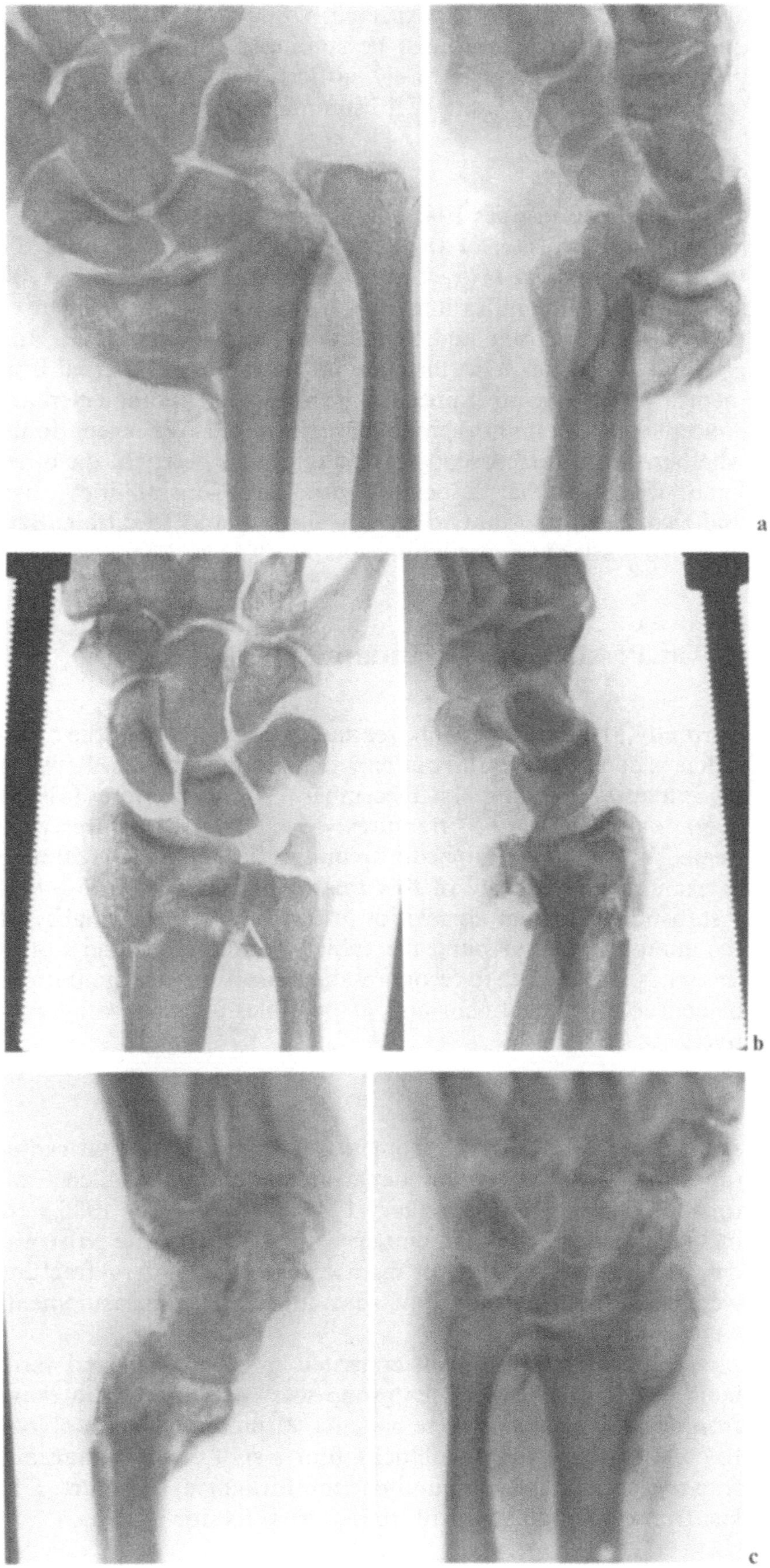

a favourable result can be expected. Otherwise, reduction is required and the fracture must be stabilized. In our experience, plaster immobilization is rarely sufficient; as we shall demonstrate subsequently. Table IV.15 summarizes our approach.

### Special Problems

Our classification does not distinguish between fractures with and without avulsion of the ulnar styloid. This is because the therapeutic outcome is practically identical. The absence of avulsion in no way signifies integrity of the ulnar compartment of the radio-carpal joint and/or the distal radio-ulnar joint, and gives no indication as to the state of the radio-ulno-carpal ligaments. What is to be gained by introducing a complementary concept of uncertain therapeutic relevance? We even doubt whether routine arthroscopy can enlighten us here. On the other hand, we know that associated intra-carpal instabilities exist, and that it is important to recognize these and to differentiate them from adaptive angulations.

## C. The Possibilities of Treatment

Currently, the most common treatment for fractures of the distal radius is conservative and our experience supports this. Between 1st January 1980 and 31st December 1982 there were only 54 operations listed for 653 fractures; over 90% of fractures were treated by simple orthopaedic splintage. Hence, it is legitimate to examine the efficacy of this treatment, since we know that a statistically proven correlation exists between the quality of the anatomical results and the subjective outcome. The aim of this study is therefore to recognize the indications and limitations of conservative treatment and, if possible, to propose alternatives.

### Choice of Patients

All the patients suffering from a fracture of the distal radius reporting to the emergency department of the St Gallen Cantonal Hospital from 1st January 1985 to 15th March 1985 were included in this study. Patients in whom the opposite wrist was deformed, either by injury or disease, or with a bilateral fracture, were excluded from the study, since no reference measurements were possible.

The series (Table IV.16) consisted of 27 women and three men. The average age of the group was 64 years, with a range from 15 to 88 years. Of these patients, 21 presented a monoblock fracture (single epiphyseal block), four a split block or marginal fracture and five a comminuted (multifragment) fracture. The last five were all treated with the external fixator.

**Table IV.16.** Treatment summary

| | | Conservative | External fixation | Total |
|---|---|---|---|---|
| Men | | 1 | 2 | 3 |
| Women | | 22 | 5 | 27 |
| | Total | 23 (76.7%) | 7 (23.3%) | 30 |
| Mean age | | 64.10 | | |
| Min. age | | 15 | | |
| Max. age | | 88 | | |

## Methods of Measurement

No satisfactory method exists for measuring the radio-ulnar index, impaction and the different frontal angles. The position of the arm and forearm will modify the results. For example, the relative length of the ulna in relation to that of the radius differs significantly between pronation and supination (Palmer et al. 1982).

Because of this, all our films were taken with the wrist and forearm in the neutral position, i.e. in mid-rotation of the forearm and with the elbow flexed to 90°. This position has been previously defined in the chapter on radiology. We also developed original methods of measuring the palmar and dorsal frontal angles as well as the radio-ulnar index (Sprenger and Sennwald 1985).

### *Measurement of Frontal Angles*

On standard PA films, two frontal angles can be defined on the radius based on three points of reference (Fig. IV.14):
1. the radial styloid,
2. the dorsal-ulnar corner of the radius,
3. the palmar-ulnar corner of the radius.

The dorsal frontal angle is defined by the intersection of the straight line connecting the dorsal-ulnar corner of the radius and the tip of the radial styloid with the perpendicular to the axis of the radius. The palmar frontal angle is defined by the intersection of the straight line drawn between the palmar-ulnar corner of the radius and the radial styloid with the perpendicular to the axis of the radius.

### *Measurement of the Radial Shortening*

The ulna serves as a fixed reference point. A straight line is drawn down its middle; 3 cm proximal to the articular plateau, a perpendicular to this is drawn which crosses the radius. Its intersection with the longitudinal axis of the radius, drawn through its geometric centre, defines the point from which the distance to the palmar or dorsal lip of the radial socket are measured. This measurement is always made on the central line along the longitudinal axis of the radius. Based on the length defined on the sound side, one can measure the degree of shortening at the time of the accident, after reduction and after treatment for 8 weeks. The method of measurement is shown diagramatically in Fig. IV.15.

Table IV.17 supplies all the results found. They are divided into two groups according to treatment, one comprising the 23 patients treated in plaster, and the other, the last 7 patients in the table, who were treated by external fixator. The different means and variances are to be found at the bottom of the table.

## Analysis of Results

### *Conservative Treatment*

*Loss of length.* Fracture of the distal radius presents an average dorsal shortening of 9.40 mm in relation to the norm. Reduction reduces this shortening to only 1.66 mm. Follow-up at 8 weeks shows a definitive residual shortening of 8.09 mm. Between reduction and the follow-up at 8 weeks, the loss of bone length is 6.42 mm for an initial gain of 7.74 mm, i.e. a loss of correction of 82.9%.

On the palmar aspect, although the telescoping of trabeculae is minimal, there is also shortening, amounting to 1.46 mm at 8 weeks. Is this associated with the instability of the epiphysis on its undermined pedestal, or is it an index of true crushing? Instability seems to be the more likely explanation.

*The angles.* Their analysis offers many more difficulties of interpretation. It is a matter of a three-dimensional system where all the points of reference are mobile in relation to each other, the opposite of what was previously the case. Theoretically one would expect the dorsal frontal angle to be altered the most,

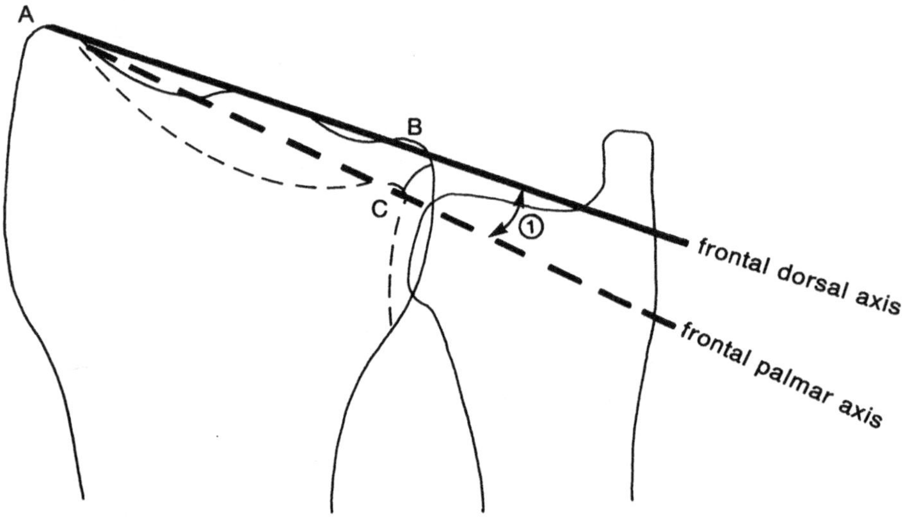


**Fig. IV.14.** Measurement of frontal angles and angular difference between dorsal and palmar frontal angles (see also Fig. II.5b, p. 52)
*1* difference approx. 7°
*A* Radial styloid
*B* Dorsal-ulnar corner
*C* Palmar-ulnar corner

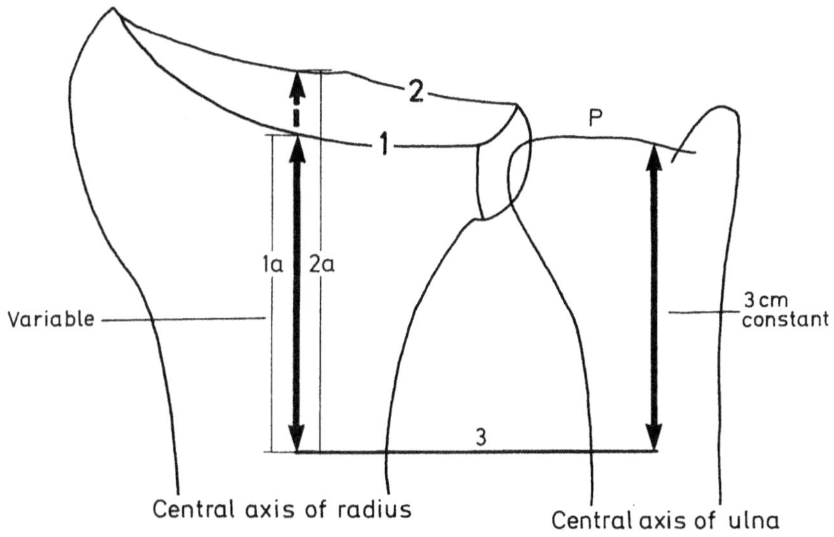


**Fig. IV.15.** Measurement of impaction;
*P* fixed point: the articular plateau of the ulna
*1* palmar lip of the radial glenoid
*2* dorsal lip of the radial glenoid
*1a* reference line for palmar glenoid distance
*2a* reference line for dorsal glenoid distance
*3* line of reference

but in fact, it is the palmar frontal angle. This can be explained as follows:

The radial styloid tilts dorsally along with the dorso-ulnar corner of the radius. These two points move more or less together since the entire dorsal mass is crushed on itself. There is therefore simultaneous translation without much angular modification. The apex of the ulnar-palmar angle remains more or less fixed, and an angular displacement appears between it and the radial styloid. The angle varies as a function of the displacement of the mobile point in relation to the fixed point. This is indicated in reality by a virtually normal dorsal frontal angle on the admission film and a plainly pathological palmar angle (−17°). Thus, we must accept that there is a correlation between the dorsal shortening and the modification of the palmar angle. Statistically, using the *gamma* test previously described, and taking the dorsal shortening and the palmar angular modification as dependent variables, we can confirm our hypothesis with a risk of 1.2% since *gamma* is 0.53 with $Z$ equal to 2.26 (Table IV.18).

It may therefore readily be concluded that:

*Conservative treatment is not suited to the management of fracture of the distal radius. A loss of 80% of the lengthening obtained by reduction is dramatic evidence of this. The dorsal shortening and changes in the palmar frontal angle occur simultaneously.*

## *Treatment by External Fixator*

This will be analysed in relation to conservative treatment (Table IV.19). We postulate, and this hypothesis will remain the same throughout our evaluation, that the fractures, the reduction and

**Table IV.17 a.** Measurement of telescoping (mm)

| Age | | | Dorsal articular margin – reference line | | | | |
|---|---|---|---|---|---|---|---|
| | | | On admission | After reduction | After 8 weeks | Normal | Difference normal – 8 weeks |
| *Conservative treatment* | | | | | | | |
| BH | 63 | F | 31 | 36 | 29 | 39 | 10 |
| BP | 63 | F | 26 | 35.5 | 28 | 35.5 | 7.5 |
| BV | 74 | F | 30.5 | 38.5 | 30 | 39 | 9 |
| CM | 72 | F | 31.5 | 40 | 34 | 39.5 | 5.5 |
| CM | 53 | F | 26.5 | 36 | 30 | 35 | 5 |
| EL | 65 | F | 31 | 31.5 | 27.5 | 38 | 10.5 |
| FH | 66 | F | 30 | 38 | 27 | 39 | 12 |
| FI | 65 | F | 32 | 40 | 29 | 39.5 | 10.5 |
| HW | 63 | F | 33 | 40 | 34 | 40 | 6 |
| KE | 69 | F | 32 | 39.5 | 34 | 37 | 3 |
| KE | 82 | F | 28 | 37 | 31 | 39 | 8 |
| KL | 81 | F | 26 | 27 | 22 | 36 | 14 |
| KB | 82 | F | 29 | 32 | 29 | 34.5 | 5.5 |
| LM | 71 | F | 25 | 39 | 30 | 39 | 9 |
| NM | 15 | ♂ | 35.5 | 42 | 34 | 41 | 7 |
| NH | 73 | F | 26 | 38 | 29 | 35 | 6 |
| PI | 67 | F | 28 | 37 | 30 | 36.5 | 6.5 |
| SE | 61 | F | 29 | 35 | 33 | 38 | 5 |
| SE | 88 | F | 34 | 36 | 32.5 | 38 | 5.5 |
| SH | 64 | F | 30 | 37 | 27 | 37.5 | 10.5 |
| SB | 55 | F | 13 | 33 | 28 | 38 | 10 |
| TI | 78 | F | 24.5 | 30.5 | 27 | 41 | 14 |
| ZJ | 39 | F | 24 | 35 | 31 | 37 | 6 |
| *Treatment by external fixation* | | | | | | | |
| AM | 56 | F | 26 | 35.5 | 31 | 38 | 7 |
| GM | 65 | F | 26 | 35.5 | 36 | 37 | 1 |
| HC | 70 | F | 24 | 35 | 32.5 | 36 | 3.5 |
| LE | 55 | ♂ | 33.5 | 36 | 36.5 | 39.5 | 3 |
| SM | 25 | ♂ | 27 | 40 | 39 | 37 | −2 |
| VE | 66 | F | 30.5 | 36.5 | 36 | 33.5 | −2.5 |
| WB | 77 | F | 28 | 33 | 31 | 36 | 5 |
| *Means* | | | | | | | |
| All cases (30) | | | 28.35 | 36.17 | 30.93 | 37.63 | 6.70 |
| Conservative (23) | | | 28.50 | 36.24 | 29.83 | 37.91 | 8.09 |
| Ext. fix. (7) | | | 27.86 | 35.93 | 34.57 | 36.71 | 2.14 |
| *Variances* | | | | | | | |
| Conservative | | | 20.28 | 12.17 | 8.25 | 3.32 | 8.43 |
| Ext. fix. | | | 8.77 | 3.82 | 8.17 | 2.99 | 10.62 |

**Table IV.17 b.** Measurement of telescoping (mm)

| | Age | | Palmar articular margin – reference line | | | | |
|---|---|---|---|---|---|---|---|
| | | | On admission | After reduction | After 8 weeks | Normal | Difference normal – 8 weeks |
| *Conservative treatment* | | | | | | | |
| BH | 63 | F | 37 | 39 | 34 | 34 | 0 |
| BP | 63 | F | 29 | 32 | 31 | 30 | −1 |
| BV | 74 | F | 34.5 | 35 | 34 | 35 | 1 |
| CM | 72 | F | 35 | 34 | 30 | 35 | 5 |
| CM | 53 | F | 33 | 31 | 26 | 31 | 5 |
| EL | 65 | F | 31 | 34.5 | 33.5 | 33.5 | 0 |
| FH | 66 | F | 35 | 33 | 32 | 33 | 1 |
| FI | 65 | F | 37 | 34 | 30.5 | 34.5 | 4 |
| HW | 63 | F | 37 | 37 | 37 | 35 | −2 |
| KE | 69 | F | 36 | 34 | 30 | 32 | 2 |
| KE | 82 | F | 34 | 34 | 28 | 34 | 6 |
| KL | 81 | F | 33 | 32.5 | 30 | 30 | 0 |
| KB | 82 | F | 34 | 36 | 32 | 29 | −3 |
| LM | 71 | F | 32 | 35 | 33 | 34 | 1 |
| NM | 15 | ♂ | 39 | 39 | 37.5 | 35 | −2.5 |
| NH | 73 | F | 24 | 32 | 35 | 31 | −4 |
| PI | 67 | F | 34.45 | 33 | 32 | 32 | 0 |
| SE | 61 | F | 35 | 32 | 30 | 34 | 4 |
| SE | 88 | F | 30 | 31 | 29.5 | 31 | 1.5 |
| SH | 64 | F | 35 | 32 | 34 | 33 | −1 |
| SB | 55 | F | 19.5 | 30 | 25 | 32 | 7 |
| TI | 78 | F | 30.5 | 33.5 | 33.5 | 35 | 1.5 |
| ZJ | 39 | F | 34 | 33 | 28 | 34 | 6 |
| *Treatment by external fixation* | | | | | | | |
| AM | 56 | F | 34 | 33 | 35 | 33.5 | −1.5 |
| GM | 65 | F | 29.5 | 31.5 | 30.5 | 32 | 1.5 |
| HC | 70 | F | 32 | 30 | 27 | 31.5 | 4.5 |
| LE | 55 | ♂ | 27.5 | 29 | 28 | 34.5 | 6.5 |
| SM | 25 | ♂ | 36 | 36 | 35 | 32 | −3 |
| VE | 66 | F | 34 | 32 | 29 | 30 | 1 |
| WB | 77 | F | 32 | 31 | 29 | 31 | 2 |
| *Means* | | | | | | | |
| All cases (30) | | | 32.80 | 33.30 | 31.30 | 32.72 | 1.42 |
| Conservative (23) | | | 33.00 | 33.76 | 31.54 | 32.91 | 1.37 |
| Ext. fix. (7) | | | 32.14 | 31.79 | 30.50 | 32.07 | 1.57 |
| *Variances* | | | | | | | |
| Conservative | | | 18.08 | 5.19 | 9.54 | 3.32 | 9.07 |
| Ext. fix. | | | 7.19 | 4.42 | 9.07 | 1.96 | 9.10 |

**Table IV.17 c.** Measurement of telescoping, dorsal frontal angle

| | Age | | Angles measured in degrees | | | | |
|---|---|---|---|---|---|---|---|
| | | | On admission | After reduction | After 8 weeks | Normal | Difference normal – 8 weeks |
| *Conservative treatment* | | | | | | | |
| BA | 63 | F | 18 | 31 | 15 | 12 | 3 |
| BP | 63 | F | 13 | 14 | 16 | 11 | 5 |
| BV | 74 | F | 19.5 | 19 | 23 | 19 | 4 |
| CM | 72 | F | 30 | 20 | 17 | 22 | −5 |
| CM | 53 | F | 13 | 12 | 11 | 15 | −4 |
| EL | 65 | F | −18 | 12 | 14 | 18 | −4 |
| FH | 66 | F | 20 | 10 | 21 | 15 | 6 |
| FI | 65 | F | 29 | 20 | 23 | 20 | 3 |
| HW | 63 | F | 23 | 26 | 27 | 19 | 8 |
| KE | 69 | F | 22 | 15 | 15 | 14 | 1 |
| KE | 82 | F | 15 | 17 | 11 | 10 | 1 |
| KL | 81 | F | 15 | 17 | 20 | 12 | 8 |
| KB | 82 | F | 22 | 25 | 27 | 18 | 9 |
| LM | 71 | F | 19 | 12 | 21 | 17 | 4 |
| NM | 15 | ♂ | 18 | 18 | 15 | 16 | −1 |
| NH | 73 | F | 13 | 18 | 19 | 14 | 5 |
| PI | 67 | F | 18 | 18 | 23 | 18 | 5 |
| SE | 61 | F | 15 | 8 | 10 | 15 | −5 |
| SE | 88 | F | 14 | 12 | 12 | 14 | −2 |
| SH | 64 | F | 26 | 16 | 19 | 19 | 0 |
| SB | 55 | F | 4 | 3 | 2 | 17 | −15 |
| TI | 78 | F | 14 | 21.5 | 16 | 21 | −5 |
| ZJ | 39 | F | 12 | 17 | 11 | 19 | −8 |
| *Treatment by external fixation* | | | | | | | |
| AM | 56 | F | 4 | 15 | 21 | 12 | 9 |
| GM | 65 | F | 12 | 21 | 17 | 17 | 0 |
| HC | 70 | F | 23 | 21 | 19 | 18 | 1 |
| LE | 55 | ♂ | 10 | 17 | 12 | 12 | 0 |
| SM | 25 | ♂ | 18 | 25 | 24 | 19 | 5 |
| VE | 66 | F | 21 | 13 | 18 | 18 | 0 |
| WB | 77 | F | 28 | 24 | 28 | 19 | 9 |
| *Means* | | | | | | | |
| All cases (30) | | | 16.35 | 17.25 | 17.50 | 16.33 | 1.23 |
| Conservative (23) | | | 16.28 | 16.59 | 16.80 | 16.30 | 0.57 |
| Ext. fix. (7) | | | 16.57 | 19.43 | 19.86 | 16.43 | 3.43 |
| *Variances* | | | | | | | |
| Conservative | | | 86.41 | 35.75 | 34.20 | 10.12 | 24.08 |
| Ext. fix. | | | 59.39 | 17.67 | 22.69 | 8.24 | 14.45 |

**Table IV.17 d.** Measurement of telescoping, palmar frontal angle

| | Age | | Angles measured in degrees | | | | |
|---|---|---|---|---|---|---|---|
| | | | On admission | After reduction | After 8 weeks | Normal | Difference normal – 8 weeks |
| *Conservative treatment* | | | | | | | |
| BA | 63 | F | 7 | 19 | 8 | 27 | 19 |
| BP | 63 | F | 29 | 17 | 6 | 21 | 15 |
| BV | 74 | F | 13 | 25 | 17 | 27.5 | 10.5 |
| CM | 72 | F | 25 | 32 | 24 | 31 | 7 |
| CM | 53 | F | 7 | 18 | 17 | 24 | 7 |
| EL | 65 | F | −35 | 8 | 9 | 26 | 17 |
| FH | 66 | F | 13 | 21 | 11 | 24 | 13 |
| FI | 65 | F | 23 | 30 | 15 | 29 | 14 |
| HW | 63 | F | 16 | 29 | 21 | 26 | 5 |
| KF | 69 | F | 16 | 30 | 25 | 25 | 0 |
| KE | 82 | F | 10 | 22 | 20 | 22 | 2 |
| KL | 81 | F | 2 | 5 | −1 | 25 | 26 |
| KB | 82 | F | 11 | 19 | 19 | 27 | 8 |
| LM | 71 | F | 6 | 24 | 15 | 23 | 8 |
| NM | 15 | ♂ | 18 | 18 | 15 | 21 | 6 |
| NH | 73 | F | 4 | 28 | 12 | 25 | 13 |
| PI | 67 | F | 13 | 24 | 17 | 17 | 0 |
| SE | 61 | F | −2 | 16 | 18 | 26 | 8 |
| SE | 88 | F | 21 | 19 | 17 | 28 | 11 |
| SH | 64 | F | 16 | 24 | −2 | 23 | 25 |
| SB | 55 | F | −3 | 8 | −13 | 29 | 42 |
| TI | 78 | F | 6 | 17 | 9.5 | 26 | 16.5 |
| ZJ | 39 | F | −7 | 21 | 18 | 22 | 4 |
| *Treatment by external fixation* | | | | | | | |
| AM | 56 | F | −2 | 26 | 10 | 24 | 14 |
| GM | 65 | F | 7 | 27 | 29 | 28 | −1 |
| HC | 70 | F | −4 | 29 | 29 | 26 | −3 |
| LE | 55 | ♂ | 23 | 32 | 28 | 25 | −3 |
| SM | 25 | ♂ | 4 | 30 | 29 | 25 | −4 |
| VE | 66 | F | 14.5 | 15 | 17 | 23.5 | 6.5 |
| WB | 77 | F | 21 | 30 | 32 | 29 | −3 |
| *Means* | | | | | | | |
| All cases (30) | | | 8.12 | 22.10 | 15.72 | 25.17 | 9.45 |
| Conservative (23) | | | 7.83 | 20.61 | 12.93 | 24.98 | 12.04 |
| Ext. fix. (7) | | | 9.07 | 27.00 | 24.86 | 25.79 | 0.93 |
| *Variances* | | | | | | | |
| Conservative | | | 151.45 | 48.59 | 75.83 | 9.53 | 87.50 |
| Ext. fix. | | | 98.46 | 27.43 | 56.41 | 3.56 | 39.46 |

**Table IV.18.** *Gamma* test (see formula and statistical analysis of results in fractures of the radius, p. 125ff.)

Agreements of dorsal shortening and palmar frontal angle

| mm | Degrees | mm | Degrees | mm | Degrees | mm | Degrees |
|---|---|---|---|---|---|---|---|
| 3 | 9 | 7.5 | 6 | 9 | 11 | 12 | 26 |
| 4 | 7 | 7.5 | 7 | 9 | 21 | 12 | 30 |
| 5 | 9 | 8 | 6 | 9 | 28 | 13 | 29 |
| 5.5 | 3 | 8 | 8 | 9.5 | 21 | 14 | 17 |
| 5.5 | 16 | 8 | 20 | 10 | 21 | 16.5 | 20 |
| 6 | 2 | 8.5 | 4 | 10 | 23 | 25 | 32 |
| 7 | 10 | 8.5 | 14.5 | 11 | 12 | | |
| 7 | 61 | 8.5 | 17 | 11 | 21 | | |

*Gamma* = 0.531
300 agreements
92 inversions
392 pairs out of 435 possible pairs
Corresponding $Z = 2.26$
$P = 0.012$ (one-tailed curve)

**Table IV.19.** Comparative efficacy of conservative treatment (23) and external fixation (7)

Shortening:

| | DAM | | PAM | |
|---|---|---|---|---|
| | Cons. | Ext. fix. | Cons. | Ext. fix. |
| Reduction | 7.74 | 8.07 | 0.76 | −0.36 |
| P | −6.41 | −1.36 | −2.22 | −1.29 |
| RS | 1.67 | 0.79 | −0.85 | −0.29 |
| RS 8 | 8.09 | 2.14 | 1.37 | 1.57 |

Shortening given in mm, angles in degrees; Reduction, gain obtained by reduction; P, loss after 8 weeks compared with reduction; RS, residual shortening after reduction; RS 8, final shortening after 8 weeks; DAM, dorsal articular margin; PAM, palmar articular margin; Cons, conservative treatment

Angulation:

| | DAA | | PAA | |
|---|---|---|---|---|
| | Cons. | Ext. fix. | Cons. | Ext. fix. |
| Reduction | 0.30 | 2.28 | 12.78 | 17.93 |
| P | 0.28 | 0.43 | − 7.67 | − 2.14 |
| R | −0.28 | −3.00 | 4.37 | − 1.21 |
| RS 8 | −0.57 | −3.43 | 12.04 | 0.93 |

DAA, articular angle at dorso-ulnar reference point; PAA, articular angle at palmar-ulnar reference point

**Table IV.20.** Student's *t* test for mean of independent samples with unequal variance and normal distribution

Comparison of two observed means where:

$n_a$ = population of a
$s_a^2$ = variance of a
$n_b$ = population of b
$s_b^2$ = variance of b
$X_a$ = observed mean of complement of a
$X_b$ = observed mean of complement of b

Hypothesis: The means of the observed samples are equal.

$$t = \frac{X_a - X_b}{\sqrt{(s_a^2/n_a - 1) + (s_b^2/n_b - 1)}}$$

Measurement of degrees of freedom (*df*):

$$df = \frac{[(s_a^2/n_a - 1) + (s_b^2/n_b - 1)]^2}{(s_a^2/n_a - 1)^2\ (1/n_a = 1) + (s_b^2/n_b - 1)^2\ (1/n_b + 1)} - 2$$

If $n > 30$, the values of $t$ follow the normal law and the standard distribution table can be used. If $n < 30$, the table of $t$ gives the response of the risk probability *alpha* in terms of the number of degrees of freedom (*df*). The values of the means and variances are defined in the table summarizing the measurements

the results of treatment are the same in the two samples considered: the 23 patients treated conservatively, and the seven patients treated by external fixator. We have had to resort to a *t* test allowing comparison of the mean of samples that are independent of one another and of unequal variance, but whose distributions are normal. Tables IV.20 and IV.21 define the test employed and give the details of the results. Statistically, the initial radiological lesions in the seven patients treated by fixator were no different from those of the 23 patients treated in plaster.

The radiological image, i.e. the quality of the reduction, did not significantly differ from one group to another although the fixator did make it possible to obtain a slightly better reduction. This confirms the generally accepted opinion that the reduction of this fracture is not difficult and fosters the misconception that these are easy fractures to treat. The results after 8 weeks are significantly better for the patients treated by external fixator; the initial hypothesis is rejected, with $P > 0.001$ for the shortening and 0.01 for the angles.

*The external fixator significantly improves the quality of the final structural results!*

Of the seven patients treated by external fixator, five had comminuted fractures. Even though the radiological measurements made immediately after reduction of these fractures did not differ significantly from the others, this group has greater

**Table IV.21.** Statistical comparison of conservative treatment and external fixation (*t* test as defined in Table IV.20)

| | Measurement of dorsal shortening | | Measurement of palmar frontal angle | | Conclusion |
|---|---|---|---|---|---|
| | Mean | Variance | Mean | Variance | |
| a) *Primary treatment* | | | | | |
| Conservative | 28.50 | 20.283 | 7.83 | 151.448 | Hypothesis |
| External fixation | 27.86 | 8.765 | 9.07 | 98.459 | confirmed |
| | $t$ (mm) = 0.353, $df = 17$ | | $t$ (angle) = 0.244, $df = 13$ | | |
| Significant at 5% if $t \geq 2.11$ ($df = 17$) or $\geq 2.16$ ($df = 13$) | | | | | |
| b) *Reduction* | | | | | |
| Conservative | 1.67 | 10.861 | 4.37 | 56.048 | Hypothesis |
| External fixation | 0.79 | 6.347 | −1.21 | 21.561 | confirmed |
| | $t$ (mm) = 0.654, $df = 14$ | | $t$ (angle) = 1.85, $df = 18$ | | |
| Significant at 5% if $t \geq 2.145$ ($df = 14$) or $\geq 2.101$ ($df = 18$) | | | | | |
| c) *After 8 weeks* | | | | | |
| Conservative | 8.09 | 8.427 | 12.04 | 87.498 | Hypothesis |
| External fixation | 2.14 | 10.622 | 0.93 | 39.459 | refuted |
| | $t$ (mm) = 4.61, $df = 10$ | | $t$ (angle) = 2.93, $df = 16$ | | |

The hypothesis tested is that the samples are similar as regards the lesion, the reduction and the result:
Sample treated by external fixation ($n = 7$)
Sample treated in plaster ($n = 23$)
Total: 30

According to the tables, the test shows a significant difference at 1‰ for the result obtained for shortening and at 1% for the result obtained for the angles. The two samples do not differ statistically as regards the original lesion; however, the outcome after 8 weeks is statistically different. The efficacy of external fixation is demonstrated

potential for progressive deformation of the fragmented epiphyseal mass. Despite this handicap, the results are statistically better, and our conclusions assume even more validity. However, doubt persists, for restoration is not complete; at 8 weeks there exists an average shortening of 2 mm relative to the opposite side. This is progress, but is it sufficient? Further study will have to determine this.

## Discussion

It is clear that conservative treatment of fractures of the distal radius cannot maintain reduction; or assure a good result, except for those cases in which the deformity on admission does not exceed 5° of tilt and 2 mm of impaction. Once these limits are exceeded, surgical management is required. In this context the external fixator marks definite progress, since it guarantees anatomical reduction to within 2 mm, even in comminuted fractures. However, secondary deformation is possible after removal of the fixator (see Fig. IV.13). Brunner et al. (1985) made similar observations, and proposed that the apparatus be kept in place for at least 8 weeks.

In fact, it is the bony gap that creates the problem, and the object of treatment is to fill it. An initial cancellous bone graft is the logical answer. It makes up for the loss of substance, remodels the articulation if this is deformed, and reduces the period of use of the external fixator. It may even permit plaster fixation alone (maintenance of the fragments and of the reduction being assured by the graft). Obviously, this analysis has taken no account of the associated intra-carpal lesions. Castaing claims that these are rare; we, on the other hand, believe that they are simply not diagnosed. It will not be possible to establish their frequency with certainty until diagnostic radiological techniques are standardized on the anatomical-pathological foundations we have endeavoured to demonstrate.

## References


Brunner R, Regazzoni P, Pfeiffer KM (1985) Distale, intraartikuläre Radiusfrakturen: Indikation für den Fixateur Externe. Annual meeting of the Société Suisse de Chirurgie de la Main, Interlaken, 14.6.85

Castaing J (1964) Les fractures récentes de l'extrémité inférieure du radius. Rev Chir Orthop 50: 581–696

Chamay A (1977) Considérations sur les limites de tolérances du traitement conservateur des fractures du poignet. Ann Chir 31: 340–342

Chamay A, Meythiaz AM, Della Santa D (1983) Le traitement des fractures instables du poignet par fixateur externe de Hoffmann. Etude d'une série de 40 cas. Rev Chir Orthop 69: 637–643

Clancey GJ (1984) Percutaneous Kirschner-wire fixation of Colles fractures. A prospective study of thirty cases. J Bone Joint Surg [Am] 66: 1008–1014

Cooney WP, Linscheid RL, Dobyns JH (1979) External pin fixation for unstable Colles fracture. J Bone Joint Surg [Am] 61: 840–845

Coquoz M (1982) Assemblée annuelle de la section suisse du collège international des chirurgiens (CIC): les fractures de l'extrémité inférieur du radius. Méd Hyg 40: 1550

Fourrier P, Bardy A, Roche G, Cisterne JP, Chambon A (1981) Approche d'une définition du cal vicieux du poignet. Int Orthop (SICOT) 4: 299–305

Frykmann G (1967) Fracture of the distal radius including sequelae, shoulder-hand-finger syndrome, disturbance in the distal radio-ulnar joint and impairment of nerve function. Acta Orthop Scand 108 [Suppl]: 5–143

Karjalainen P, Alhava EM (1977) Bone mineral content of the forearm in a healthy population. Acta Radiol Ther Phys Biol 16: 199–208

Kurtz NR (1983) Introduction to social statistics. McGraw-Hill, New York

Mayfield JK, Johnson RP, Kilcoyne RK (1980) Carpal dislocations: pathomechanics and progressive perilunar instability. J Hand Surg 5: 226–241

Mazess RB, Cameron JR (1973) Bone mineral content in normal U.S whites. In: Intercontinental conference on bone mineral measurement. U.S. Department, Chicago, Illinois, HEW, pp 228–238

Moore WT, Schapiro JR, Jorgensen H, Reid J, Epps CH, Whedon GD (1975) The evaluation of bone density findings in normal populations and osteoporosis. Trans Am Clin Assoc 86:128–138

Palmer AK, Glisson RR, Werner FW (1982) Ulnar variance determination. J Hand Surg 7:376–379

Sennwald G, Segmüller G (1984) De l'attitude du médecin praticien face à la fracture de Pouteau-Colles (fractures distales du radius). Méd Hyg 42:1500–1508

Sprenger FB, Sennwald G (1985) Der Teleskopeffekt der distalen Radiusfraktur. Annual meeting of the Société Suisse de Chirurgie de la Main, Interlaken, 14.6.85

CHAPTER V

# Operative Techniques and Indications

"There are two ways of being ignorant, to have learned nothing or to have forgotten everything, and they are not the same."
G. Cesbron
Un Désespoir Allègre, Laffont, Paris 1983.

### Introduction

It is difficult to deal with this topic; several steps are involved:

- a review of the known techniques,
- an analysis of tested techniques,
- an explanation of the reasons for our choices,
- suggestion of new techniques.

Present knowledge, experience already gained and our concept of carpal stability have allowed us to sketch the main lines of treatment. No doubt, the surgical procedures described will not all resist the test of time; the reader will note our unfavourable opinion of Silastic and our reluctance to use it. Many factors induce us to remain very cautious in this field. In any case, to fill a cavity for fear of a void is rarely a solution.

Here, we present rational bases for treatment. There is always more than one possible solution, but it is important to choose the best for that situation. It is for the surgeon to make this choice on the bases of the problems confronted and of personal temperament. We shall sometimes refer the reader to the examples already presented to indicate the alternatives or to specify the techniques adopted. Our desire is that this work should be a working tool, a base for therapeutic dialogue, rather than a cookbook of recipes; recipes vary too greatly from one country to another, and the dishes produced are not necessarily to one's neighbour's taste.

## A. The Avascular Osteonecroses

### Kienböck's Disease (Avascular Osteonecrosis of the Lunate)

According to Delcoulx, the four stages of avascular osteonecrosis of the lunate are:

Stage I: uniform density, shape preserved
Stage II: bone mottled, shape preserved (Fig. V.1 a)
Stage III: deformation, limited arthrosis (Fig. V.1 b)
Stage IV: deformation, radio-carpal arthrosis

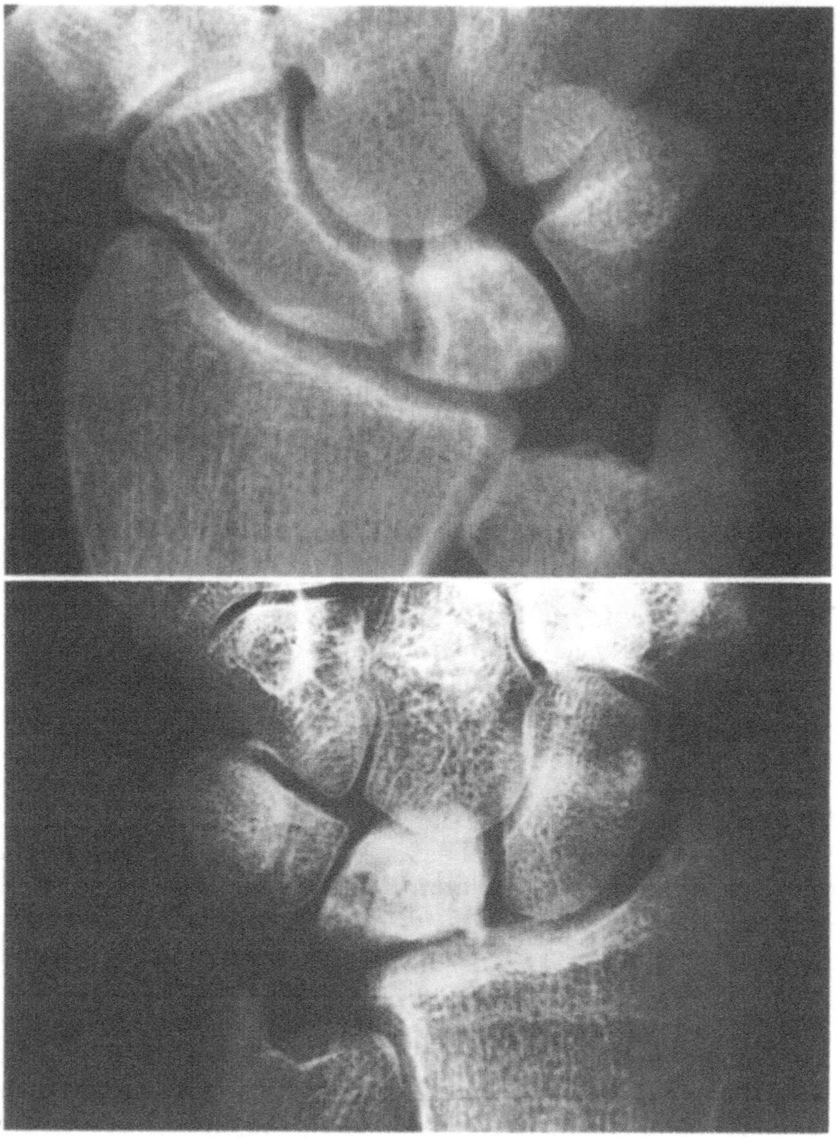

a

b

**Fig. V.1. a** Mottled appearance of lunate, shape retained, Delcoulx's stage II. **b** Lunate deformed, sclerosis of ulnar border of radius and incipient local arthrosis, Delcoulx's stage III

*Suggested Treatments*

These are many, controversial, and often related to the stage of the disease. Conservative treatment (immobilization of the wrist for 2 or 3 months) offers no guarantees (Stähl 1947). Decompression of the carpal tunnel (Codega and Iselin 1967) is also unpredictable. Denervation, a purely symptomatic treatment, in no way modifies the course of the disease and is not a true therapeutic modality.

Simple resection of the lunate creates a mechanical disequilibrium which, in the long term, *must* end in collapse of the carpus. Replacement of the bone by a prosthesis or tendon does not correct the mechanical disorder following resection since neither the prosthesis (Fig. V.2) nor the tendon can compensate the lack of support. Besides, the prosthesis carries the risk of synovitis, more so if not protected from stress, since abrasion may be rapid and extensive.

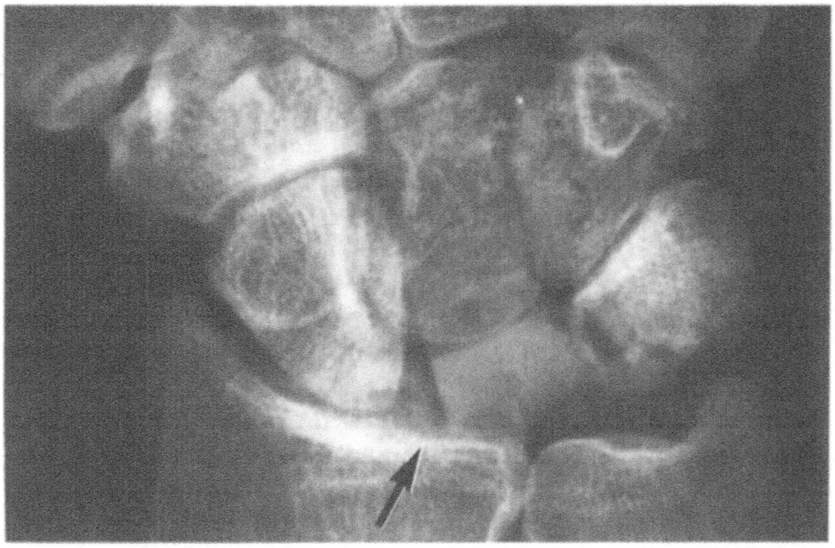

**Fig. V.2.** Proof of inability of Silastic to restore the anatomy: scaphoid vertical, gap between prosthesis and scaphoid, early synovitis

Resection of the proximal row (Clayton 1982; Inglis and Jones 1977; Jorgensen 1969; Steinhäuser 1974) is a mutilating operation, and its results are controversial. The operation of Graner et al. (1966) does not seem physiological; the proximal pole of the capitate is devascularized by the osteotomy with consequent necrosis and deformation.

New methods are now available for study: the vascularized graft (Kühlmann and Guerin-Surville 1980) and scapho-trapezo-trapezoid (STT) arthrodesis (Watson 1982), with or without prosthesis. Radio-lunate arthrodesis, which gives good results in rheumatoid disease, has disappointed us in post-traumatic surgery.

*Author's Personal Choice*

The solution proposed for the disease must be safe, simple and reliably give satisfactory results. It must control the pain, and arrest the collapse and progression of the arthrosis for at least 15 years. We are still satisfied with operations modifying the level of the radius in relation to that of the ulna. Axelson and Moberg (1983), Razemon (1983) and, recently, Kübler and Segmüller (1985) have demonstrated its efficacy, and Kenesi et al. (1973) have supplied mechanical proof of the merits of the method.

*Operative technique of radial shortening.* We prefer to perform shortening of the radius within the cancellous bone using a dorsal approach and stable osteosynthesis, because:

- the cancellous region consolidates rapidly,
- the dorsal route avoids nerve damage,
- stable osteosynthesis permits mobilization as soon as the operative incision is healed,
- the operative technique is simple and rapid.

*Description.* The operative procedure is as follows:

1. For the incision, the reference points (Fig. V.3) are the radial styloid, the head of the ulna, and the muscle bellies of the extensor pollicis brevis and abductor pollicis longus. The incision is centred between the radial styloid and the head of the ulna, and is extended along the muscles.
2. In the subcutaneous plane (Fig. V.4a); exposure of the proximal and distal margins of the extensor retinaculum is performed. Lister's tubercle should be identified. The extensor pollicis longus (Fig. V.4b) passes over the ulnar slope of this tubercle, in the third compartment, which is opened to free the tendon.
3. The tendon and corresponding muscle are elevated; the dorsal interosseous nerve is identified and then resected (Fig. V.5).
4. From the third compartment, Lister's tubercle is removed with a chisel (the blade parallel to the dorsal plane of the radius) and the periosteum and ligamentous substance on the dorsum of the radius is elevated radially and ulnarly (Fig. V.6).
5. The epiphyseal mass is now bare (Fig. V.7). A 2.7 mm or 3.5 mm dynamic compression plate is placed on the mass to plan the level of the osteotomy, and to mark rotation by means of a longitudinal notch (Fig. V.8a, b). We no longer use wires; they are poor markers, and bend or tear out, sometimes injuring the surgeon or the assistant. A longitudinal groove at the osteotomy site ensures alignment of the axes. It remains visible throughout the operation, if placed to one side of the future site of the plate, and long enough not to disappear with the excised disc of bone.
6. The plate and screws are removed, and a disc of bone about 4 mm thick is excised (Fig. V.9a, b). The plate is then reattached to the now free epiphyseal mass, using the previously prepared holes, and this construct is fixed to the shaft with due regard for the correct rotation (Fig. V.10a).
7. Closure of the extensor retinaculum is performed without returning the extensor pollicis longus (EPL) tendon to its compartment (Fig. V.10b). This avoids tendon-plate friction and the risk of bowstringing of the common extensors, the latter never having been exposed. Function of the EPL remains normal despite its new position.
8. The patient leaves the operating theatre with a small palmar plaster splint, which is removed on the 14th day together with the sutures. The hand is then used for activities of daily living, although full stress is not allowed until after 6 weeks.

*Note.* Osteotomy of the distal radius by the dorsal route is done using the same approach and in much the same way (see also p. 234). In fresh comminuted fractures of the radius, it is essential not to open the extensor retinaculum, for this holds the bony fragments together. The plate must be adapted to the patient. We use the 2.7 mm dynamic compression plate in a frail

**Fig. V.4a, b.** Dorsal approach ▷ to distal radius. **a** Definition of extensor retinaculum, identification of Lister's tubercle. **b** Third compartment opened, exposure and release of belly and tendon of extensor pollicis longus (EPL)
*1* Lister's tubercle (radial side)
*2* extensor retinaculum
*3* line of incision (on ulnar side of tubercle)
*4* EPL

**Fig. V.3.** Landmarks:
*1* radial styloid
*2* head of ulna
*3* muscle mass of extensor pollicis brevis and abductor pollicis longus

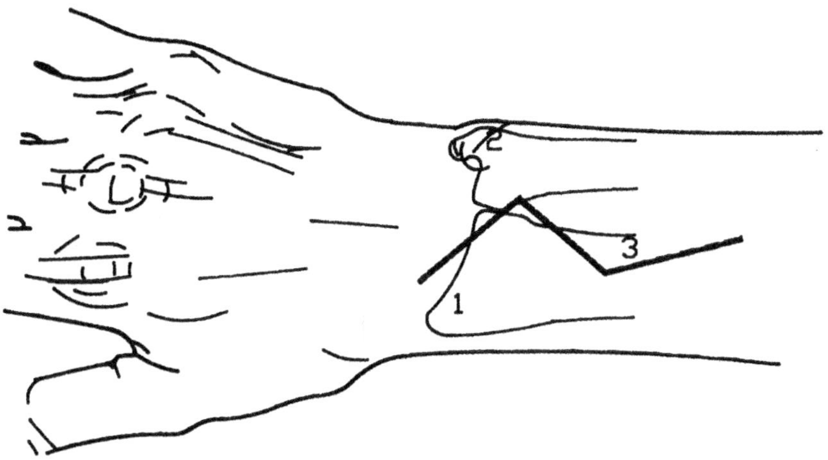


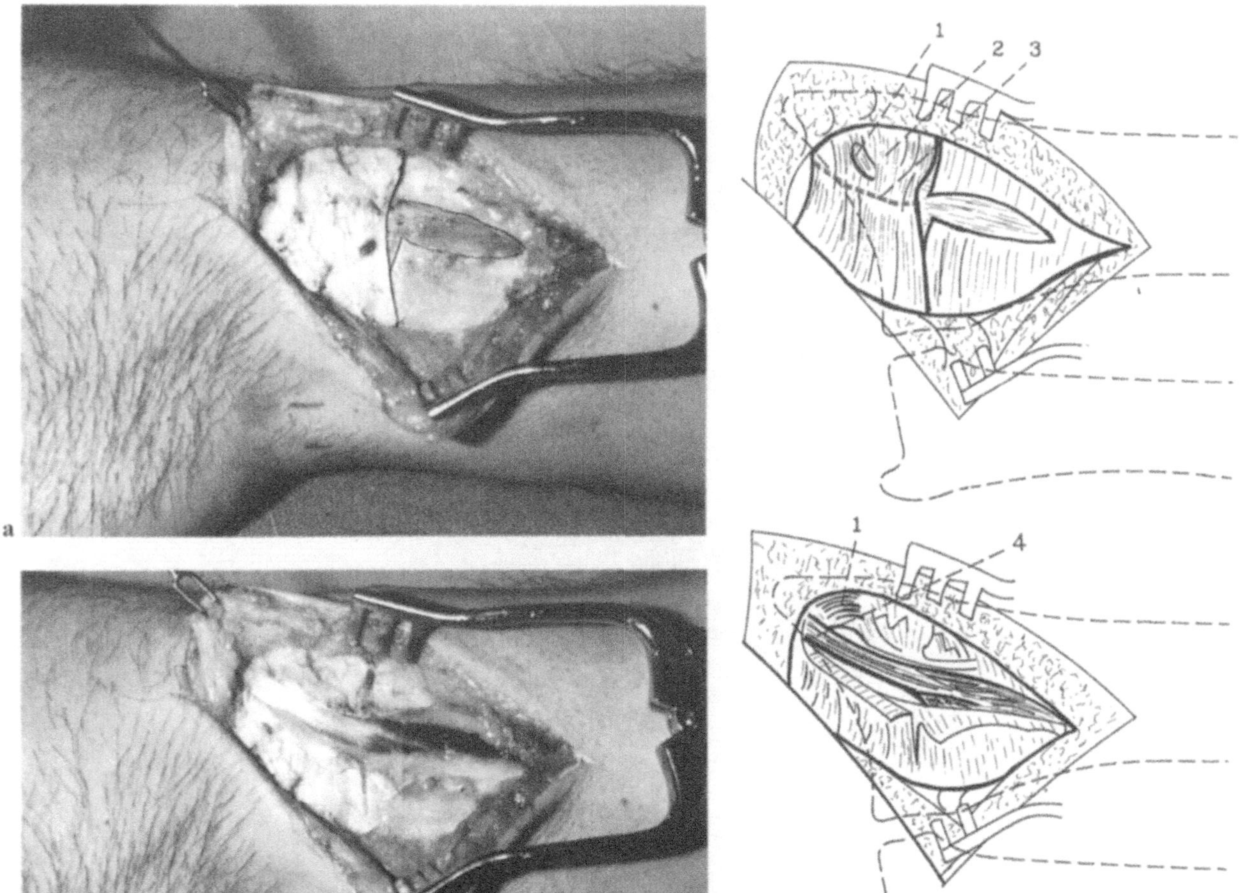

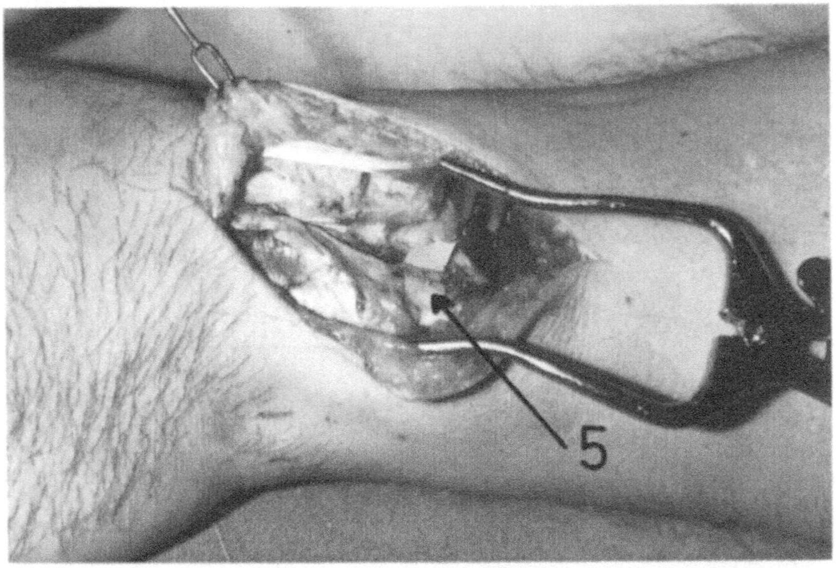


**Fig. V.5.** Display and high resection of dorsal interosseous nerve (*5*)

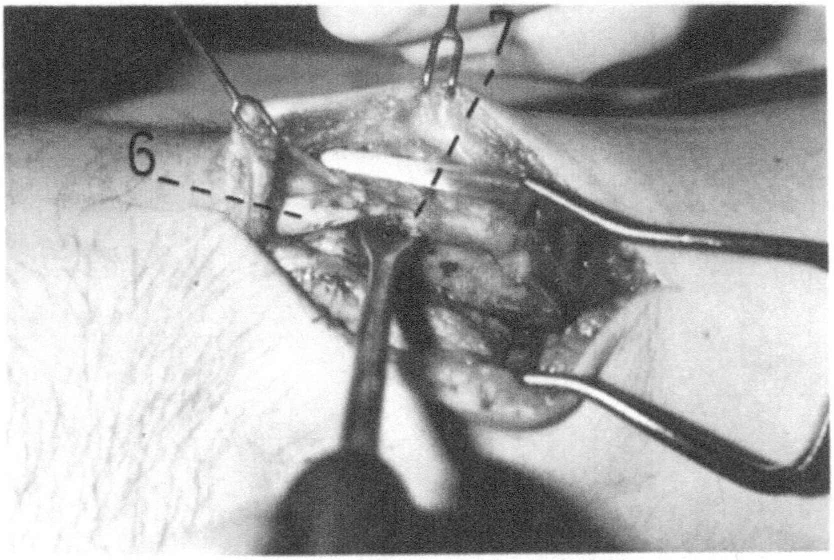


**Fig. V.6.** Decapitation of Lister's tubercle (*7*). Extensor carpi radialis brevis is easily identified.
*6* third compartment opened with extensor pollicis longus visible

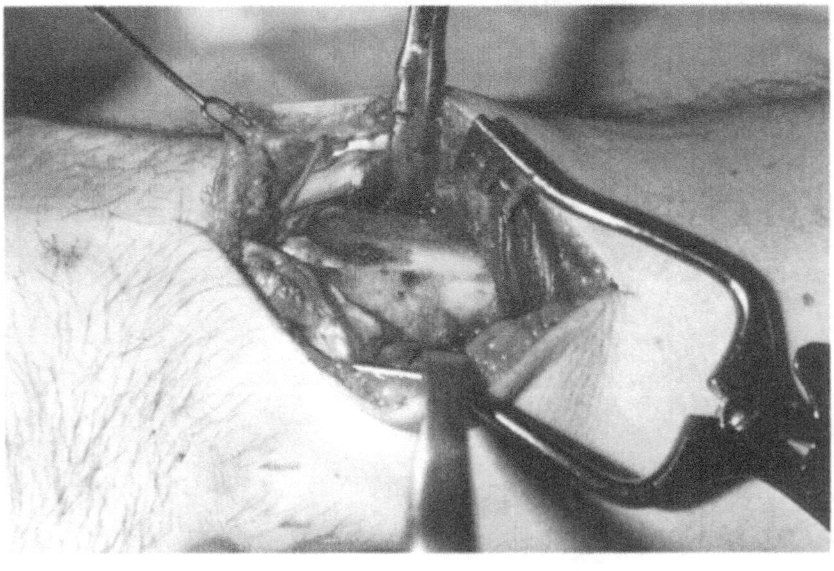

**Fig. V.7.** Epiphyseal segment exposed, introduction of two Hohmann retractors

**Fig. V.8a, b.** Drilling of holes and application of plate to distal epiphyseal segment. **a** Marking of rotation. **b** Diagrammatic lateral view; *red line*, level of osteotomy

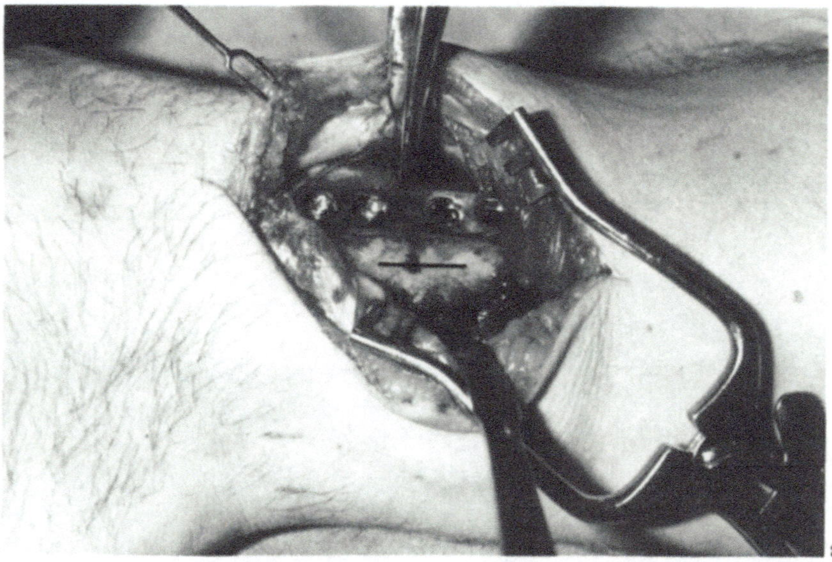

a

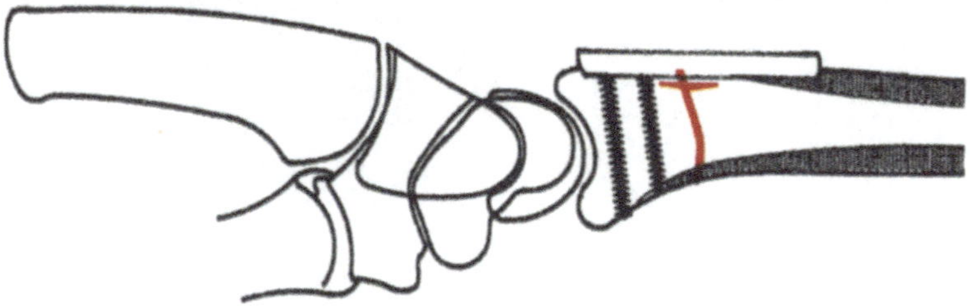

b

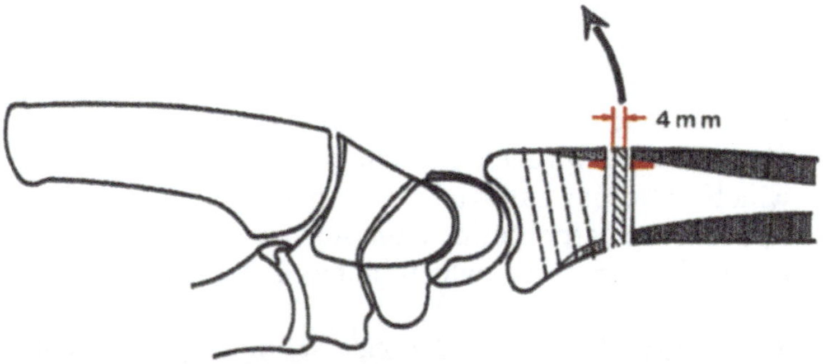


a

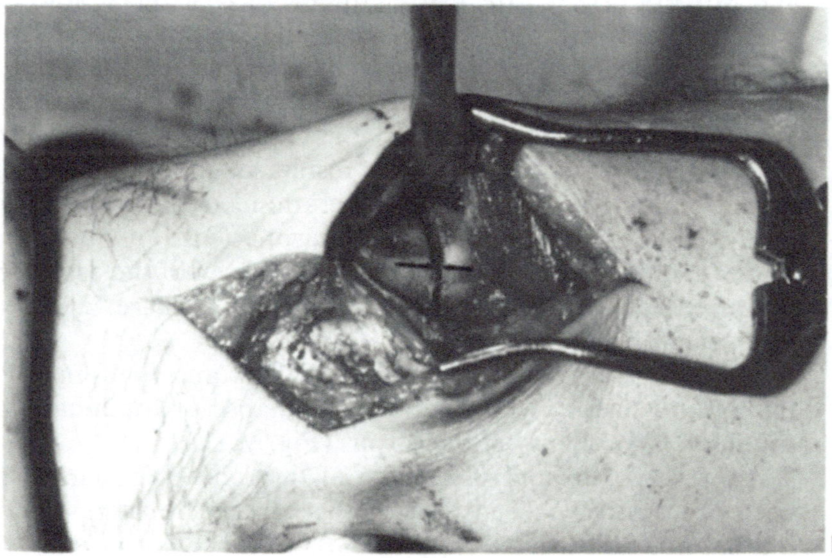

b

**Fig. V.9. a** Excision of a 4 mm disc. **b** Gap visible after excision

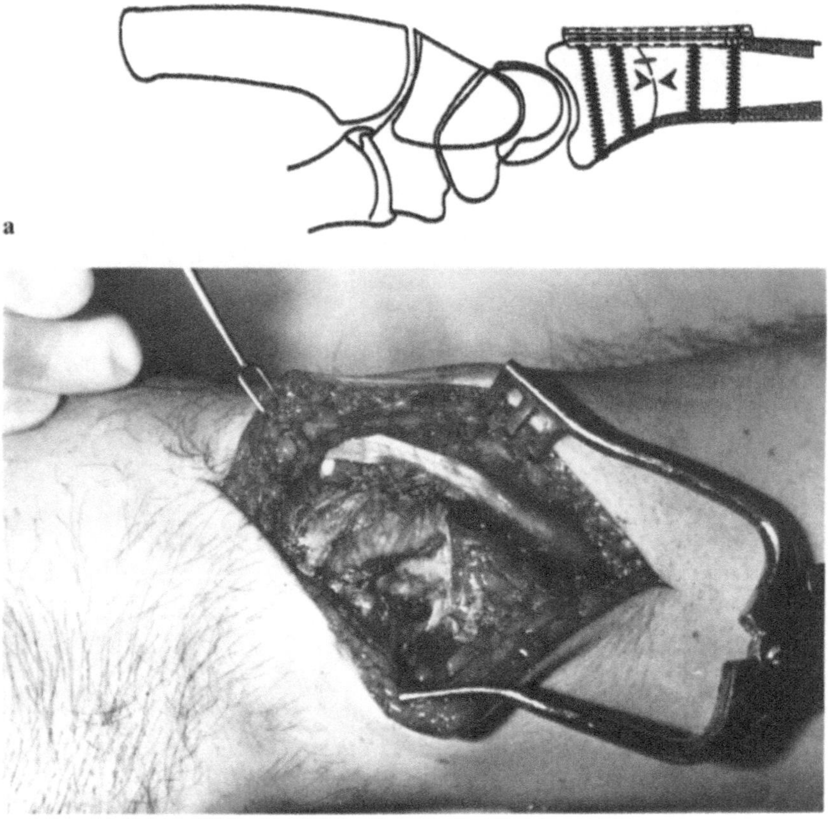

a

b

**Fig. V.10 a, b.** Operation concluded by refixing the plate distally, then proximally; the shortening is easy. **a** Attention to rotation. **b** Closure of third compartment, allowing tendon of extensor pollicis longus to glide freely on retinaculum

woman, but prefer a 3.5 mm AO plate in men (Fig. V.12a, b). The palmar approach is more traumatic and calls for a T-plate, which is somewhat trickier to manage. It sometimes requires opening the carpal tunnel, and may cause direct or indirect injury of the median nerve, which increases the risk of causalgia.

*Discussion.* Nigst (1981, 1982), starting from the work of Axelson and Moberg (1983), stressed the importance of the "radio-carpal" ligament, without exactly specifying the anatomical structures to which this term refers, and emphasized the need to make the osteotomy in the radius very distal. These assertions are counter to the methods and the clinical results of Kenesi, since elongation of the ulna gives results as good as shortening of the radius. We perform the operation on the distal radius (Fig. V.12) for purely anatomical reasons (ease of operation). In our own series, we did not note that the level of the osteotomy produced subjective or objective differences. Figure V.11 illustrates our point.

– The disease was already obvious in 1974, and the films show the natural history with progressive collapse of the lunate and simultaneous collapse of the carpus (Fig. V.11 a).

– After very proximal shortening of the radius, the lunate has been progressively reconstituted; the collapse remains obvious but has not deteriorated (Fig. V.11 b).

**Fig. V.11.** **a** Kienböck's disease: progressive crushing of lunate and collapse of carpus. **b** Progress after shortening of radius in distal third; serial remodelling of lunate, no further collapse. **c** Favourable outcome (disappearance of pain and normalization of function despite a very proximal osteotomy) ▷

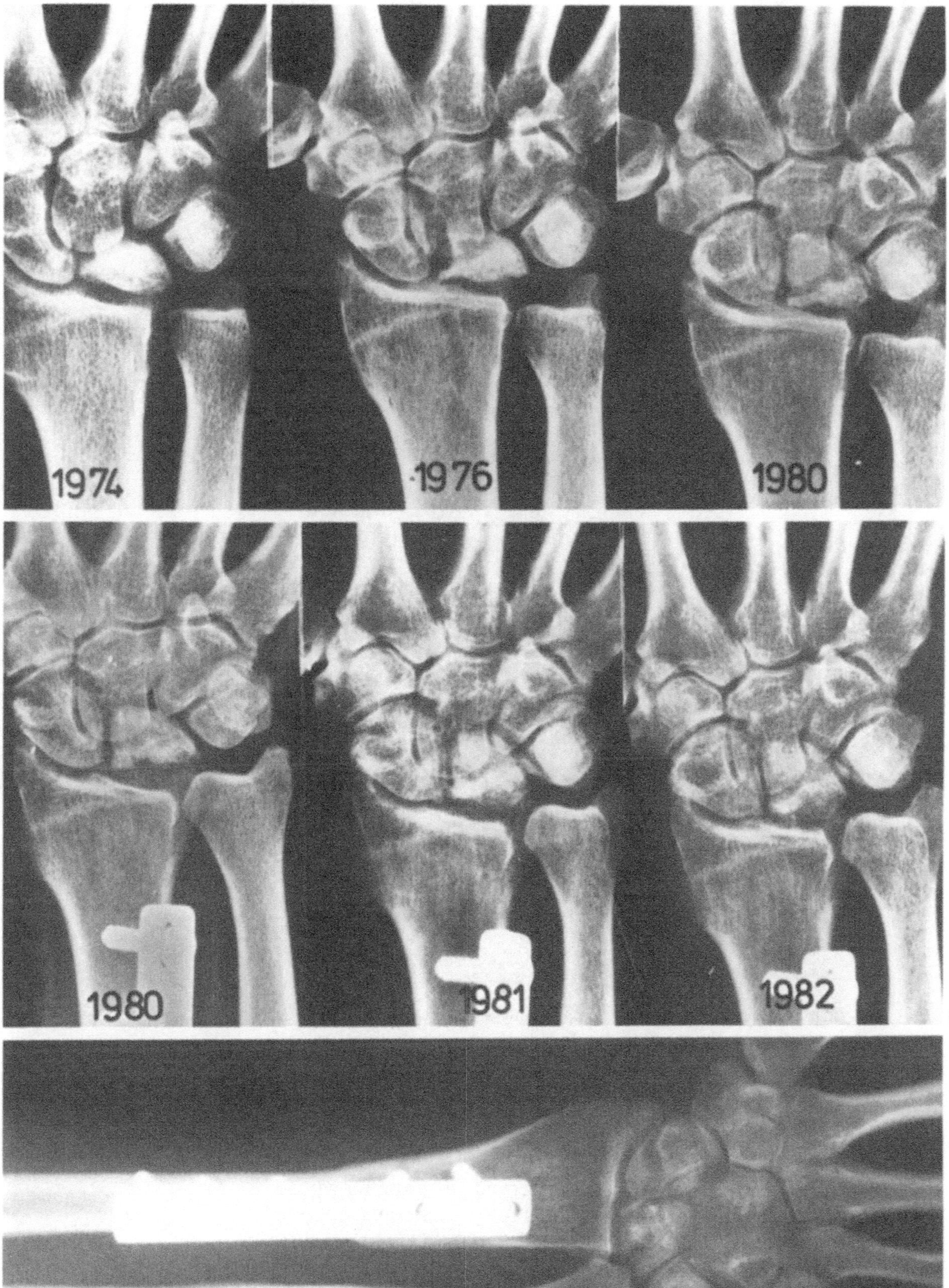

a
b
c

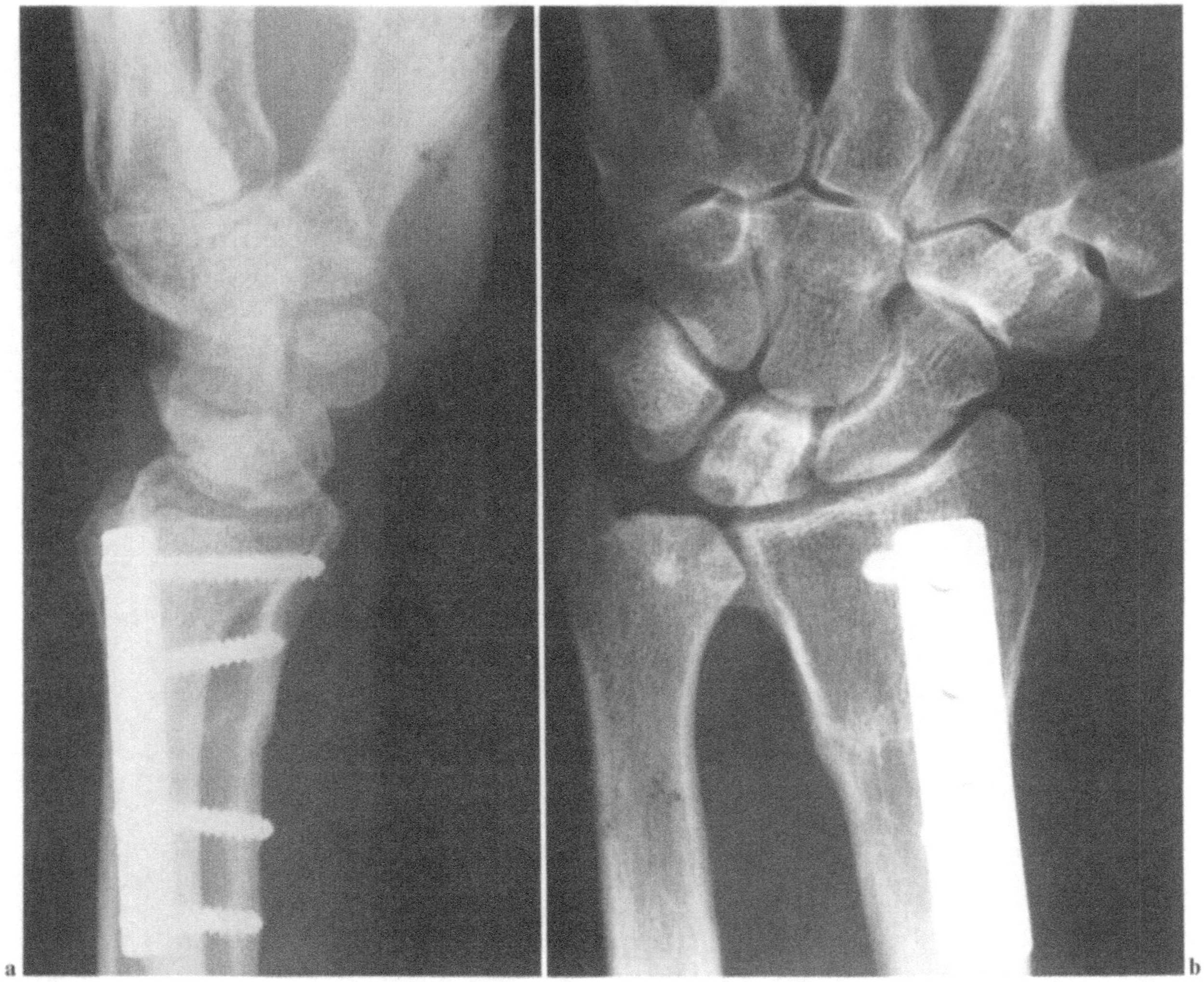

**Fig. V.12 a, b.** Rapid union of osteotomy at cancellous site: PA (**a**) and lateral (**b**) films taken 3 months after shortening

This clinical observation negates Nigst's concept. While this case allows observation of the effects of revascularization of the bone, it raises another problem: the evident persistence of collapse (Fig. V.12).

*Lengthening of the Ulna*

This is not our usual technique; it is reserved for patients whose arms are already relatively short. It calls for a cortico-cancellous graft resistant to pressure (iliac bone), a 3.5 mm AO compression plate and a modern articulated tension device. This device has a double function; in the first stage of the operation it permits the desired lengthening, and in the second it compresses the interposed fragment and creates a perfectly stable assembly.

*Technique*

Figure V.13 illustrates this technique, which involves the following stages:

1. For access, the ulnar crest, situated between the extensor carpi ulnaris and the flexor carpi ulnaris, is easily palpable. The incision is the length of the plate to be employed (6 or 7 holes) plus a quarter, this quarter being the room required for use of the tightener.
2. The bone is exposed and the level of osteotomy is chosen, marking rotation with a groove (Fig. V.13a). Choice of placement of the plate and its adaptation to the shape of the bone with platebenders is made, though minimal shaping of the plate is necessary if it is applied on the ulnar-palmar surface.
3. The plate is applied distally, and fixed with at least two screws. At the proximal end of the plate, the tension device is applied with due regard for its useful excursion. Fixation is in the axis of the plate (Fig. V.13b).
4. Removal of the osteosynthesis material is performed, with osteotomy exactly at right angles to the axis of the bone (Fig. V.13c).
5. The plate is re-fixed distally. The tension device, used as a distractor, is opened to the desired elongation (average +7 mm, Fig. V.13d), followed by placement of a graft corresponding in size to the calculated lengthening, then reversal of the position of the tension device hook and application of 60–70 kg compression (Fig. V.13e). Insertion of screws is performed with a neutral guide-drill, beginning with the hole nearest the osteotomy.
6. A check of pronation-supination is carried out, possibly with intra-operative X-ray. After wound closure, a small plaster splint is applied until the removal of sutures, when the hand may be used for everyday activities, with progressive loading after 6 weeks.

*Other Techniques*

*Z-lengthening of the ulna* is a difficult technique, which we do not recommend.

*Hemi-epiphyseal lengthening,* as described by Comtet et al. (1981), seems an interesting technique. It is done in a well-vascularized zone, and does not alter the level of the ulnar styloid, but it does carry a risk of fracture above the osteotomy, and is tricky to perform (Fig. V.14). Moreover, opening the distal radio-ulnar joint is unavoidable, which is why we do not utilize this method.

*STT arthrodesis,* as proposed by Watson (1982), has the same aim as lengthening of the ulna, i.e. to de-stress the lunate. However, there is a trade-off, the unloading is performed at the expense of the scaphoid and the radial compartment, which is already burdened by the collapse. After this operation all the

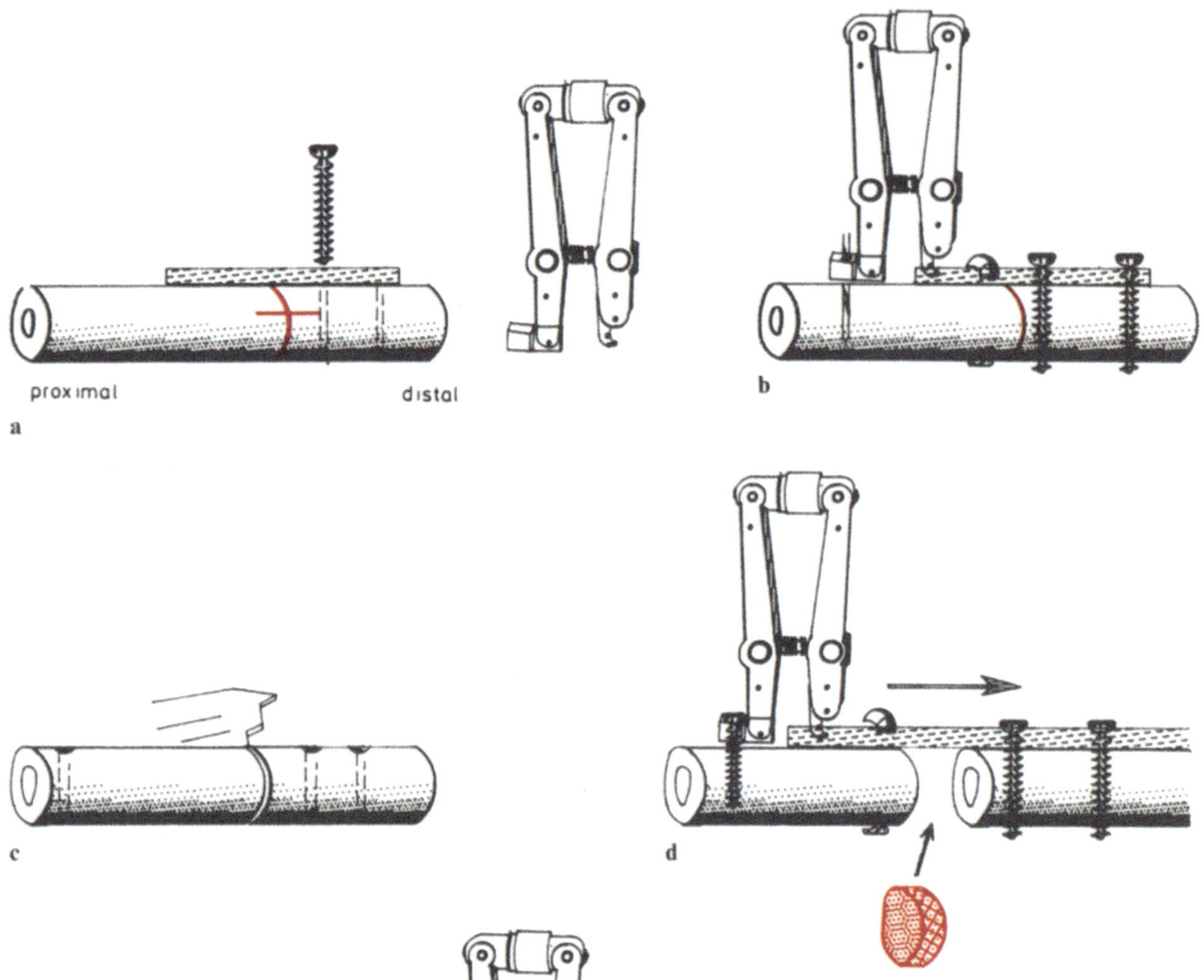


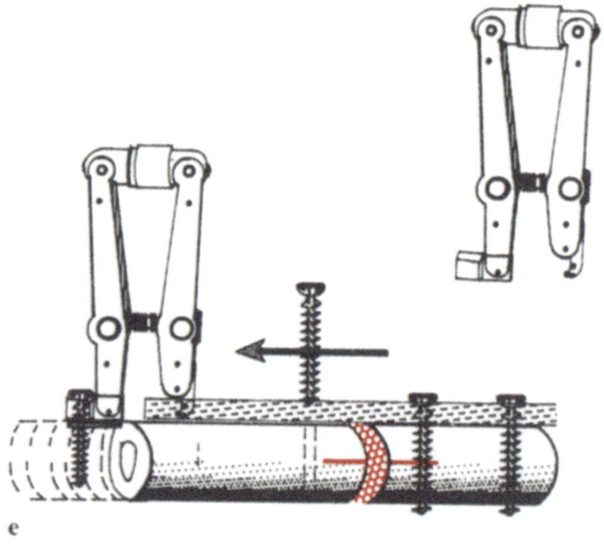


**Fig. V.13a–e.** Technique of lengthening of the ulna. **a** Marking of osteotomy site (in *red*); rotation guided by a *red horizontal line* on either side of the *vertical osteotomy line*; provisional fixation of plate distally. **b** Choice of placement of plate, application of distractor (in axis of plate). **c** Removal of osteosynthesis material. The osteotomy is perpendicular to the axis of the bone. **d** Definitive fixation of plate and alteration of shape if necessary, placing of tension device, sliding of plate onto bone controlled with forceps, lengthening by 5–7 mm, insertion of graft into space created. **e** Reversal of position of hook of tension device, application of 60–70 kg compression, fixation of screws beginning with the one nearest the osteotomy

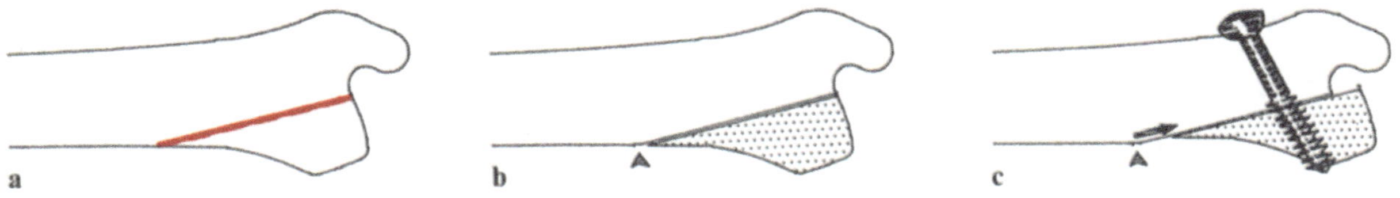


**Fig. V.14a–c.** Comtet's method of hemi-epiphyseal lengthening

load passes through the scaphoid and the radial styloid. For these mechanical reasons we do not use this fusion in Kienböck's disease. Techniques of measurement like those of Kenesi are also needed to understand the true effects of this novel technique.

*Conclusions*

The last word remains to be said on the treatment of avascular necrosis of the lunate. It seems logical to envisage the future combination of an old and tested method with a new and very promising method: perhaps the combination of radial shortening with a vascularized graft. The shortening would give the mechanical guarantees and the vascularization would ensure rapidity of healing and possible remodelling of the collapsed lunate.

## Avascular Necrosis of the Scaphoid

According to Häuptli (1954), this disorder was first recognized by Preiser in 1910, hence it is also known as Preiser's disease. It is a rare condition, and one we have not yet encountered in our department. Nigst (1982) reported only one case.

*Aetiology*

This is still unknown.

*Treatment*

This is difficult. Nigst suggests a scaphoid prosthesis. In our view, a pedicled graft, as described by Kühlmann, ought to be tried in every case before resorting to solutions as radical and irreversible as prosthetic replacement or resection of the proximal row of the carpus. On several occasions we have prepared a graft of this type. The artery is not easy to preserve, and even when one has succeeded the graft must not be devascularized. Finally, the pedicle must be of sufficient length. We have had valuable success with this procedure. One certainty is the constancy of this palmar carpal arterial branch, which was found whenever we sought it.

*Conclusion*

The rarity of this disorder and the long wait required for final assessment of the results leaves us unsure of the correct approach. However, progress in microsurgery gives hope of a rational and satisfactory solution.

## References


Axelson R, Moberg E (1983) Le traitement de la maladie de Kienböck et le rôle des interventions de rééquilibration radio-cubitale. In: Razemon JP, Fisk GR (eds) Le poignet. Expansion Scientifique Française, Paris, pp 210–217

Clayton ML (1982) The caput ulnae syndrome: update. In: Strickland JW, Steichen JB (eds) Difficult problems in hand surgery. Mosby, St Louis Toronto London

Codega G, Iselin M (1967) Thérapeutique de la maladie de Kienböck. Mém Acad Chir 703–706

Comtet JJ, Moyen B, Machenaud A (1981) Allongement du cubitus et raccourcissement du radius dans le traitement de la maladie de Kienböck. In: Simon L, Allieu Y (eds) Poignet et médecine de rééducation. Masson, Paris, pp 150–155

Delcoulx P, Marchand M, Minet P, Razemon JP (1957) La maladie de Kienböck chez le mineur. Lille Chir 12:65–81

Graner O, Lopes EI, Carvalho BC, Atlas S (1966) Arthrodesis of the carpal bones in the treatment of Kienböck's disease, painful ununited fractures of the navicular and lunate bones with avascular necrosis and old fracture-dislocations of carpal bones. J Bone Joint Surg [Am] 48:767–774

Häuptli O (1954) Die aseptischen Chondro-Osteonekrosen. De Gruyter, Berlin, pp 95–101

Inglis AE, Jones EC (1977) Proximal row-carpectomy. J Bone Joint Surg [Am] 59:460–463

Jorgensen ED (1969) Proximal row carpectomy. An end result study of twenty-two cases. J Bone Joint Surg [Am] 51:104–111

Kenesi C, Gastambide D, Lesage JP (1973) Le syndrome de Kienboeck, étude biomécanique. Rev Chir Orthop [suppl 1] 59:126–131

Kübler JU, Segmüller G (1985) Niveau-Operation bei Lunatum-Malazie. 72nd annual meeting of the Société suisse de médecine des accidents et des maladies professionnelles and the Société suisse de chirurgie de la main. Interlaken, 14 June 1985

Kühlmann JN, Guerin-Surville H (1980) Greffon osseux pédiculé sur l'artère transverse du carpe (ramus carpeus palmaris) Bull Assoc Anat 64:243–252

Nigst H (1982) Aseptische Nekrosen der Karpalknochen. In: Buck-Gramcko D, Nigst H (eds) Frakturen, Luxationen und Dissoziationen der Karpalknochen. Hippokrates, Stuttgart, pp 133–138

Nigst H (1981) Erkrankungen der Knochen. In: Nigst H, Buck-Gramcko D, Millesi H (eds) Handchirurgie, vol I. Thieme, Stuttgart, pp 19.24–19.25

Razemon JP (1983) La maladie de Kienböck. Etude radiologique et thérapeutique à propos de 22 cas de raccourcissement du radius. In: Razemon JP, Fisk GR (eds) Le poignet. Expansion Scientifique Française, Paris, pp 204–209

Stähl F (1947) On lunatomalacia (Kienböcks disease). A clinical and röntgenological study, especially on its pathogenesis and the late results of immobilization treatment. Acta Chir Scand 95 [suppl] 126

Steinhäuser J (1974) Langzeitergebnisse mit der transnaviculolunaeren Resektionsarthroplastik (Steinhäuser-Operation) bei fortgeschrittener Mondbeinnekrose. Arch Orthop Unfallchir 78:237–247

Watson HK (1982) Limited wrist arthrodesis. In: Strickland JW, Steichen JB (eds) Difficult problems in hand surgery. Mosby, St Louis, p 337

## B. Pseudarthrosis of the Scaphoid

### Introduction

Pseudarthrosis of the scaphoid may be stable or unstable. Instability can be:

1. Ligamentous, due to inadequacy of the strap ligament (proximal V)
2. Bony, due to lack of bulk and/or angulation
3. Combined, with associated bony and ligamentous problems.

Treatment is determined by the type of pseudarthrosis and technical considerations. We shall consider, in order: the inset cortico-cancellous graft, with and without Kirschner wiring, and with and without ligamentoplasty; and the sandwich operation.

### Treatment by Inset Cortico-Cancellous Graft

*Pseudarthrosis Without Ligamentous Instability*

*Surgical approaches.* The various radio-palmar approaches are shown in Fig. V.15. For the Matti-Russe procedure, we use the incision of Fig. V.15a:

1. The landmarks are the flexor carpi radialis and the tubercle of the scaphoid.
2. A zig-zag incision gives excellent exposure and identification, but there is a risk of skin damage due to devascularization, and of damage to branches of the radial and musculocutaneous nerves and the palmar branch of the median nerve.
3. The superficial aponeurosis is displayed (Fig. V.16), and then divided longitudinally between the sheath of the flexor carpi radialis and the neurovascular bundle (the classical penetration through the tendon sheath is often easier and sometimes unavoidable).
4. The pronator quadratus (Fig. V.17) and the distal edge of the radius are exposed; as is the proximal V ligament, which is incised longitudinally.

*Note.* It is important to clearly identify the cut ligaments, so that they may be carefully sutured after the operation; otherwise there is a risk of secondary ligamentous instability (Fig. V.18). Also, the proximal pole of the scaphoid or the lunate should not be exposed as there is a risk of damaging the radio-scaphoid ligament and its vessels, and hence of necrosis.

*Operative procedure.* The pseudarthrosis is localized and analysed with the wrist in hyperextension. Bone stability is assessed by ulnar and radial deviation. The choice of procedure depends on the degree of stability.

*Good stability.* There is virtually no detectable movement at the site of the pseudarthrosis.

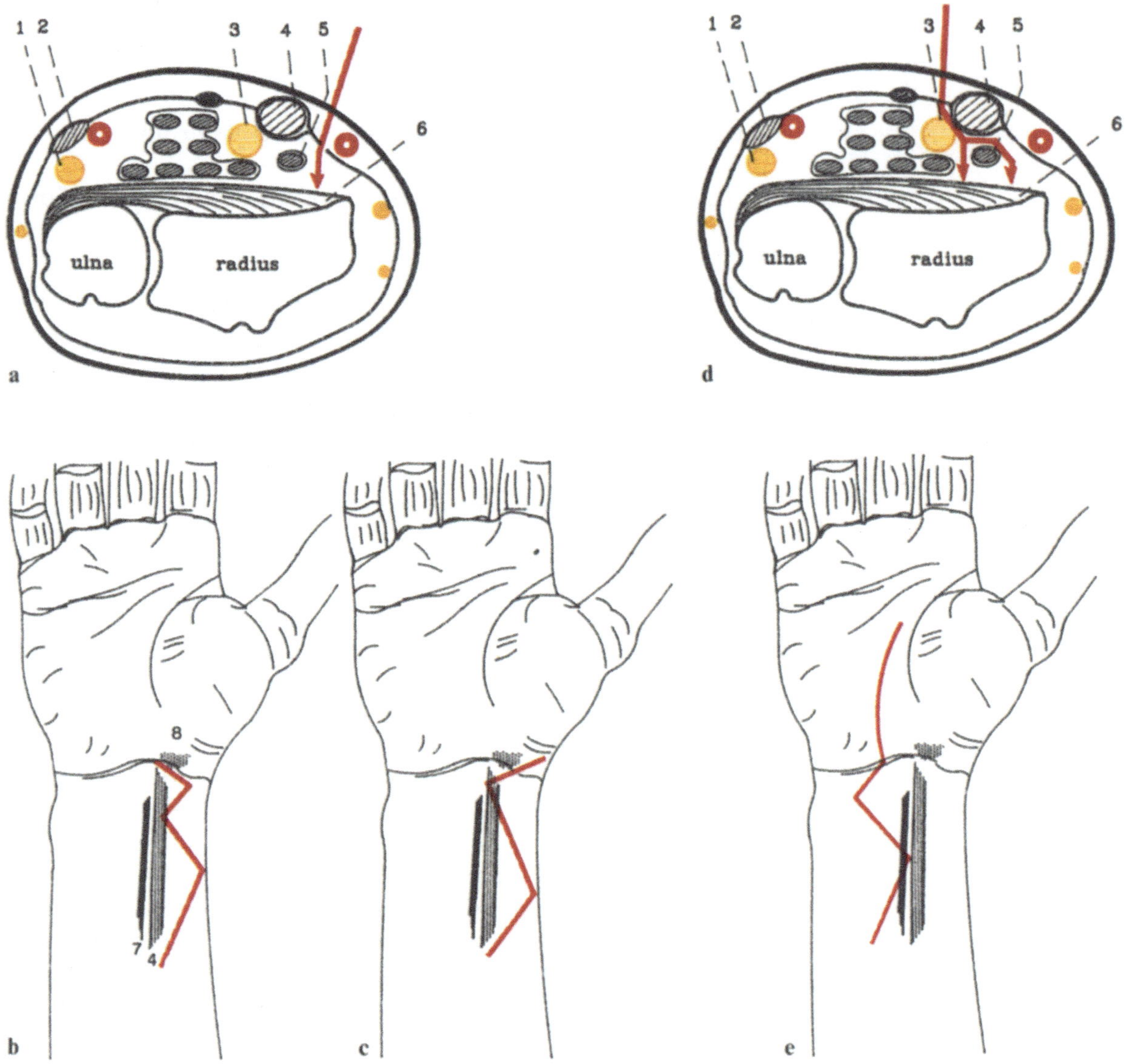


**Fig. V.15a–e.** Palmar incisions. **a** Dissection between flexor carpi radialis (FCR) and radial artery. **b** Classical Matti-Russe (MR) approach. Three landmarks are used: FCR (*4*), palmaris longus (*7*) and tuberosity of scaphoid (*8*). **c** Extended palmar approach for sandwich operation: penetration in depth similar to that of MR, but incision extended along the radial border of the scaphoid tuberosity; this approach is used for vascularized grafts and corrective radial osteotomy by palmar approach. **d–e** Dissection between FCR and median nerve with a view to achieving a vascularized graft, corrective radial osteotomy or ligamentoplasty of the carpus by the palmar route

*1* ulnar nerve
*2* flexor carpi ulnaris (FCU)
*3* median nerve
*4* FCR
*5* flexor pollicis longus
*6* pronator quadratus
*7* palmaris longus
*8* scaphoid tuberosity

**Fig. V.16 a, b.** The superficial aponeurosis stretches between the radial artery and the FCR. The coagulation of perforators is necessary.
*1* FCR
*2* radial artery
*3* site of scaphoid tuberosity
*4* aponeurosis

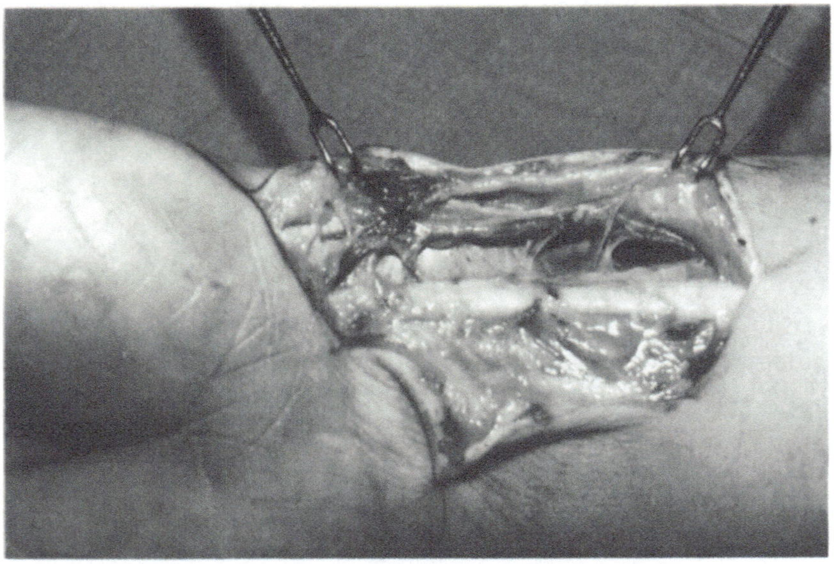

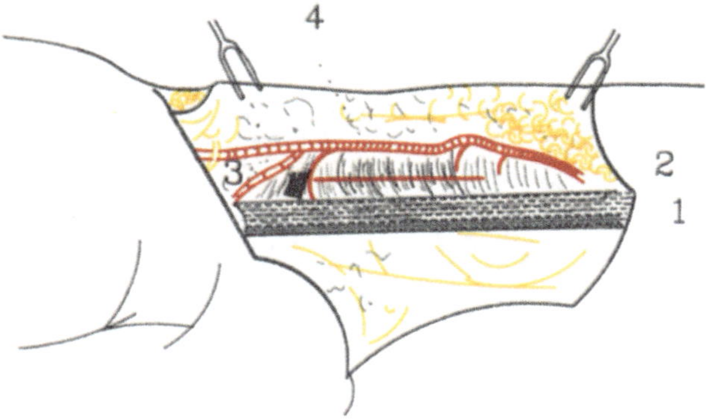


*Procedure.* A mortice is dug, first using a bone chisel and then a curette or a mini-drill (Fig. V.19 a) and a cortico-cancellous graft is countersunk (Fig. V.19 b).

*Note.* In these cases, simple cancellous grafting is sufficient, as the aim of the operation is to encourage revascularization and not stability, which is not compromised.

*Doubtful stability.* There is definite movement of the fragments on one another, but a cartilaginous bridge is still present.

*Procedure.* A mortice is dug as in the previous case, the use of a cortico-cancellous graft is essential, as the cortex is required for stability (Fig. V.20). The graft is removed from the metaphyseal region of the radius, under the pronator quadratus, with the aid of an oscillating saw; with a chisel, the risks of impaction are significant.

Although the radial cortex is of good quality, its spongy bone is loose and compressible, and the graft must be embedded without pressure on the radial spongiosa; additional cancellous chips will wedge the graft in place. If necessary, they can be

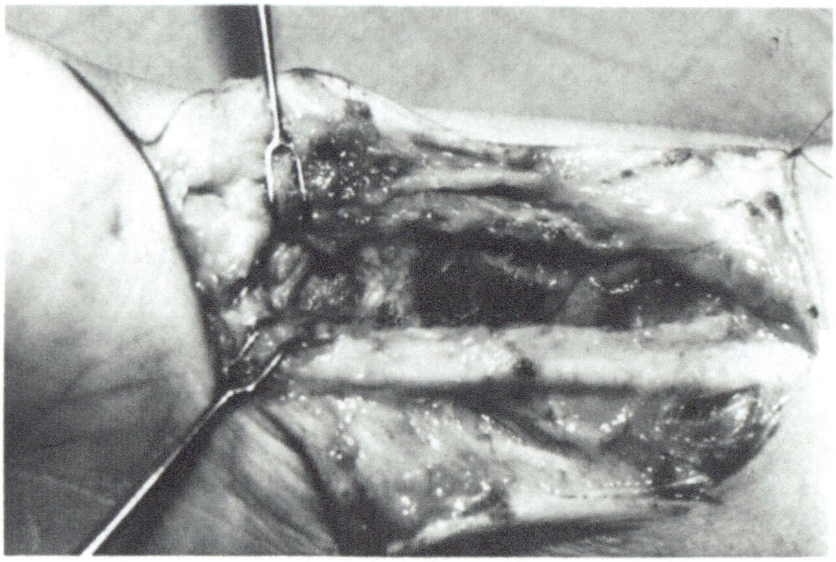

**Fig. V.17.** The aponeurosis has been incised, allowing identification of pronator quadratus, distal edge of radius and attachment of proximal V ligaments. The *longitudinal red* line shows incision of V ligaments.
*1* FCR
*2* flexor pollicis longus (FPL)
*3* radial artery
*4* radial nerve
*5* scaphoid
*6* pronator quadratus
*7* proximal and distal V ligaments

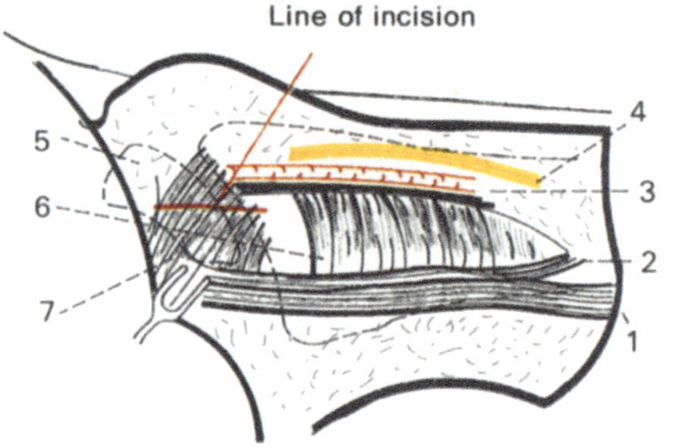


**Fig. V.18.** Inspection of hyperextended wrist, with carpal ligaments drawn apart, to localize pseudarthrosis and assess stability.
*1* scaphoid
*2* radius
*3* loss of bone substance

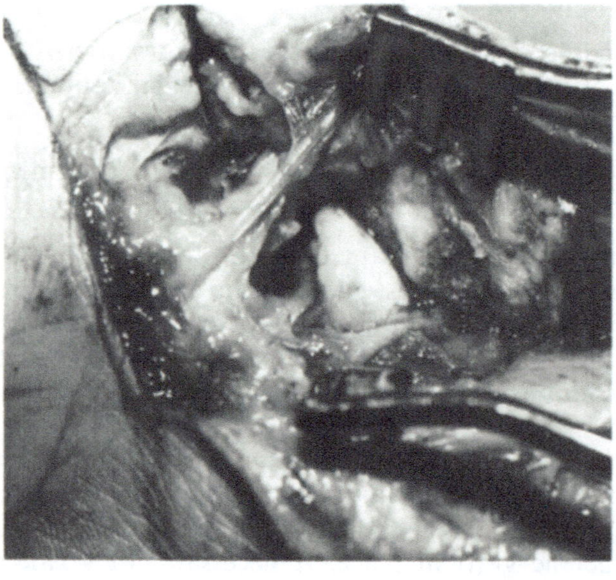

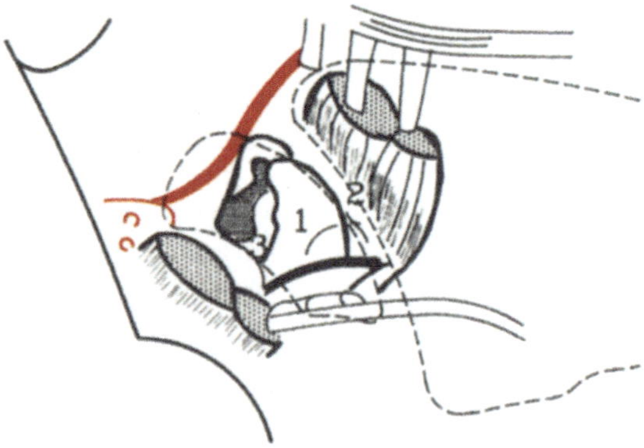

held at the surface by tissue glue. It seems unimportant whether the cortex is superficial or deep, its role being to stabilize the reduction of the fragments.

*Marked instability.* The two fragments are independent and very mobile with respect to each other; angulation is obvious, but can be corrected.

*Procedure.* The proximal and distal surfaces of the pseudarthrosis are freshened. The graft is shaped in the form of a wedge, as advised by Fernandez (1984), in such a way as to correct the axis of the scaphoid. Stabilization is obtained by one or two Kirschner wires, either within or alongside the bone; they replace or supplement the plugging of the graft in the mortice we have just described.

The example in Fig. V.21 shows the possibilities of correction by the bone-graft alone. Reduction is not perfect but seems ac-

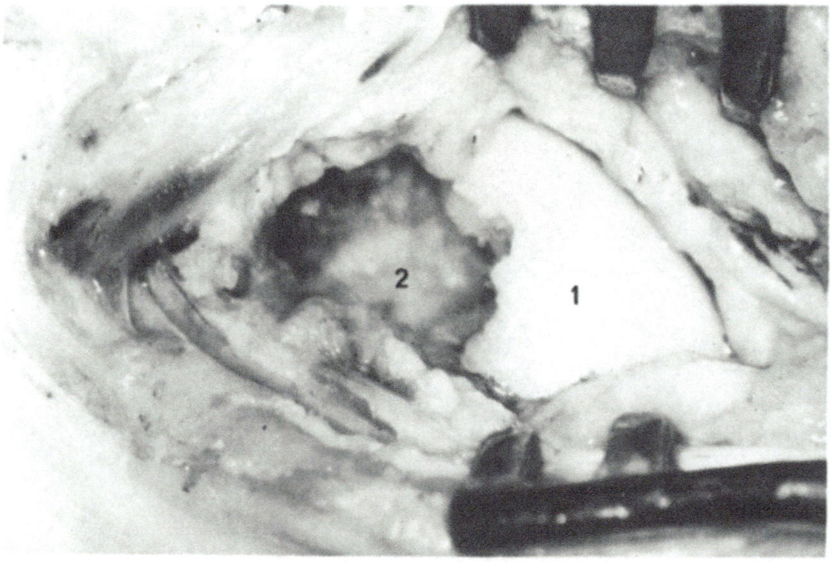


a[1]

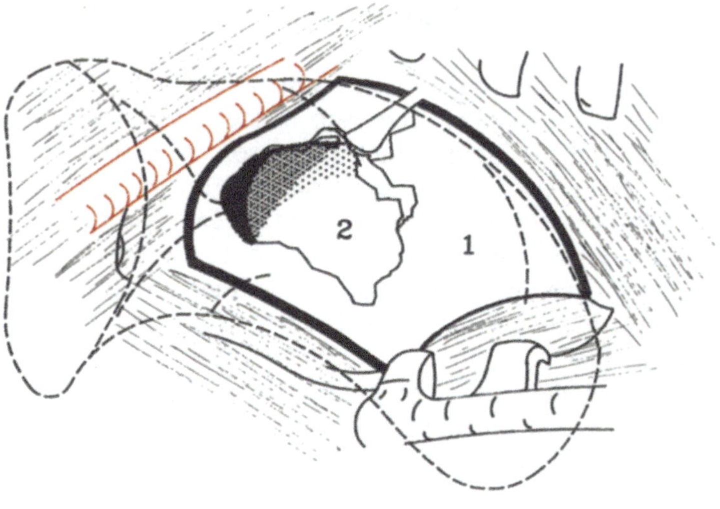


a[2]

**Fig. V.19. a** Creation of mortice to embed graft
*1* scaphoid
*2* mortice

**Fig. V.19b** see p. 174

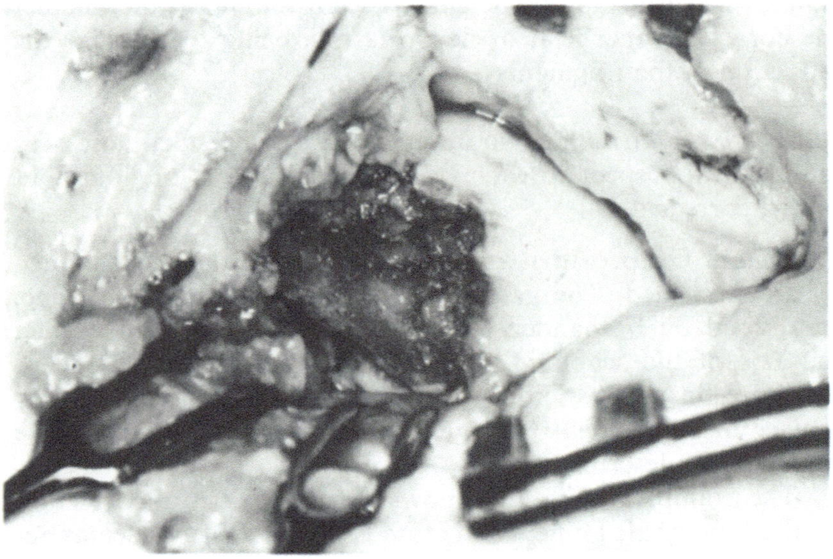

b[1]

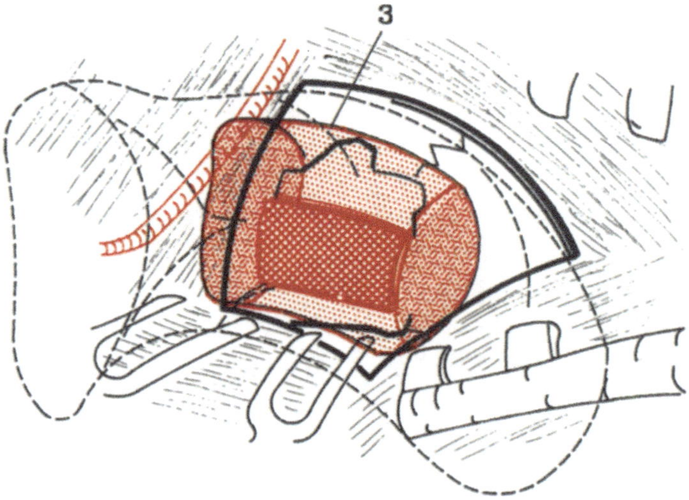


b[2]

**Fig. V.19. b** embedded graft
*3* graft in place

ceptable, as the lunate is in the neutral position. Union is present by the 11th week (Fig. V.21d).

*Note.* Insertion of the wires is difficult, and it may be helpful to introduce them via the first web space. They then fix the trapezium to the scaphoid, which increases the stability of the set-up. As far as possible, penetration into the radius must be avoided, for there is a risk of the wire fracturing, and movements of the radio-carpal joint are transmitted to the graft. In our opinion, driving the wires into the radius does not aid stability; on the contrary, it increases the observed frequency of translation movements.

Small fragments cannot be excavated, so stabilization often requires one or two para-osseous wires. An intra-osseous wire can provoke a tilt or inopportune displacement of the small proximal fragment.

**Fig. V.20. a** The cortico-cancellous graft is still easily recognizable. **b** The graft is incorporated after 2 years (in young patients)

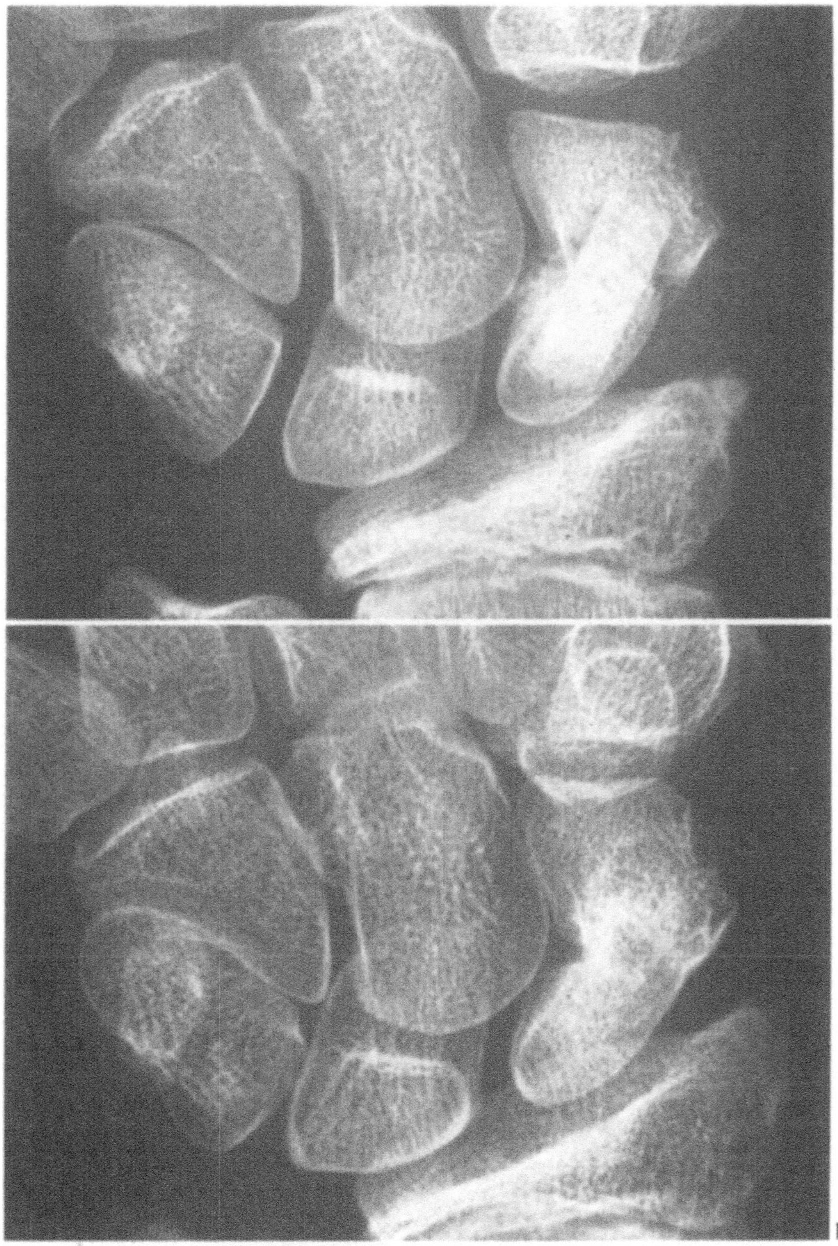

a

b

*Pseudarthrosis Combined with Ligamentous Instability*

This requires two procedures, a ligamentoplasty and insertion of graft, but there are several considerations:

- The dorsal approach for the ligamentoplasty seems preferable as there is less threat to the vascularization of the proximal fragment, whose blood-supply depends essentially on the radio-scaphoid ligament.
- The ligamentoplasty must be done before the scaphoid grafting for, once this is grafted, it is no longer possible to proceed to the often strenuous manipulations required for correction of palmar subluxation of the lunate.

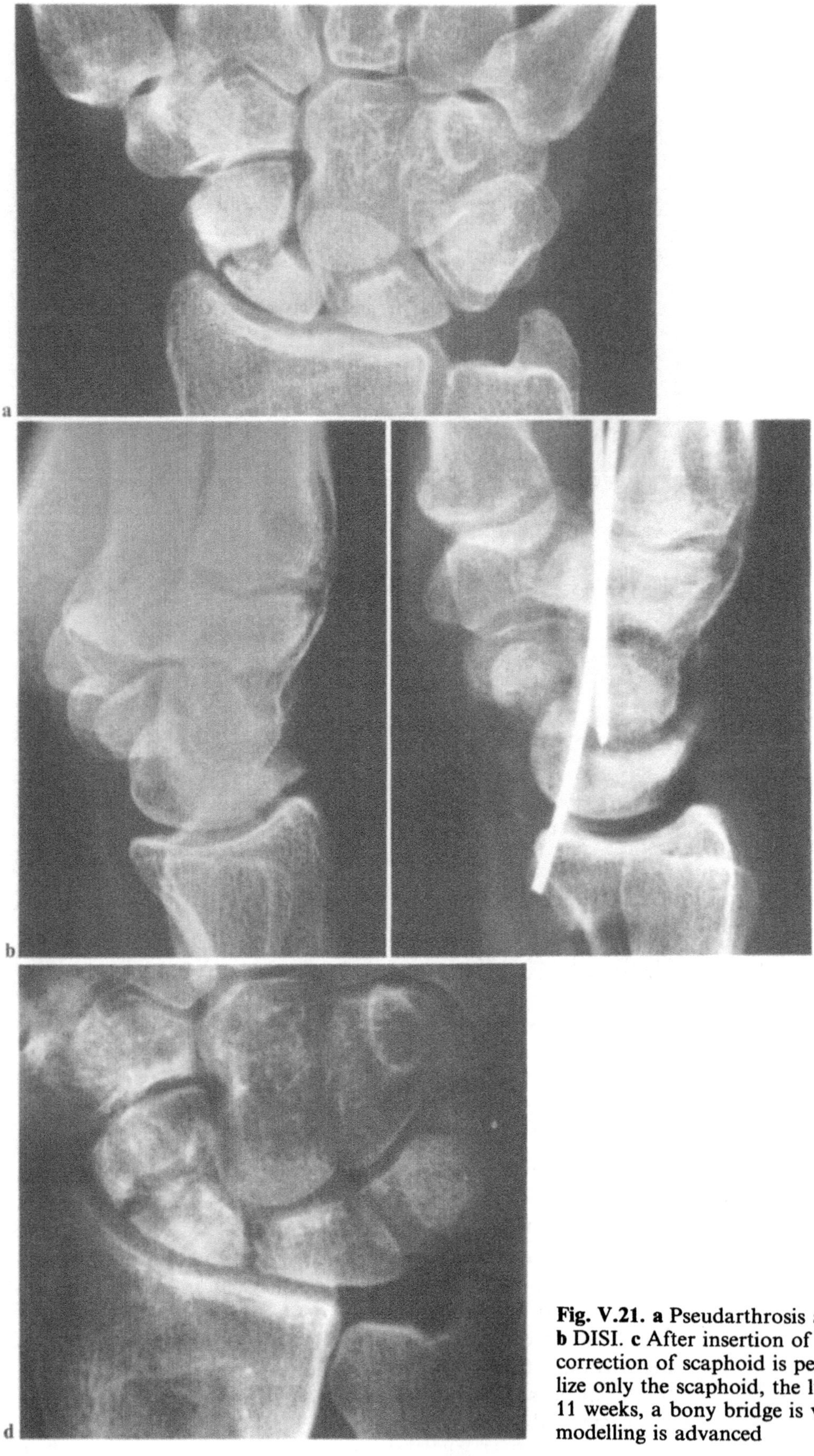

a b c d

**Fig. V.21. a** Pseudarthrosis and bony instability. **b** DISI. **c** After insertion of polyhedral graft, correction of scaphoid is performed (wires stabilize only the scaphoid, the lunate is free). **d** At 11 weeks, a bony bridge is visible and graft remodelling is advanced

The aim of ligamentoplasty is to realign the lunate while stabilizing it. This results in lengthening of the central column of the carpus; the stresses on the scaphoid decrease and the chances of union increase.

*Ligamentoplasty by dorsal approach.* Procedure (see Figs. V.2–V.5):

1. Zig-zag incision, or longitudinal incision with a break at the wrist
2. Identification of the extensor retinaculum
3. Opening of the third tunnel and freeing of the extensor pollicis longus
4. Stripping of part of the extensor retinaculum from the ulnar side
5. Partial detachment of the radio-triquetral ligament
6. Longitudinal incision of the connective fatty tissue in the axis of the second web space along the extensor carpi radialis brevis, and exposure of the carpal bones (see Fig. V.39d).

Most often, the capitate is almost in contact with the radius and hides the subluxated lunate (Fig. V.22a). By maximal flexion of the wrist, a dorsal translation movement and moderate palmar-flexion of the lunate is obtained, as determined by the pre-operative films (Fig. V.22b).

The lunate is fixed in this position with a Kirschner wire (1.6 mm diameter) transfixing both radius and lunate. The wrist is then extended into the desired position. The blocked lunate cannot escape, and is then fixed to the capitate with a second Kirschner wire (1.6 mm diameter) passed from the third web space. It is important that this should not penetrate the radius, or it will be impossible to mobilize the wrist (Fig. V.22c, d).

According to Linscheid's technique (Palmer et al. 1978), it is possible to suspend the lunate from the capitate (Fig. V.23b), using the tendon of the palmaris longus (Fig. V.24a, b) or of the extensor carpi radialis brevis (Fig. V.24c). This technique permits replacement of the defective proximal V without vascular risk, either to the lunate or to the proximal pole of the scaphoid (see Figs. V.23, 24).

The lunate is fixed either by a graft passed through a channel drilled in its dorsal pole or directly to the dorsal part of the scapho-lunate ligament. The distal anchorage can be made without difficulty in the capitate itself, using a bony channel. Using Linscheid's technique, the distal attachment of the extensor carpi radialis brevis is one of the points of anchorage, the second being in the lunate or, as we suggest, in the dorsal part of the scapho-lunar ligament. The free portion of the tendon must be interlaced carefully in order to avoid secondary loosening when the wires are removed after 6 weeks.

*Ligamentoplasty by palmar approach.* The stages in this procedure (see Fig. V.15) are:

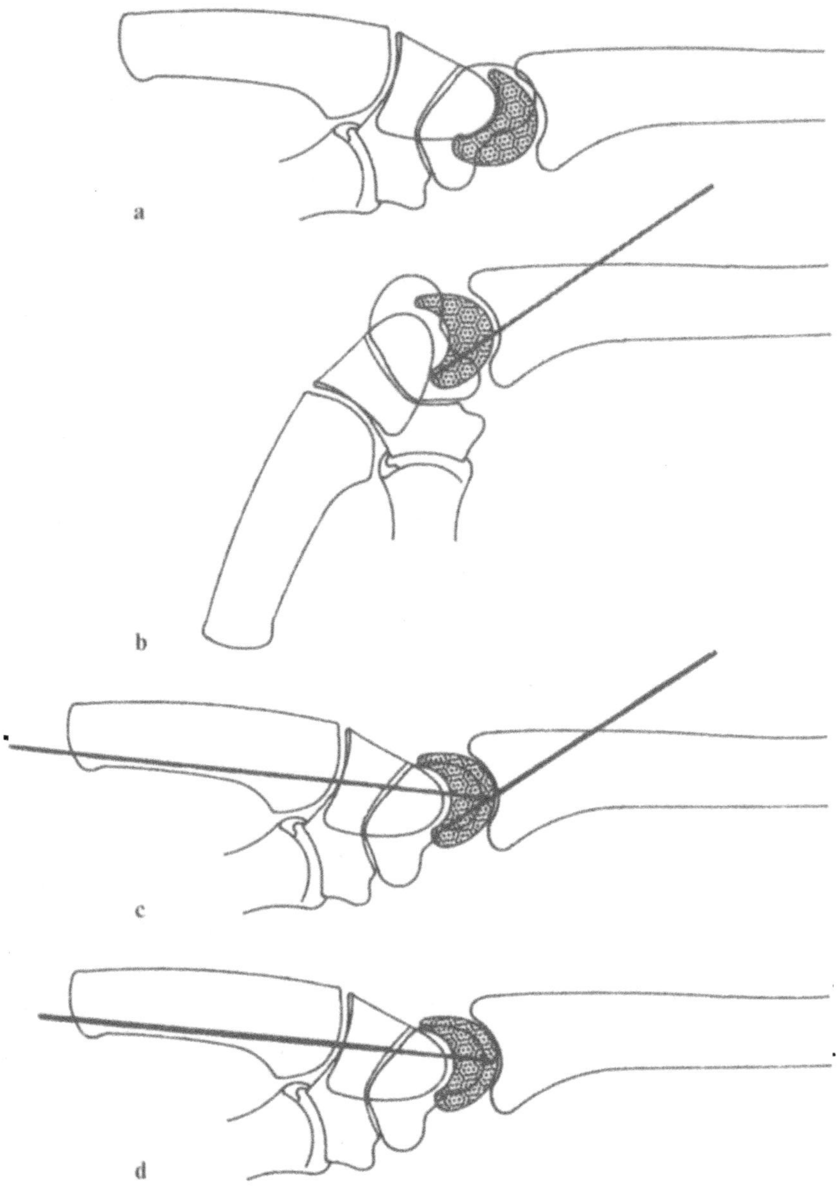

a b c d

**Fig. V.22 a–d.** Technique of reduction of lunate (*shaded*) in DISI. **a** Initial situation: lunate in palmar subluxation, capitate subluxated dorsally and almost in contact with radius. **b** Maximal palmar flexion, with more or less satisfactory reduction of lunate (generally in neutral position, hence the importance of preoperative films). Fixation of reduction is obtained with a wire. **c** Correction of capitate and fixation of capitate and lunate with wire inserted from third web space. **d** Withdrawal of first wire, ensuring reduction of lunate

1. To avoid restriction, a generous incision is made crossing the tendons of the flexor carpi radialis (FCR) and palmaris longus, with due care for the palmar branch of the median nerve. Moderate palmar flexion relaxes the flexors and allows detailed examination of the palmar capsulo-ligamentous apparatus. If it is necessary to open the carpal tunnel we perform a Z-shaped incision in the flexor retinaculum so as to be able to close it later. This is the only certain way to avoid subluxation of the median nerve into the scar (Fig. V.30).
2. The proximal palmar V is identified, in particular the radio-scapho-lunate ligament (RSL) carrying the vessels.
3. A channel is made in the radial epiphysis *after* taking the bone-graft. This channel is situated opposite the palmar pole of the lunate (Fig. V.23c).

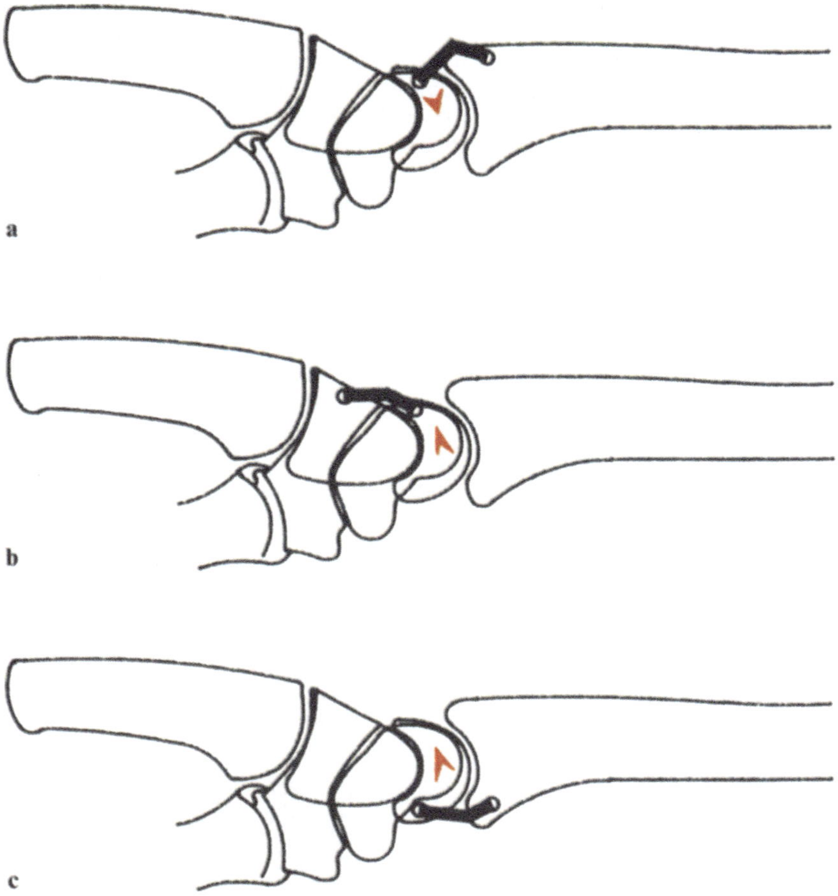

**Fig. V.23a–c.** Ligamentoplasties. **a** Dorsal radio-lunate ligamentoplasty (as in Fig. V.24c or d) directs lunate to palm, and is indicated in PISI. *Arrow*, direction of movement of lunate. **b** Dorsal capitate-lunate ligamentoplasty (as in Fig. V.24a or b) suspends palmar-subluxated lunate, and is indicated in DISI. **c** Palmar (radio-lunate) ligamentoplasty involves the same principle as dorsal plasty, and is indicated in DISI

4. The palmar V is interlaced with a tendon graft (either the tendon of the palmaris longus or half the FCR), while safeguarding the RSL. We advise against drilling an intra-osseous channel, since vascularization of the lunate is essentially, sometimes even exclusively, through the palmar pole.
5. The subluxated lunate is reduced, and the reduction held with a Kirschner wire passing from radius to lunate (Fig. V.22). An antero-posterior wire temporarily transfixing the lunate may aid reduction.
6. The ligamentoplasty is completed and the unnecessary wires extracted. Wire immobilization need not exceed 6 weeks. An example is given in Fig. III.7a–c, p. 76, with the relevant history.

*Post-operative Treatment*

*Post-operative immobilization.* This period (12–16 weeks in all) comprises:
1. In the first 15 days: a long-arm splint including the thumb and forearm
2. From 2 to 6 weeks: a long-arm plaster with the elbow flexed at 90°, the thumb included, leaving the interphalangeal (IP) joint free, in opposition and ante-position (palmar abduction), with neutral forearm rotation

**Fig. V.24 a–e.** Dorsal ligamentoplasties: *red diagrams* show course of tendon graft (palmaris longus or plantaris). If these are absent, use half the FCR for palmar grafts or half the extensor carpi radialis brevis (ECRB) for dorsal grafts, but ensure a tendon of adequate length.
**a** Lunate (scaphoid or triquetrum) – capitate, using palmaris longus.
**b** If the instability is localized between the lunate and the triquetrum, the attachment is made between the lunate, capitate and triquetrum. Additional oblique fixation of ECRB (*2*) theoretically introduces a favourable dynamic component.
**c** Using ECRB (Linscheid), an adequately long segment of tendon is vital. This pedicled graft is equally applicable in SL or LT (lunate-triquetrum) instability.
**d** In PISI, the palmar tilt of the lunate must be restricted. This may be achieved via a free graft fixed to the radius and the scapho-lunate couple across the bone, or in the SL ligament alone (**e**)
*1* ECRL, *2* ECRB

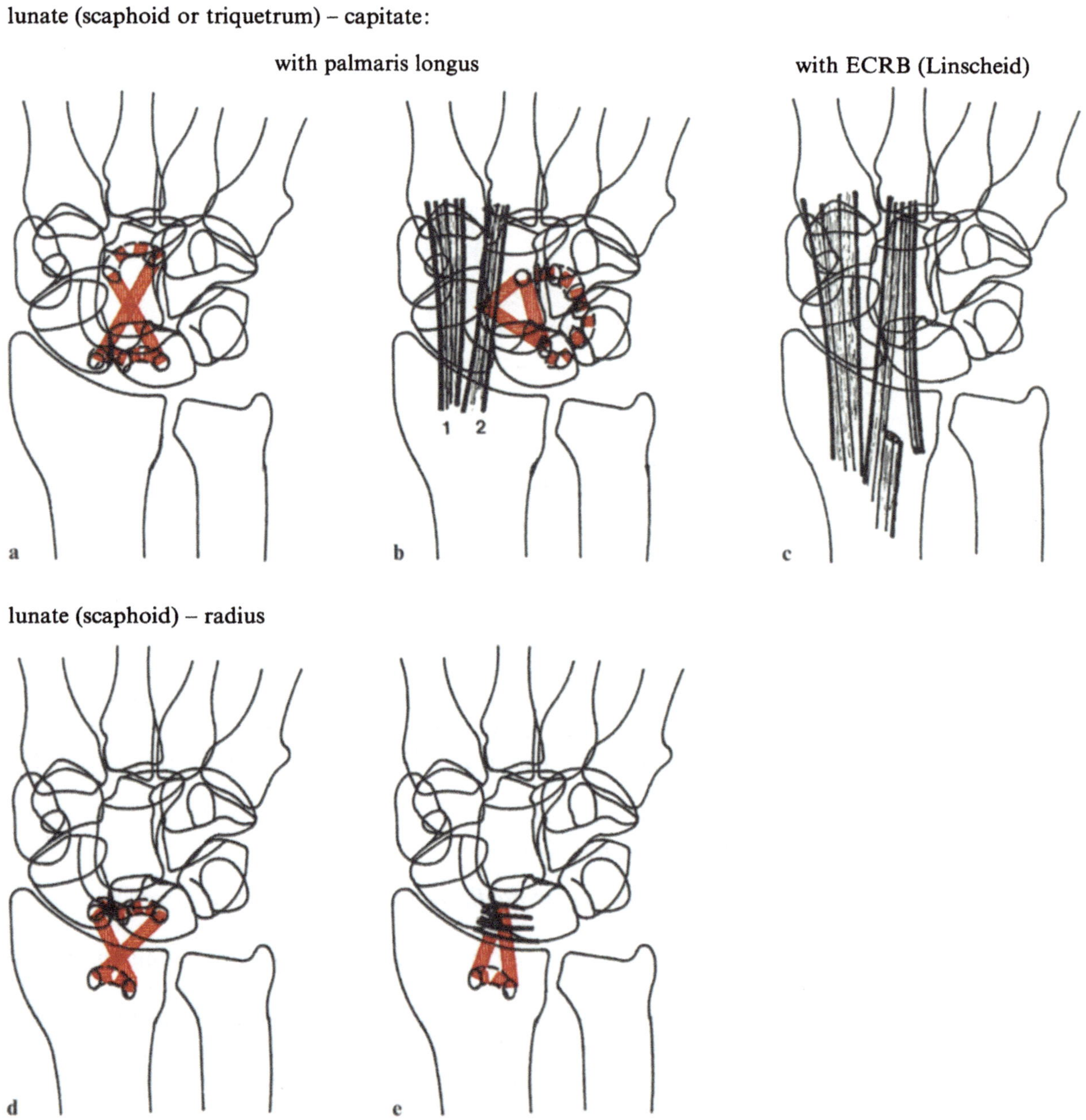

3. From 7 to 12–16 weeks: short-arm plaster, with the thumb included to the IP joint and in opposition; flexion-extension of the IP joint must be possible, as must thumb-index pinching
4. Then a removable plaster splint and progressive mobilization of the wrist with the aid of warm baths

*Note.* No aggressive physiotherapy is indicated at this stage because of fear of over-constraint of demineralised bone undergoing consolidation. Gentle mobilization allows progressive re-calcification over 2 months. After that all exertion is permitted and physiotherapy can begin in earnest if the mobility and power are still inadequate.

*Duration of wiring.* This lasts 6 weeks, i.e. as long as the long-arm plaster is worn.

### Osteosynthesis (OS)

There are two types of OS:
1. Stable OS, with or without a (sandwich) graft
2. Unstable (adaptation) OS

### Stable OS Without Graft

An osteosynthesis is stable when the bony fragments joined by compression exhibit no mobility, whatever the circumstances. As a general rule, this type of osteosynthesis requires no ancillary plaster immobilization (Fig. III.15b).

Pseudarthrosis of the scaphoid can be treated by lag-screws without auxiliary plaster immobilization, provided the compression is perfect. As demonstrated earlier, the success rate of this technique is mediocre; moreover, a stable pseudarthrosis can be easily treated by classical grafting with union in 8 weeks. Thus, stable osteosynthesis, a subtle and difficult procedure, is indicated only exceptionally, more often because of patient factors than because of the clinical conditions.

### Stable OS with Sandwich Graft

The sandwich procedure is a stable osteosynthesis fixing a cortico-cancellous graft between the proximal and distal poles of the scaphoid. This technique was described and advocated by Segmüller (1973).

*Indications.* These are limited by the site and axis of the fracture line (screw placement may be impossible), the size of the cysts and the skill of the surgeon.

*Conditions.* The graft must be resistant to compression. The axis of the screws should be at right angles to the line of osteotomy. Both rotation and shearing forces must be neutralized (two screws or one screw plus a wire are required).

*Approaches.* We use two approaches: a radial and a palmar.

For the *radial approach,* the landmarks (Fig. V.25) are the distal margin of the radius and the anatomical snuffbox bounded by the extensor pollicis longus and abductor pollicis longus. The incision crosses the terminal branches of the radial nerve and the radial artery (Fig. V.26), structures which must be dealt with very carefully. It also requires partial detachment of the crest of the scaphoid, which is rich in nutrient vessels. However, devascularization does not seem to be a problem; we have not observed even transient vascular disturbance after the radial approach for the sandwich operation.

*Palmar access* is the same as for the Matti-Russe graft (Fig. V.15). However, in order to place the screws correctly, the incision must be extended beyond the radial margin of the tuberosity of the scaphoid, which is partly denuded.

The great advantage of this approach is that it avoids the radial nerve, which is so vulnerable to manipulation. It also makes it possible to abandon the sandwich procedure if the anatomic conditions are unexpected or unfavourable, without prejudicing other forms of surgery.

*Equipment.* Two cortical screws of 2.0 or 2.7 mm are used, or possibly a 2.7 mm screw and a Kirschner wire to neutralize rotatory forces. We feel that cancellous screws are contraindicated. Their bulk is a nuisance and it may prove impossible to extract them if left in place too long. Screws of 1.5 mm are not sufficiently resistant.

The example of osteosynthesis shown in Fig. V.27 demonstrates the possibilities of the palmar approach for a fracture of the distal third of the scaphoid. The configuration of the bone prevents insertion of a second screw. In this example the screw is eccentric; the pressure is spread unevenly over the distal pole, and there is significant risk of its fracturing during compression.

*Difficulties.* Obtaining enough cortical support for the screwheads is essential for compression. The screws must be correctly aligned, i.e. with their axes at right angles to the fracture line. It is difficult to secure a sufficient grip on the distal fragment without encroaching on the joint space or adjacent bone. Overly eccentric insertion of the screw must be avoided, due to the risk of marginal fracture at the screw-head, irregular compression and secondary instability.

*Note.* During the exposure it is important to strip the subcutaneous tissue from the aponeurotic plane properly to ensure mobility of the skin and its nerve branches, which should not be subjected to tension. The cortico-cancellous graft must be very resistant to compression; only the iliac crest supplies adequate bone.

Fig. V.25. Radial approach through anatomical snuffbox. Landmarks are:
*1* extensor pollicis longus (EPL)
*2* extensor pollicis brevis (EPB) and abductor pollicis longus
*3* articular margin of radius
*4* incision, which begins parallel to the distal border of the radius and extends between the tendons of EPL and EPB

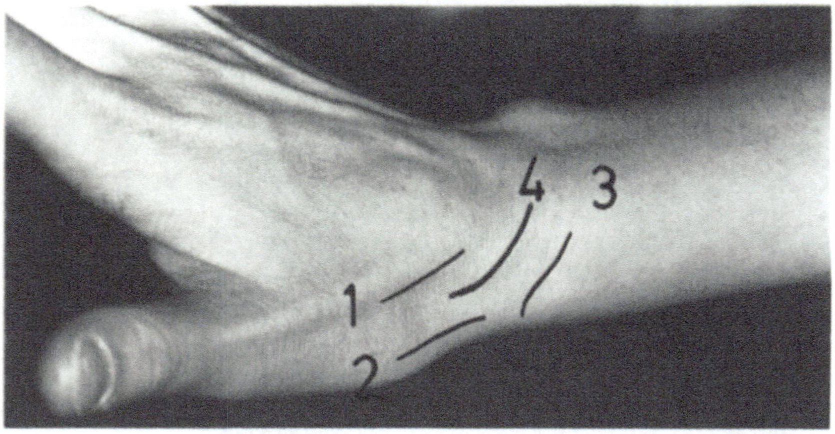


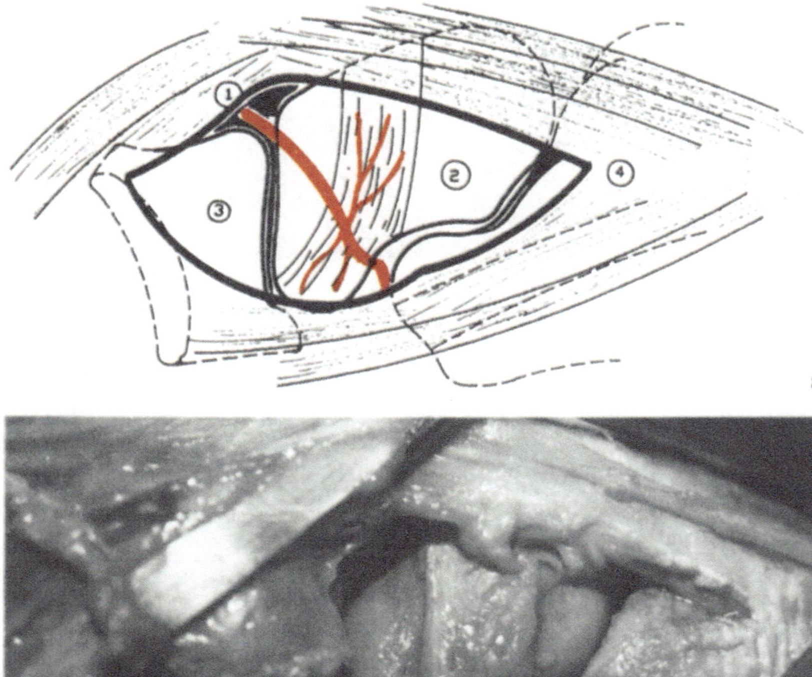

a

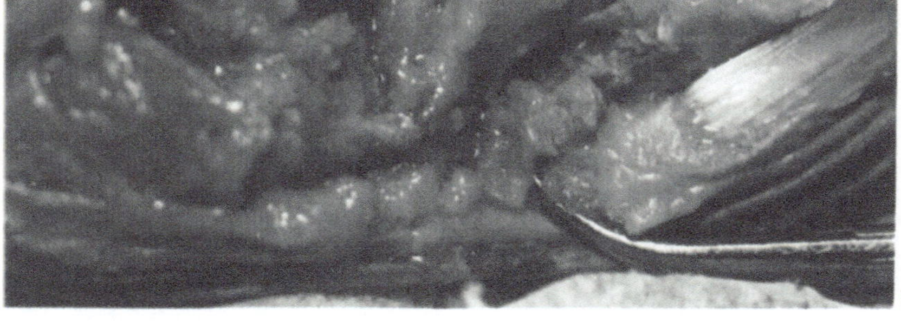
b

**Fig. V.26a, b.** Anatomy of radial aspect of opened anatomical snuffbox. **a** The radial artery traverses the snuffbox, and supplies the scaphoid via the capsulo-ligamentous system (ramification in *red*).
**b** White vertical ligamentous band clearly visible.
*1* radial artery
*2* scaphoid
*3* trapezium
*4* radius

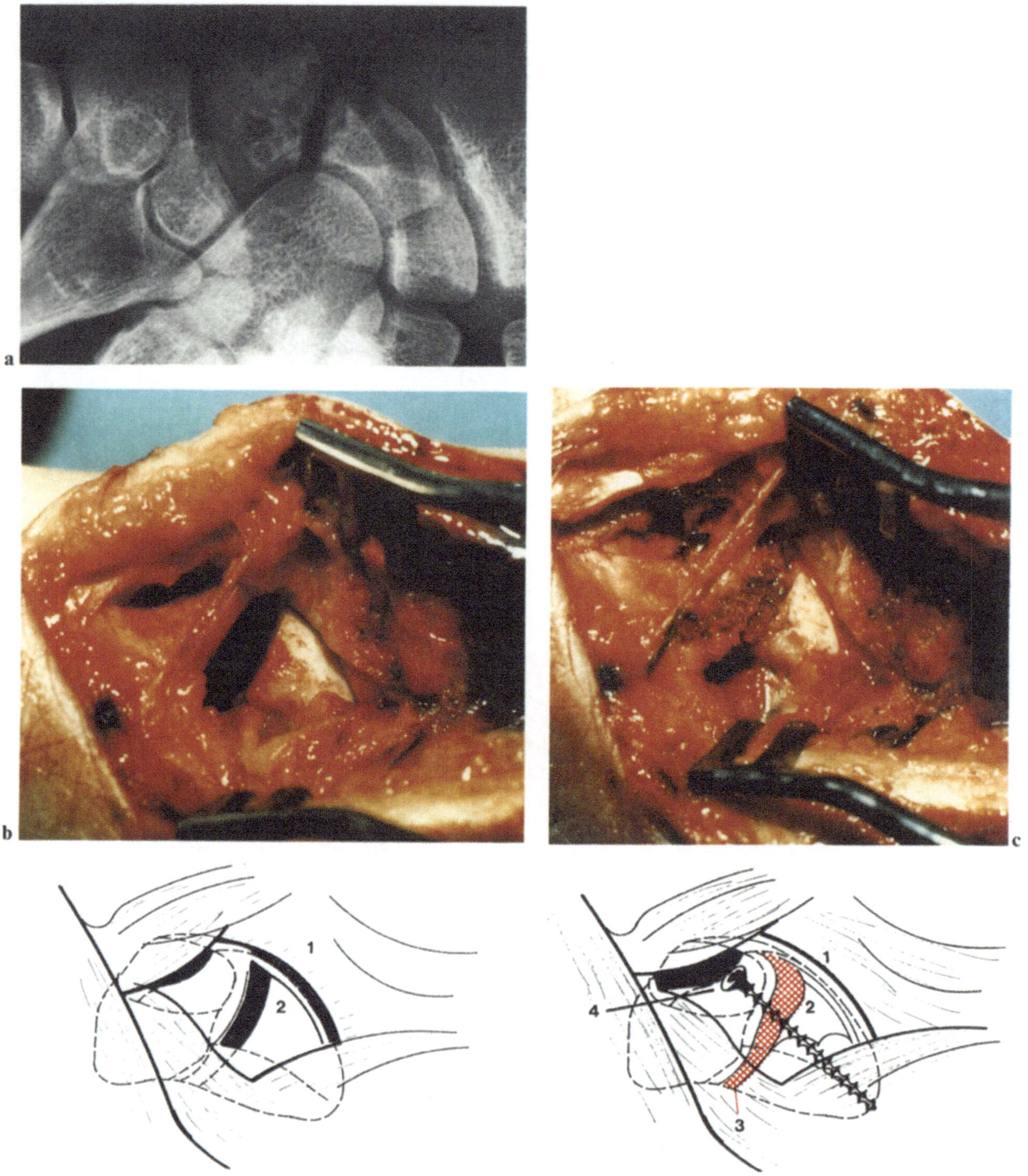


**Fig. V.27 a–e.** Sandwich operation for scaphoid pseudarthrosis. **a** Pre-operative X-ray. **b** After resection of the sclerosed tissue it is possible to assess the bony gap. **c** Graft and screw in place; the axis of the screw is correct (almost perpendicular to the resected bony surfaces)

*1* radius
*2* scaphoid
*3* graft
*4* head of screw

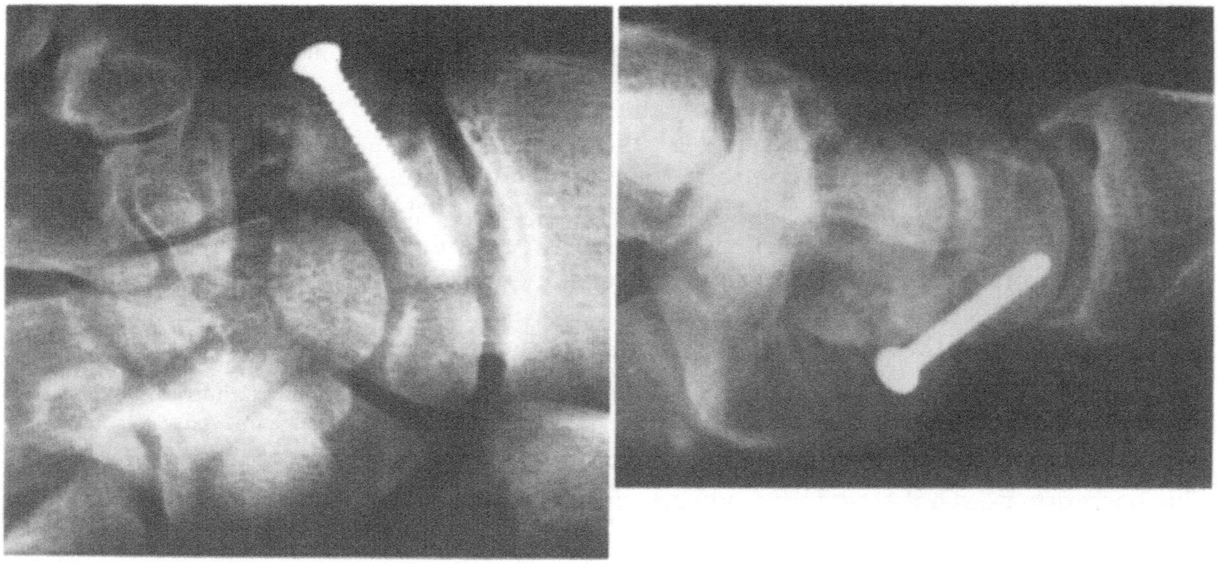

d e

**Fig. V.27 d, e** Corresponding PA and lateral films

*Post-operative management.* Immobilization is necessary until wound healing. After the 15th day, mobilization is commenced if the conditions of stability are satisfied. Exertion is allowed after 6–8 weeks. However, if the assembly is inadequate and the osteosynthesis not regarded as stable, the conditions and protocols of treatment for an "improved" Matti-Russe procedure apply.

### *Adaptation Osteosynthesis*

This exists when, after reduction, the fragments are held side by side without the immobilization being rigid. Some degree of interfragmentary motion persists so it is necessary for the fixation to be supplemented by plaster splintage. We have demonstrated the use of this form of stabilization for combined bony and ligamentous instability. It does not seem to have any other indications, even though Gallucio and Gallucio (1985) claim to have cured 100% of scaphoid pseudarthroses, some of long standing, by simple percutaneous wiring under the image intensifier.

## Special Problems

### *The Styloid Process*

Resection of the styloid process is not generally necessary, especially if the Matti-Russe procedure has corrected the collapse. On the other hand, malunion (Fig. V.28) may render such resection inevitable. This was the case in this 25-year-old woman, in whom the angulation of the scaphoid was not sufficiently corrected by the cortico-cancellous graft.

*Scaphoid Prostheses*

A prosthesis, whether partial or complete, is an inert foreign body disrupting the integrity of an intricate modular system. It cannot be expected to be functional, since the ligaments cannot play their normal roles. On the contrary, the insertion of a prosthesis, because of the additional lesions it produces, further weakens the proximal row, and does not prevent collapse of the carpus. Finally, these implants have no resistance to shear, and major wear is the forerunner of foreign-body synovitis. We have no use for prostheses as a means of treating pseudarthrosis.

*Resection of the Proximal Row of the Carpus*

Although the work of Inglis and Jones (1977) is encouraging, this operation does not seem to be indicated in this context.

**Conclusions**

The treatment of pseudarthroses of the scaphoid may require several complementary operative techniques. Success of the operation depends on the quality of the diagnosis, since this determines which complementary procedures ensure union of the pseudarthrosis. Carpal collapse, angulation of the scaphoid fragments, bony or ligamentous instability, arthrosis and age are not contraindications to cortico-cancellous grafting; they merely determine which therapeutic measures are required for good consolidation. The proximal avascular fragment constitutes the sole remaining problem. Here, a vascularized graft, as suggested by Kühlmann, may be the solution.

**Fig. V.28a–d.** A case of resection of the radial styloid. **a** Pseudarthrosis of the scaphoid with shortening of the scaphoid and radio-scaphoid arthrosis. **b** After the Matti-Russe procedure, there is union of the pseudarthrosis but with irregularity and persistence of pain. **c, d** After resection of the styloid (as limited as possible) and smoothing off the scaphoid, a good clinical and radiological result was achieved ▷

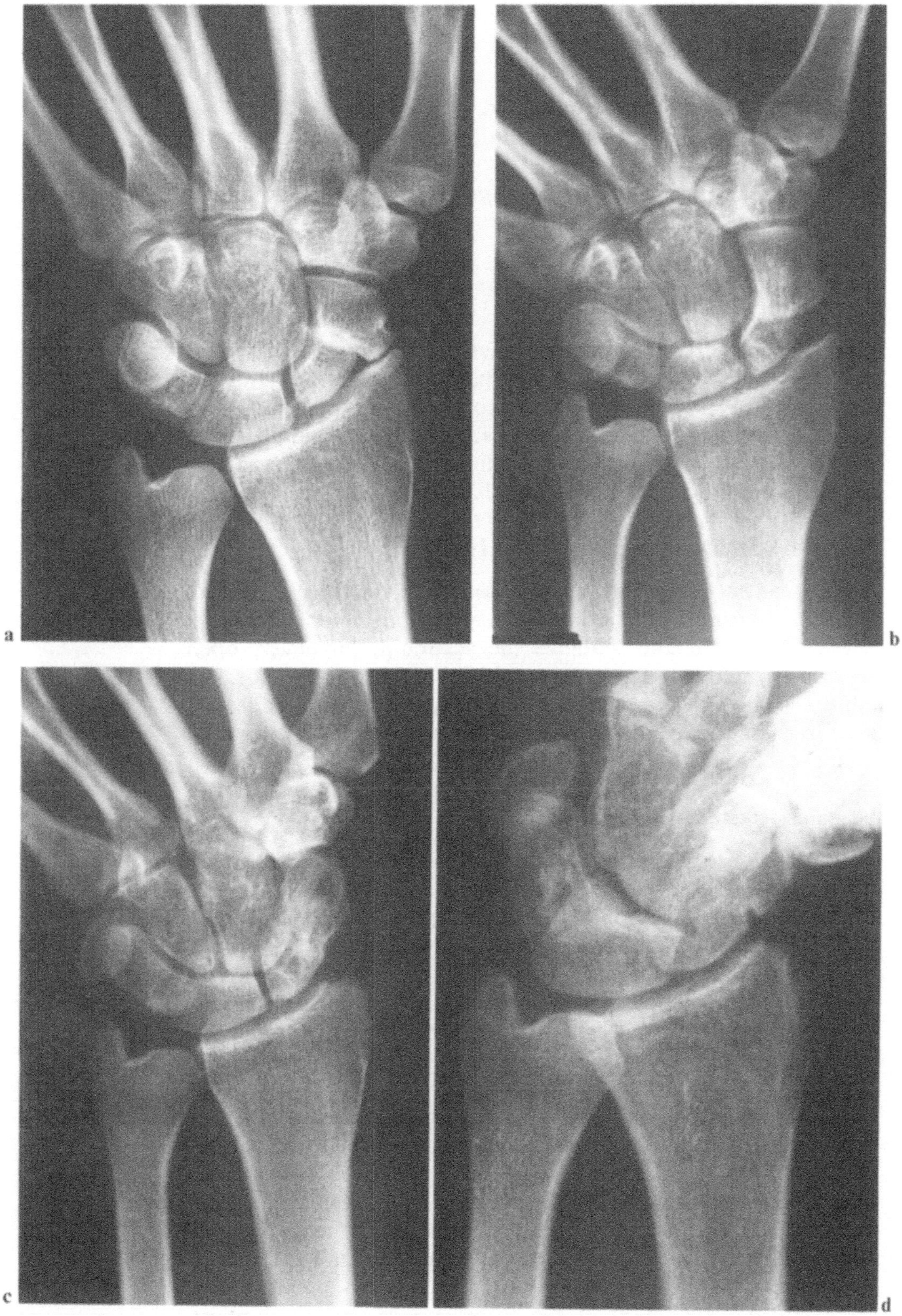

Fig. V.28 a–d

## C. Recent Fractures of the Scaphoid

These may be:
1. Stable, without displacement, and a normal lunate axis
2. Minimally stable, with minimal displacement, and a normal lunate axis
3. Unstable, with greater than 1 mm displacement, and tilting of the lunate.

Radiological diagnosis is essential.

### Stable Fractures

Union is ensured by a forearm plaster extending to the interphalangeal joint, with the thumb in palmar opposition. Dickson and Leslie (1983) have shown that consolidation takes an average of 8 weeks, with two exceptions: fractures of the proximal pole and those of the neck, where union takes 13 weeks. These figures dictate the period of immobilization.

### Minimally Stable Fractures Without Lunate Tilt

There is an increased risk that conservative treatment will fail. Kirschner wiring of the scaphoid may be considered, to permit perfect reduction and stabilize the scaphoid. However, open screwing would appear to be contraindicated, for the surgical approach may weaken a previously adequate ligamentous system. In these cases, osteosynthesis is not a more reliable method than conservative treatment.

### Unstable Fractures With Lunate Tilt

As we have seen, the unstable fracture is one of the initial stages of a de Quervain's fracture-dislocation. However, it is not known to what extent the instability is of ligamentous or of bony origin.

Reduction of the displacement is imperative, and osteosynthesis is required to maintain it. Whether it is stable or unstable matters little; with the scaphoid reduced, the position of the other carpal bones must be assured by intra-operative radiography. If simple reduction of the scaphoid restores the normal bony configuration, it may be accepted that the ligamentous lesions are minimal, and that complementary exploration may be dispensed with. The decision to perform a stable osteosynthesis or to be content with wiring of the scaphoid will depend on the surgeon's routine. If the surgeon does wish to perform stable osteosynthesis, we advise the dorso-radial approach, which has the advantage of not weakening the ligamentous system.

Abnormal alignment of the carpal bones on the standard films, or pathological mobility when examined under the image intensifier, is a definite indication for surgical inspection; only this will allow identification of the lesions and, what is more, their correction. The surgical approach is dictated by the anatomy. The supporting structures are palmar. It is these that must be restored, so a palmar approach is imperative. If a dorsal ligamentoplasty is contemplated, a double approach, palmar and dorsal, is indicated.

## D. Perilunate Dislocations, With or Without Fracture

The object of treatment is simple: to obtain union of the fractured bones and healing of the torn ligaments in anatomic position. This determines the therapeutic approach; it seems neither useful nor necessary to differentiate between simple perilunar dislocations and fracture-dislocations.

As opposed to the majority of authors, we believe that the prognostic assessment of pure dislocations should be more guarded than that of fracture-dislocations. Reduction of a fractured bone can be verified radiologically, whereas it is impossible to know the position and state of a ruptured ligament, especially when treatment is conservative. Ligamentous healing requires perfect apposition and immobilization for at least 8 weeks. The anatomy teaches us that precise reduction is difficult. However, it is precisely these cases without fractures that most authors treat by closed reduction and plaster immobilization. The efficacy of this method is doubtful (Fig. V.29). In our opinion, perfect apposition of the interosseous ligaments of the proximal row can be ensured only *under direct vision*. Therefore, *all* perilunar lesions, with or without fractures, must be routinely explored and reduced by open operation, provided the surgeon is familiar with the anatomy.

Surgery allows routine decompression of the carpal tunnel. We make a Z-incision in the flexor retinaculum (Fig. V.30a, b), which it is possible to close in every case. Closure (Fig. V.30c) prevents secondary displacement of the median nerve into the scar tissue of the retinaculum, while promoting restoration of grip strength by good reattachment of the muscle insertions. It also ensures adequate enlargement of the diameter of the carpal tunnel.

### Therapeutic Approach

#### *Open Reduction*

The palmar approach is logical, even if controversial (Campbell et al. 1964; Dobyns and Swanson 1973; Green 1982; Taleisnik 1978). It is often adequate by itself, but can be supplemented by a dorsal approach if necessary. However, it must be clear that the dorsal approach, alone, is not adequate for precise assessment of the positions of the carpal bones.

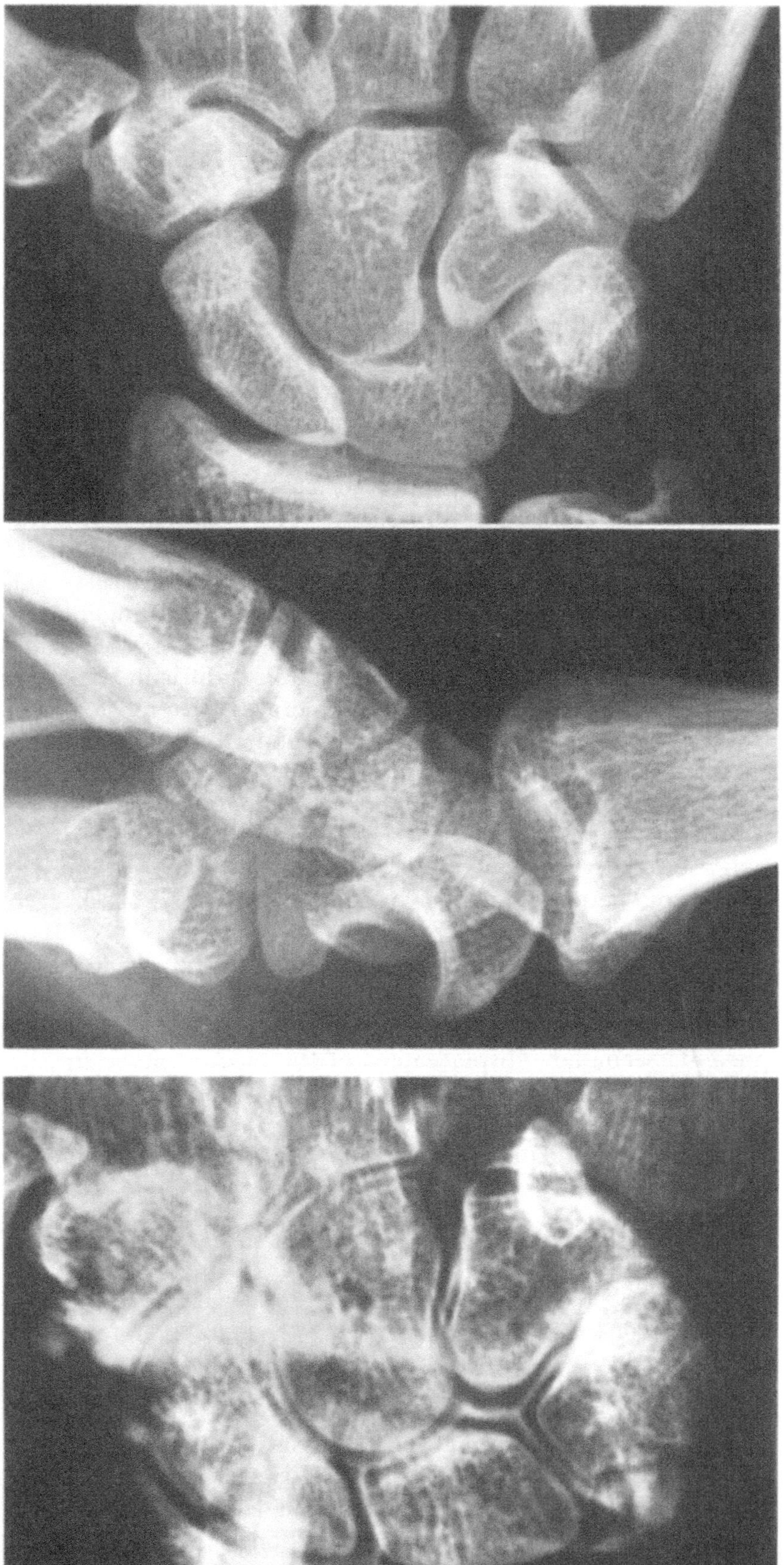

**Fig. V.29 a, b.** De Quervain's fracture-dislocation, treated conservatively, with persistent pain, clicking on exertion and triquetro-lunate instability. **a** AP and lateral films of injury. **b** Arthrogram shows rupture of triquetro-lunate (TL) ligament (for treatment, see Fig. V.44)

### Stabilization

*Stabilization of a pure ligamentous lesion.* Perilunar dislocation implies a lesion of the scapho-lunate (SL) and triquetro-lunate (TL) ligaments. These ligaments are strong and short; the bones must be perfectly reduced if perfect contact, essential for cure, is to be obtained. This is possible only under direct vision. Reduction must be ensured: by fixing the lunate to the capitate with an axial wire inserted from the third web space, and by maintaining coaptation, either by direct suture or by suture plus ancillary wiring. However, the latter may tear the suture, and we do not usually employ it. The reconstruction is completed by suture of the proximal and distal V ligaments.

*Stabilization of a fracture-dislocation.* The first stage of the operation is reduction of the fractured bones. A Kirschner wire is not only a means of fixation; it can be used as a lever arm, though the manipulation is tricky, and forcing may produce a fracture. The value of wires, as opposed to screws, is that they can be inserted without additional dissection. Screwing should not be attempted unless it is really easy to perform; it is not an end in itself (Fig. III.9b).

## Special Problems

### Scapho-Lunate Dissociation

This ligamentous lesion is equivalent to a fracture of the scaphoid and, like that, requires surgical treatment. Suture of the ligament via a palmar approach is our preference.

### Associated Fracture of the Capitate

The fracture line passes beneath the neck, leaving the proximal fragment devascularized. The risk of necrosis justifies primary arthrodesis between the lunate and capitate. However, Pfeiffer (1982) has noted healing of the proximal avascular pole of the capitate, and suggests reduction and osteosynthesis in every case.

## Conclusions

Perilunar dislocations or fracture-dislocations must be treated by open reduction. This allows correct diagnosis and anatomical reduction, and ensures perfect ligamentous coaptation.

## References


Campbell RD Jr, Lance EM, Yeoh CB (1964) Lunate and perilunar dislocations. J Bone Joint Surg [Br] 46:55–72

Dickson RA, Leslie JJ (1983) Traitement orthopédique des fractures du scaphoïde carpien. In: Razemon JP, Fisk GR (eds) Le poignet. Expansion Scientifique Française, Paris, p 90

Dobyns JH, Swanson GE (1973) Fracture conference: a 19 year-old man with multiple fractures. Minn Med 56:143–149

Fernandez DL (1984) A technique for anterior wedge-shaped grafts for scaphoid non-unions with carpal instability. J Hand Surg 9A:733–737
Gallucio D, Gallucio P (1985) L'osteosintesi minima nel tratamento della pseudarthrosi del scafoide carpale. Jornadas internacionales de cirurgía de la mano y microcirurgia, Sitges 30 May 1985
Green DP (1982) Carpal dislocations. In: Green DP (ed) Operative hand surgery, vol 1. Churchill Livingstone, New York, pp 716–733
Inglis AE, Jones EC (1977) Proximal row-carpectomy. J Bone Joint Surg [Am] 59:460–464
Pfeiffer KM (1982) Perilunäre, transskaphoidale Luxationsfrakturen (naviculo-capitate fracture syndrome) In: Buck-Gramcko D, Nigst H (eds) Frakturen, Luxationen und Dissoziationen der Karpalknochen. Hippokrates, Stuttgart, pp 163–165
Kühlmann JN, Mimoun M (1984) Greffon osseux d'aide vasculaire. Pédicule sur l'artère transverse du carpe. GEM, Paris 6–8 December 1984
Palmer AK, Dobyns JH, Linscheid RL (1978) Management of post-traumatic instability of the wrist secondary to ligament rupture. J Hand Surg 3:507–532
Segmüller G (1973) Operative Stabilisierung am Handskelett. Huber, Bern, p 104
Taleisnik J (1978) Wrist: anatomy, function and injury. AAOS Instructional Course Lect 27:61–87

## E. Operative Technique for Opening the Carpal Tunnel

*Skin Incision* (Fig. V.15)

The incision follows the creases of the hand; in general, it is parallel to the life line. It begins in the mid-palm and ends in the depression between the thenar and hypothenar eminences. If it has to be extended to the forearm, a zig-zag line is followed, with the base of the flaps on the radial or ulnar side as required.

A radial base is used for corrective osteotomies of the radius by palmar approach, for the normal approach to the carpus, for access to the anterior interosseous nerve and for procedures on the median nerve or extended procedures on the carpal tunnel. An ulnar hinge is used for procedures on the scaphoid and, if so desired, for palmar ligamentoplasty.

The palmar branch of the median nerve must be respected, especially if the incision crosses the flexion crease of the wrist opposite the flexor carpi radialis.

*Subcutaneous Levels* (Fig. V.30)

Incision of the volar ligament is followed by decompression of the ulnar nerve. The latter, hidden by the artery, is neither exposed nor dissected. Incision of the flexor retinaculum is begun distally, over the radial border of the hook of the hamate. A Z-incision allows the creation of two flaps which can be closed without risk, the increase in diameter being considerable. This closure also ensures that the median nerve remains in the carpal tunnel. Suturing is performed using a 4-0 absorbable material.

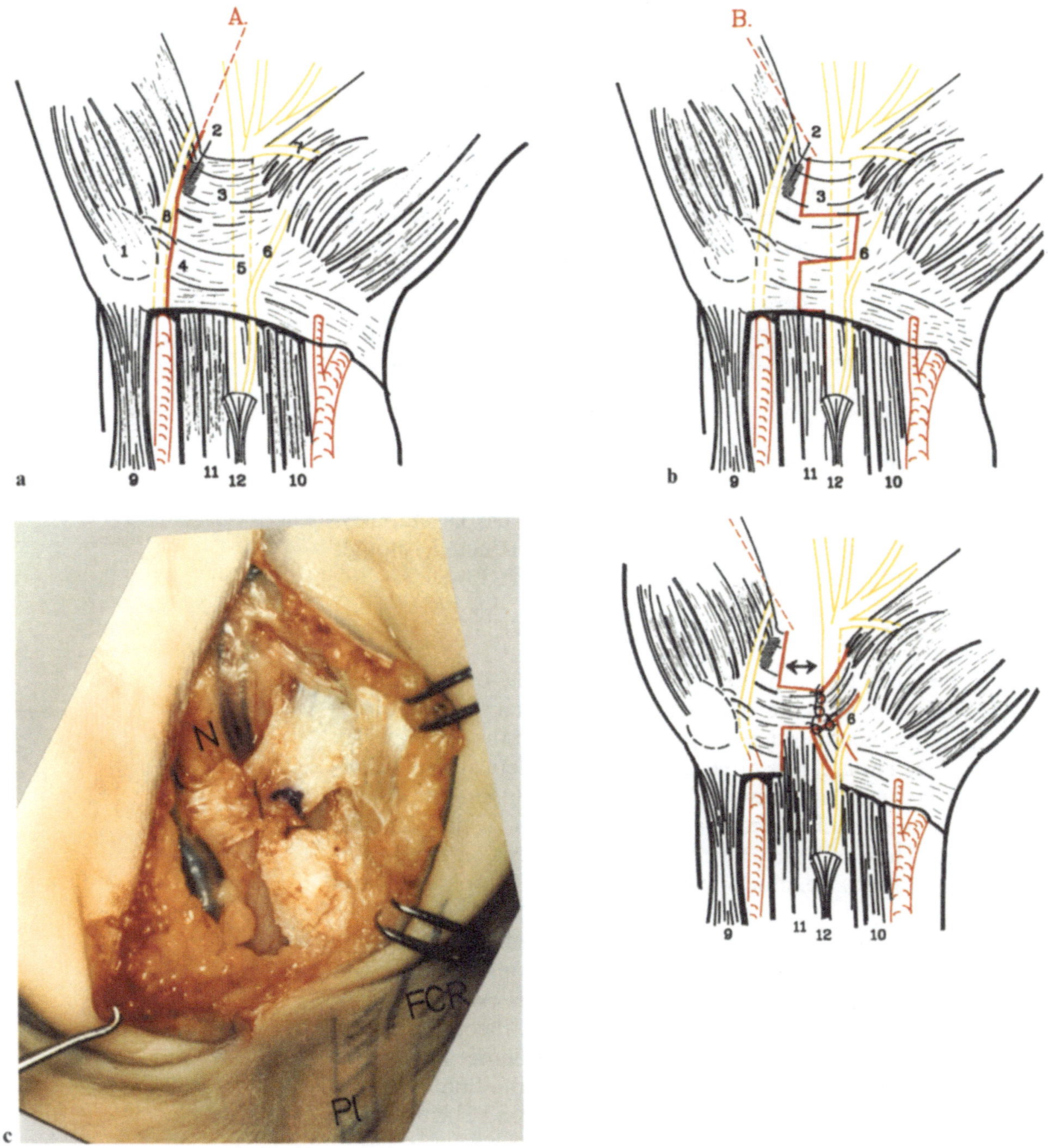


**Fig. V.30 a–c.** Technique of opening carpal tunnel. **a** Incision and opening of volar ligament. **b** Z-incision of flexor retinaculum. **c** Closure with absorbable suture.

*1* pisiform
*2* hook of hamate
*3* flexor retinaculum
*4* volar ligament
*5* median nerve
*6* palmar branch of median nerve
*7* motor branch
*8* ulnar nerve
*9* FCU
*10* FCR
*11* flexor digitorum superficialis
*12* palmaris longus

## F. Partial Arthrodeses of the Wrist, Arthroplasties and Ligamentous Reconstructions

The concept of partial arthrodesis is discussed in the appropriate chapter (p. 102). Here we devote ourselves mainly to the surgical approach and technical problems, based on clinical experience. We also emphasize the alternatives (arthroplasties or ligamentoplasties), which are all the more important since the long-term consequences of the constraints imposed by partial fusion are still unknown. It is particularly true for the scapho-trapezo-trapezoid (STT) arthrodesis described by Watson et al. (1986).

### Indications

These are not completely defined. Table V.1 summarizes the diagnoses with the therapeutic possibilites that we advise, based on our clinical experience and our concept of carpal stability. The use of Silastic is mentioned, only to be rejected, though we have used it exceptionally in the past (Fig. III.33).

### Technical Problems

It is a challenge to fix the carpal bones by stable osteosynthesis as the forces are difficult to neutralize. Their intensity and direction are unpredictable since they vary in relation to very complex movements. Though it is often possible to create a stable assembly with cortical lag-screws of 2.7 or 3.5 mm, this is not the case with the small plates for 2.7 mm screws, which are too malleable. These will only be effective if the "tension band principle" is utilized, i.e. the direction of forces is predicted and neutralized.

A good quality autogenous graft is required. It restores the volume of the damaged bones, and promotes consolidation. Determination of correct alignment of the bones is extremely difficult, because of their asymmetrical shapes, the incomplete view of the surgeon and the limited points of reference. However, the most favourable position for fusion is, in the final analysis, hypothetical, i.e. orientation of the scaphoid in STT arthrodesis or of the lunate in radio-lunate (RL) fusion.

### Approaches

Access to the carpal bones is possible by the dorsal or palmar routes. The palmar route is basically reserved for ligamentoplasties and for monitoring the position of the bones. It is always the same, but three dorsal routes of access may be distinguished, according to the bones or joints to be reached: radial, purely dorsal or dorso-ulnar.

**Table V.1.** Indications for carpal ligamentoplasty and arthrodesis

| Diagnosis | Possible treatments advised[c] |
|---|---|
| Radio-scaphoid (RS) arthrosis (traumatic or not) | RS fusion<br>Radio-scapho-lunate fusion |
| Isolated SL dissociation | Ligamentoplasty; STT or LC arthrodesis in event of failure |
| Complex SL dissociation | STT arthrodesis or<br>LC arthrodesis |
| Isolated LT dissociation | Ligamentoplasty<br>LT arthrodesis |
| Radio-carpal instability and progressive rheumatoid arthritis | RL arthrodesis<br>(except in traumatic cases) |
| Post-traumatic radio-carpal instability | RLS arthrodesis<br>RS arthrodesis |
| Carpal collapse | LC (or LCHT) arthrodesis<br>LC ligamentoplasty |
| Carpal collapse and scaphoid pseudarthrosis[a] | LC (or LCHT) arthrodesis<br>Matti-Russe + LC ligamentoplasty |
| STT arthrosis | STT arthrodesis<br>Resection/arthroplasty<br>T/T resection<br>(with or without prosthesis) |
| TP[b] arthrosis | Pisiform resection |
| Kienböck's disease | Generally, shortening of radius<br>Exceptionally, STT arthrodesis |

RS, radio-scaphoid; TP, triquetro-pisiform; SL, scapho-lunate; LT, lunate-triquetrum; LC, lunate-capitate; LT, lunate-triquetrum; RL, radio-lunate; RLS, radio-lunate-scaphoid; LCHT, lunate-capitate-hamate-triquetrum; T/T, trapezium/trapezoid

[a] Pseudarthrosis of the scaphoid should always be grafted, with or without ligamentoplasty; it is rarely an indication for a partial arthrodesis

[b] Piso-triquetral arthrosis is simply treated by resection of the pisiform. The operation is simple, with little risk, and is accompanied by denervation of the FCU. We have never noted any subsequent disturbance of mobility of the proximal row. Theoretically, arthrodesis preserves one of the dynamic controls of the proximal carpal row via the triquetrum, and on this basis it remains an alternative line of treatment

[c] We do not perform Graner's operation because of the risk of necrosis of the proximal pole of the capitate

### *Radial Approaches*

These allow access to the scaphoid, the trapezo-scaphoid joint, the trapezium and the first carpo-metacarpal joint. The route may be entirely radial, i.e. centred on the anatomical snuffbox (Figs. V.25 and V.26), or dorso-radial (Figs. V.31 and V.32), i.e. bisecting the angle between the axes of the first and second metacarpals, the thumb being in palmar opposition.

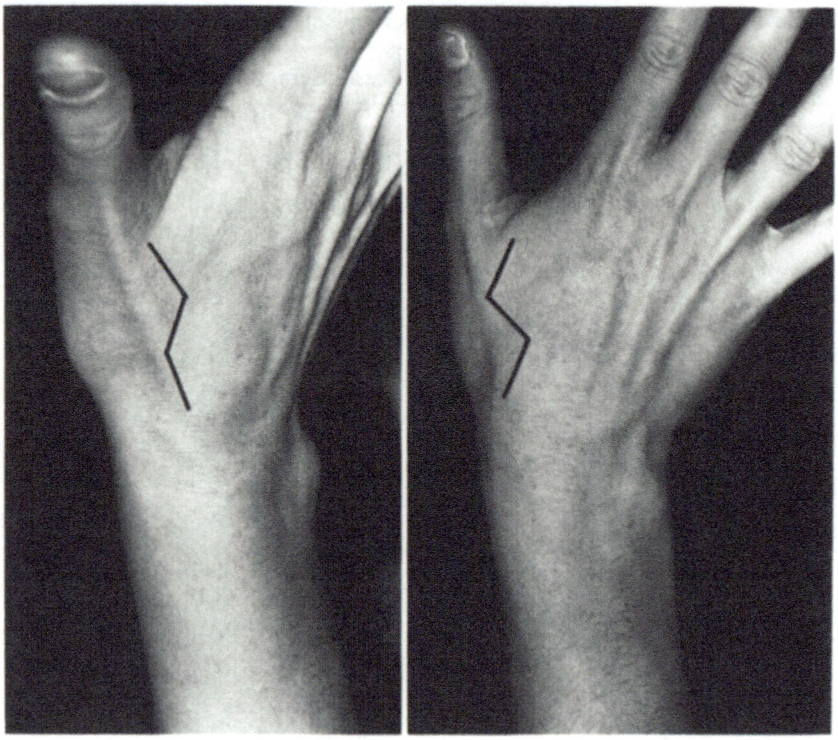

**Fig. V.31.** Dorso-radial approach. The line of incision (*black line*), in relation to extensor pollicis longus, is centred on the bisector of the angle formed by the axes of the first and second metacarpals, the thumb being in palmar opposition

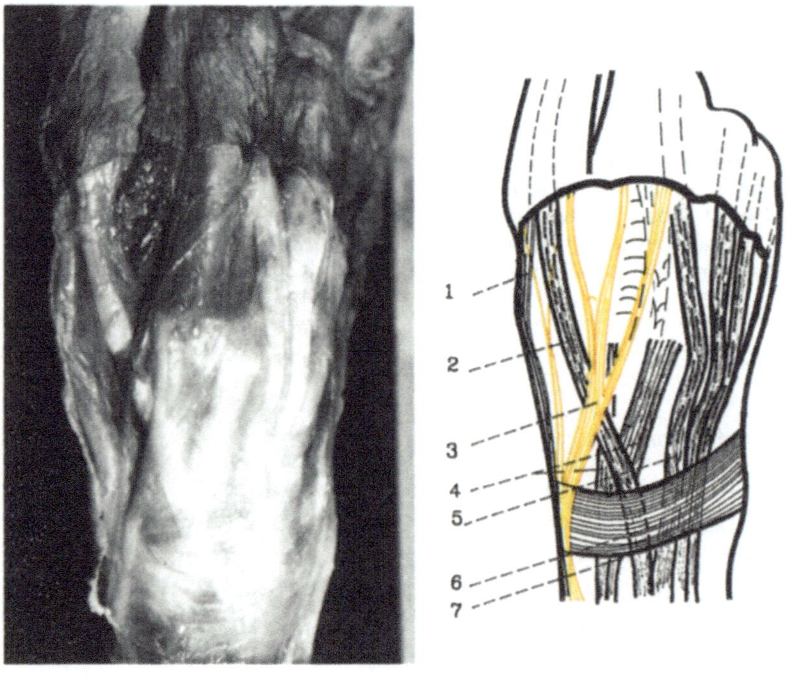


**Fig. V.32.** Anatomy of the dorso-radial approach to the carpus. Note the size of the cutaneous branches of the radial nerve and the importance of individual variations.
*1* EP brevis
*2* EP longus
*3* terminal branches of radial nerve
*4* ECR longus and brevis
*5* extensor digitorum communis
*6* extensor retinaculum
*7* third compartment

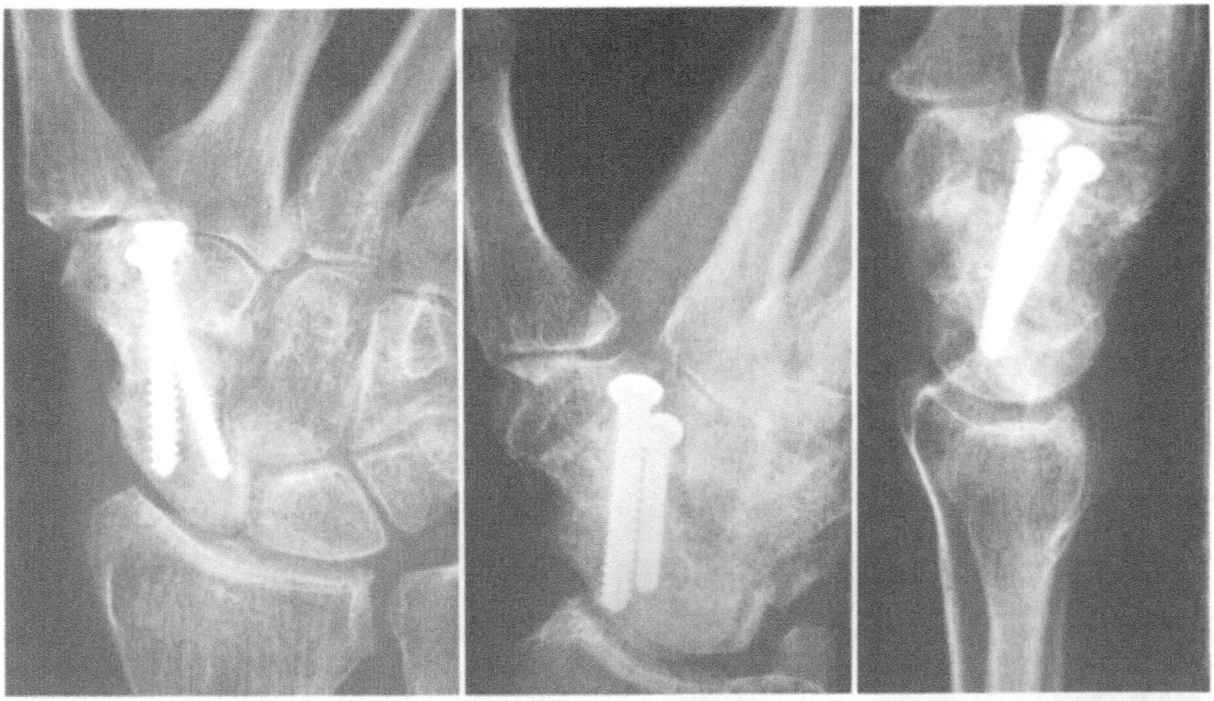

V.33

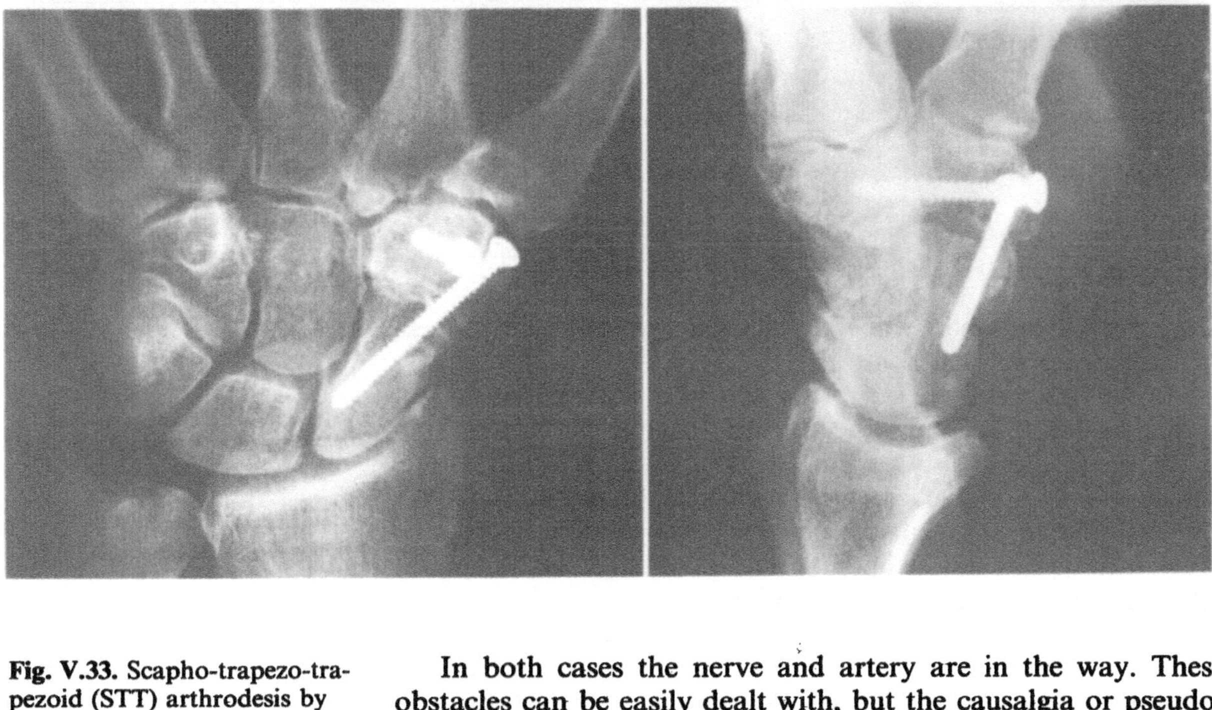

V.34

**Fig. V.33.** Scapho-trapezo-trapezoid (STT) arthrodesis by dorso-radial approach. The axes of the screws are perfect. Union has been achieved

**Fig. V.34.** STT arthrodesis by radial approach: screw axis eccentric, stability dubious

In both cases the nerve and artery are in the way. These obstacles can be easily dealt with, but the causalgia or pseudo-causalgia that may result from irritation of the radial nerve make this approach undesirable, especially if an alternative procedure is available. Therefore, the radial approach should be used only if essential: for peritrapezial arthrosis and isolated arthroses of the scapho-trapezial and scapho-trapezoid joints that are resistant to medication. Both these radial approaches allow performance of either an STT arthrodesis or a resection-arthroplasty.

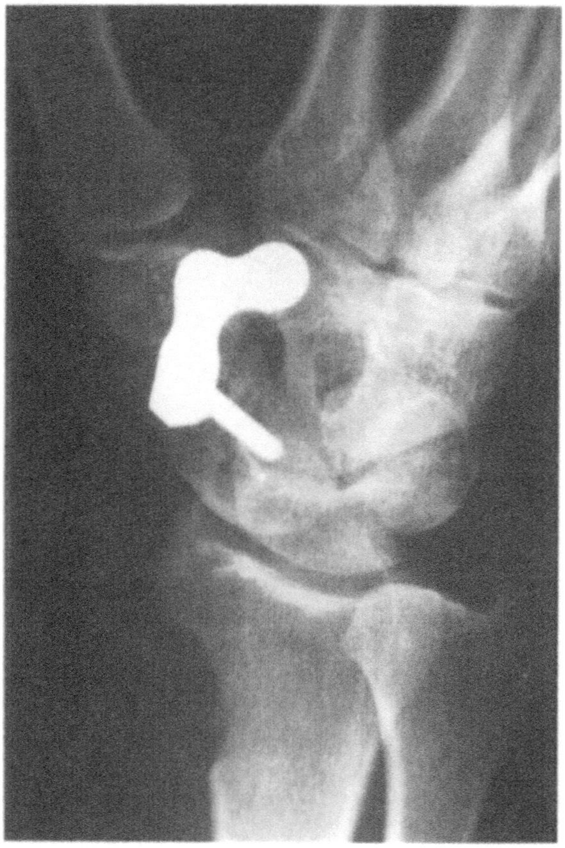

**Fig. V.35.** STT arthrodesis: an alternative method with an L-plate for 2.7 mm screws

*STT arthrodesis*

Two clinical examples will illustrate the respective advantages of these two approaches.

In the first case, the axis of the screws is perfect (Fig. V.33); in the second (Fig. V.34), the eccentric axis of the screw raises doubt as to the quality of the osteosynthesis. We believe that the dorso-radial approach is ideal for a reinforced graft, as was the case in the first example, in which consolidation occurred uneventfully. The failure in the second example, using the purely radial approach, supports our opinion.

The major obstacle in the dorso-radial approach is the radial nerve. It requires a generous incision that allows tendons and nerve branches to be mobilized and retracted without traction. Incision of the capsulo-ligamentous apparatus along the radial border of the extensor carpi radialis longus gives access to the scapho-trapezo-trapezoid joints. The joint surfaces are resected with the wrist in the neutral position, in order to place the scaphoid in an intermediate position. A cortico-cancellous graft is used as it resists compression. It should be slightly larger than the space created by the articular resections (including the scapho-trapezoid joint). Exposure of the non-articular border of the trapezium allows optimal alignment of the screw. The

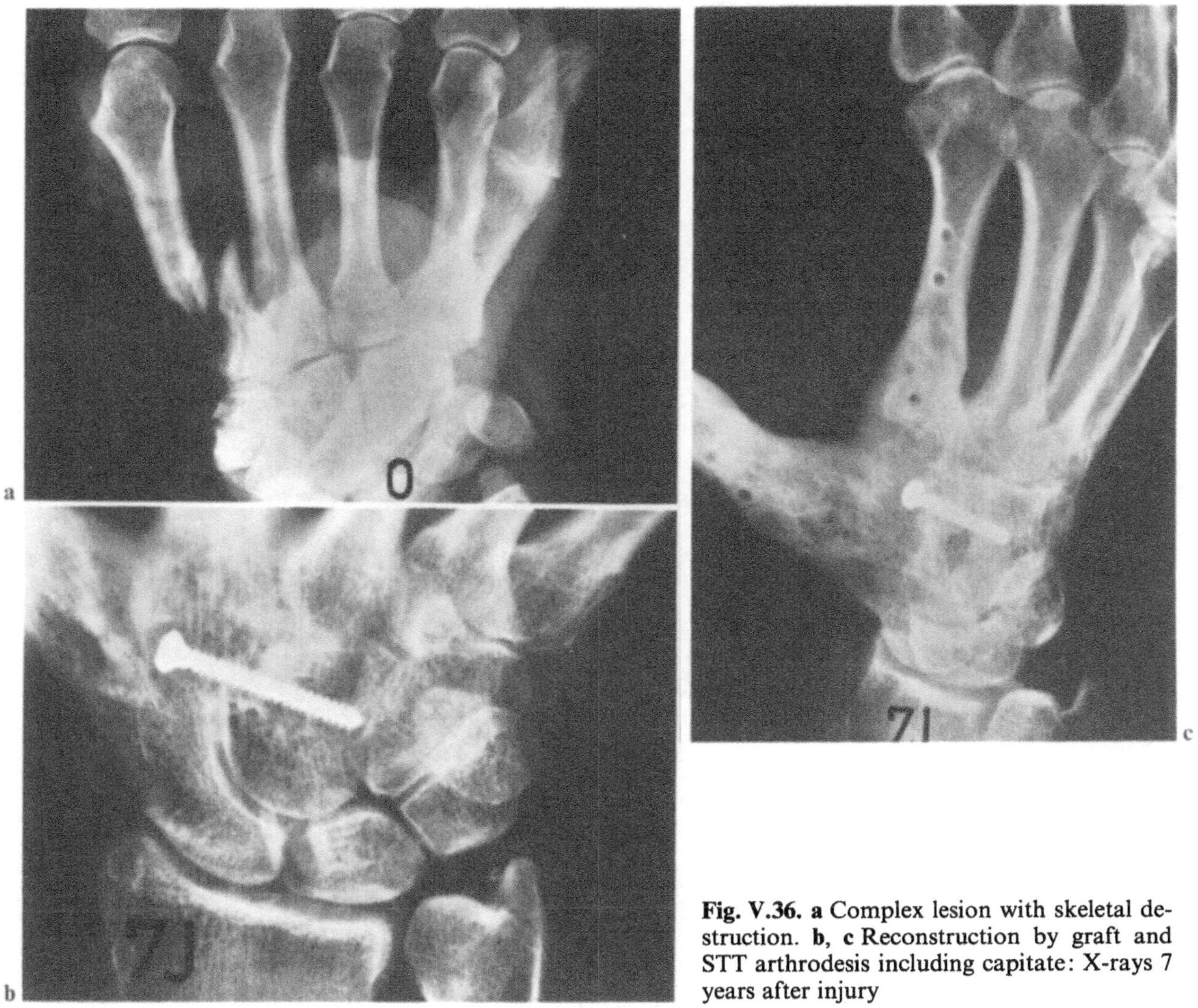

**Fig. V.36. a** Complex lesion with skeletal destruction. **b, c** Reconstruction by graft and STT arthrodesis including capitate: X-rays 7 years after injury

stabilization of the trapezium and scaphoid is enough to ensure union, and a supplementary arthrodesis including the trapezoid is unnecessary. Osteosynthesis with an L-plate for 2.7 mm screws (Fig. V.35) is certainly an interesting, but possibly a less elegant, alternative.

In traumatic cases such an arthrodesis may be the only reasonable solution, as in the 50-year-old patient in Fig. V.36. Here there is destruction of the base of the first metacarpal, devascularization of the trapezium and trapezoid, and loss of substance at the base of the second metacarpal. Function, 7 years after the accident, is satisfactory, and the patient experiences no pain or handicap with the use of the hand (Fig. V.37).

*Resection-arthroplasty*

Simple resection of the articular surfaces, combined with interposition of the capsule or an adjacent tendon, is a very attractive alternative to arthrodesis. The operation is simple, rapid and

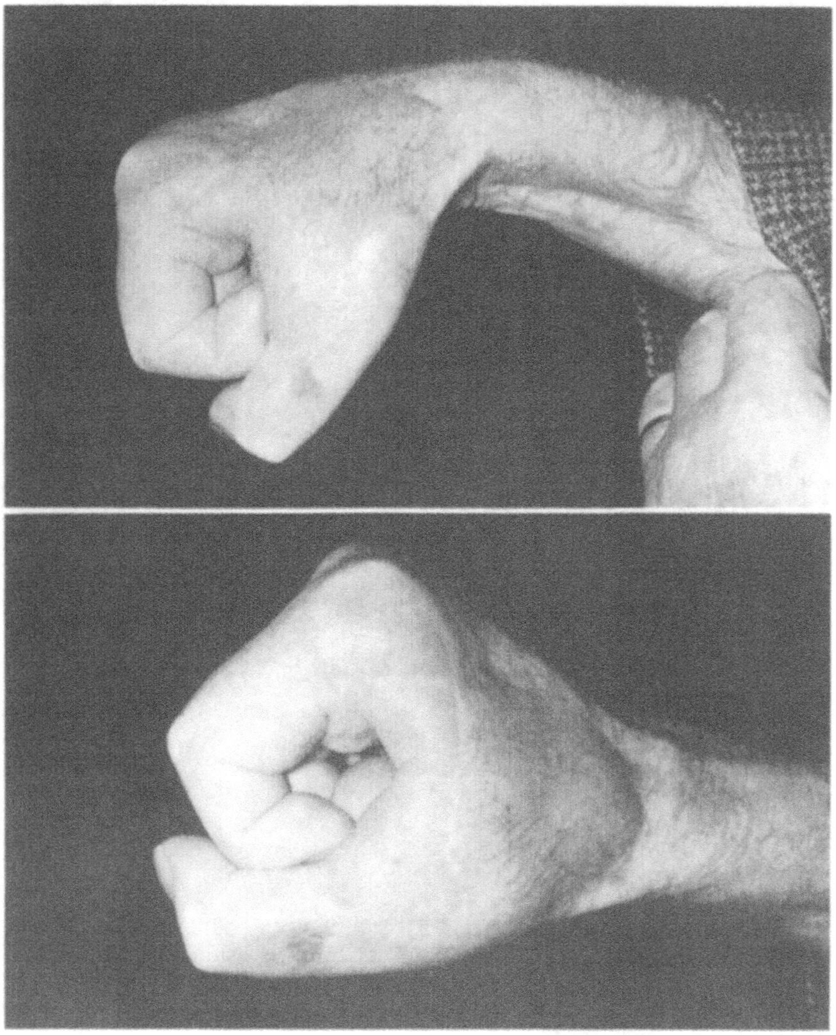

Fig. V.37. Previous case: range of movement at the wrist is 50°

effective, and causes little or no disturbance of carpal mechanics. The incision can be made in the anatomical snuffbox (bordered by the extensors pollicis longus and brevis and the distal radial border of the scaphoid); the trauma to both the nerve and the artery is trivial, and it is unnecessary to bare a large expanse of bone for orientation. A subsequent arthrodesis is always possible.

The 63-year-old man in Fig. V.38, handicapped by a severe STT arthrosis, rapidly recovered after an STT resection-arthroplasty. Six months later, despite the unencouraging radiological appearance (Fig. V.38b), he had recovered normal power and complete use of the hand. The grip strength here is now twice that of the opposite side, where there is no pathology!

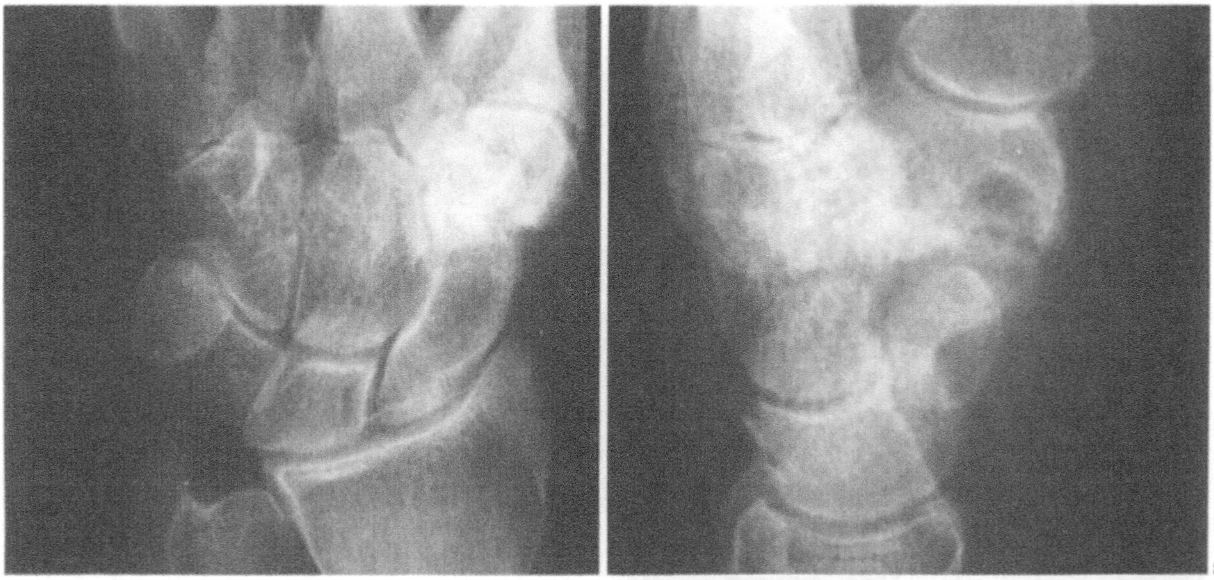

a

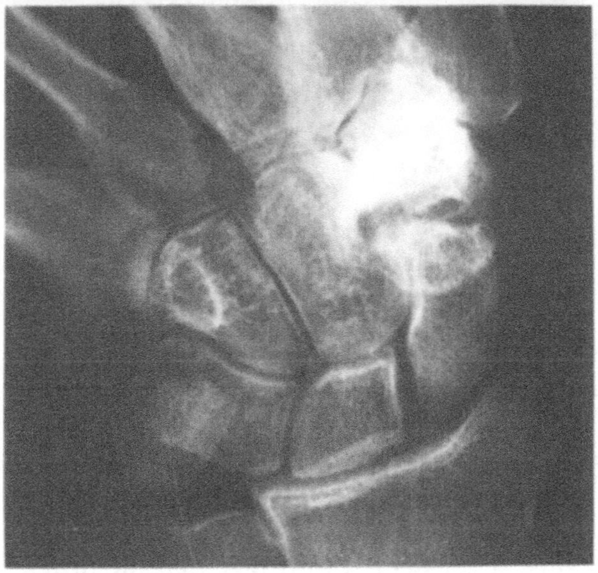

b

**Fig. V.38 a, b.** Resection-arthroplasty, an alternative to arthrodesis. **a** STT arthrosis with absorption cyst in trapezium. **b** After resection-arthroplasty, the X-ray appearance is not encouraging, but there is full movement at the wrist and normal power in the hand

*Dorsal Approach* (Fig. V.39)

This gives access to the lunate and the perilunar articulations to perform:

1. Ligamentoplasties between:
   (a) the lunate, scaphoid and capitate
   (b) the lunate, triquetrum and capitate
   (c) the lunate, scaphoid and radius
   (d) the scapho-lunate ligament and the radius
2. Arthrodeses between:
   (a) the scaphoid and capitate
   (b) the scaphoid and radius
   (c) the scaphoid, lunate and capitate
   (d) the lunate and capitate
   (e) the lunate and radius
   (f) the lunate, scaphoid and radius

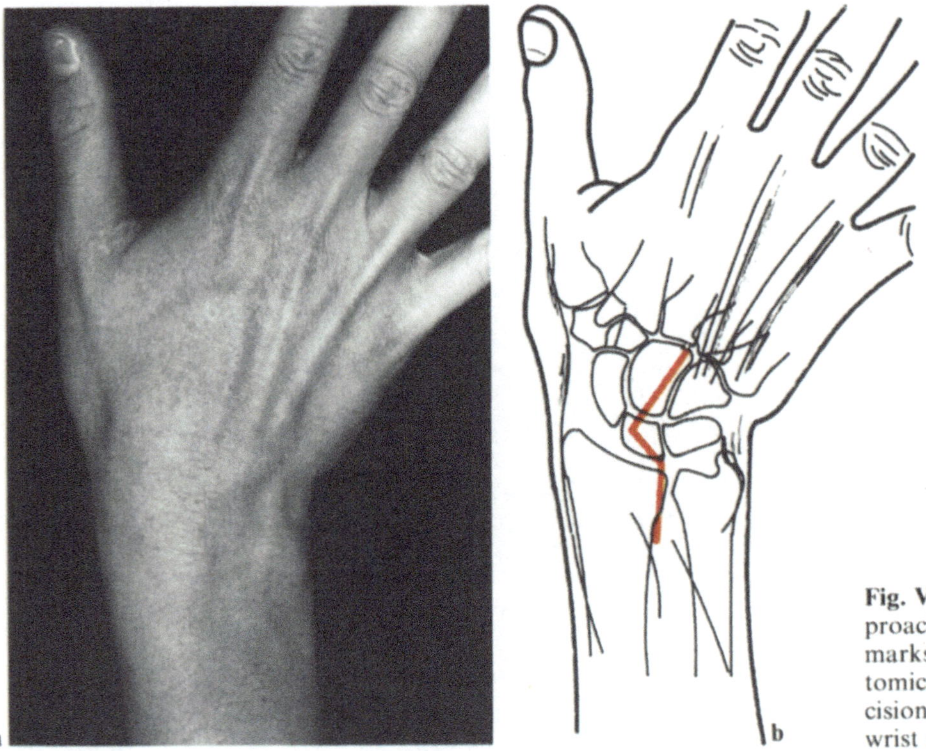

a b

Fig. V.39 a–d. Dorsal approach to carpus. **a** Landmarks. **b** Skin incision. **c** Anatomical features. **d** Line of incision in retinaculum and wrist capsule

It is unsuitable for arthrodeses or ligamentoplasties involving the triquetrum and hamate; in such cases a dorso-ulnar approach is required.

We have already detailed the approach to the distal radial epiphysis (Fig. V.3–V.6). For access to the carpus, it is enough to prolong the incision distally along the ulnar border of the extensor carpi radialis brevis, the tendon that gives entry into the carpal articulation (Fig. V.39d).

*Note.* It is essential to realize that the proximal pole of the capitate usually hides the dorsal pole of the palmar-subluxated lunate. The latter appears as soon as the wrist is placed in forced flexion. Also, before fixing the reduced lunate, the various articulations must be carefully inspected. The operative tactics are dictated by the anatomical lesions.

*Surgical Options*

*Intact radio-lunate articulation with DISI.* Reconstruction of the central column is performed by ligamentoplasty if the adjacent articulations are free from arthrosis, the patient is young, and the lesion limited (pre-operative diagnosis is essential).

Otherwise reconstruction is by arthrodesis of the central column, even in the presence of arthrosis of the radial compartment. The reduction of the lunate corrects the height of the carpus, decompresses the radial compartment and, despite the arthrosis, gets rid of the pain (see Fig. III.32a–c). Arthrodesis of the central

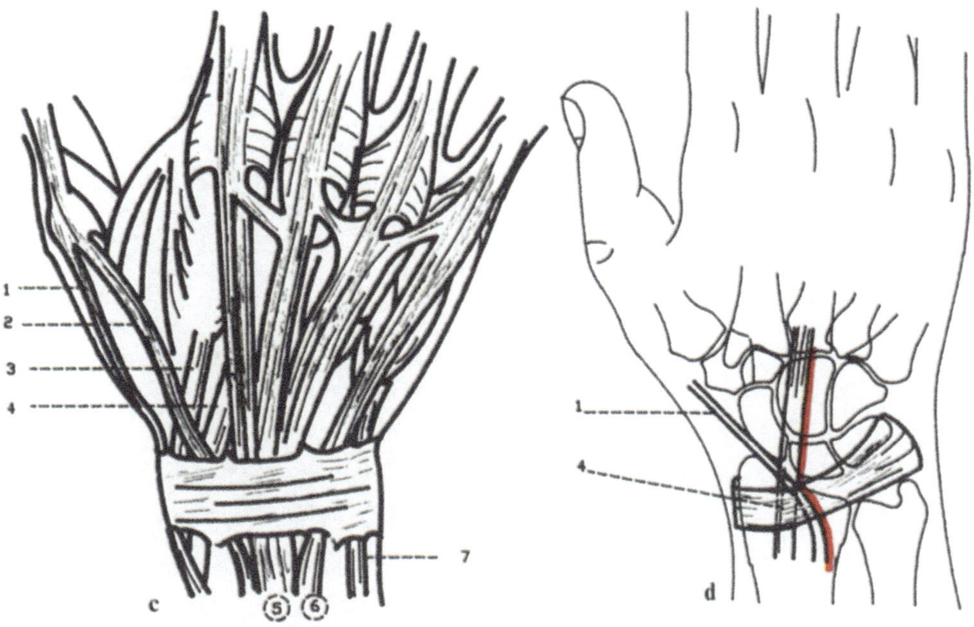


*1* EP brevis
*2* EP longus
*3* ECR longus
*4* ECR brevis
*5* extensor digitorum communis and extensor indicis proprius
*6* extensor digiti minimi proprius
*7* ECU

column primarily involves the lunate and capitate, but may include the triquetrum and hamate without affecting mobility. Including these two bones increases the contact area which simplifies the procedure and increases the union rate. The 47-year-old man with two plates, shown in Fig. V.40, has a painless left wrist, even with arthrosis, after resection of the proximal pole of the scaphoid, correction of the DISI and extended arthrodesis of the central column. The mobility will undoubtedly improve after removal of the osteosynthesis material.

*Arthrosis of the radial compartment, other articulations intact.* Treatment is by radio-scaphoid or radio-scapho-lunate arthrodesis. We have discussed two techniques (Fig. III.28 and Fig. III.29). That of Fig. III.28a can be criticized for not neutralizing the flexion forces. Use of the tension band principle seems essential to us. That is why, even if retrograde insertion of the screws is no longer done (because of distal articular embarrassment and poor proximal grip), we think it useful to offer this alternative. The screw protrusion is well tolerated, probably due to the minor residual mobility of the midcarpal joint. The rupture of the cerclage wire demonstrates the elasticity of the bone; but the arrangement has served its purpose perfectly, as demonstrated by the success of the arthrodesis.

*Lesion of SL ligament and DISI without arthrosis.* Ligamentoplasty is performed (see case S.F., Fig. IIIb, c). If the intraoperative X-ray shows inadequate scapho-lunate reduction, a supplementary palmar approach is imperative in order to stabilize the palmar poles of the lunate and scaphoid in the correct position. In young patients a partial arthrodesis should be done only in the event of obvious failure of the ligamentoplasty, or if there are extensive and complex ligamentous lesions.

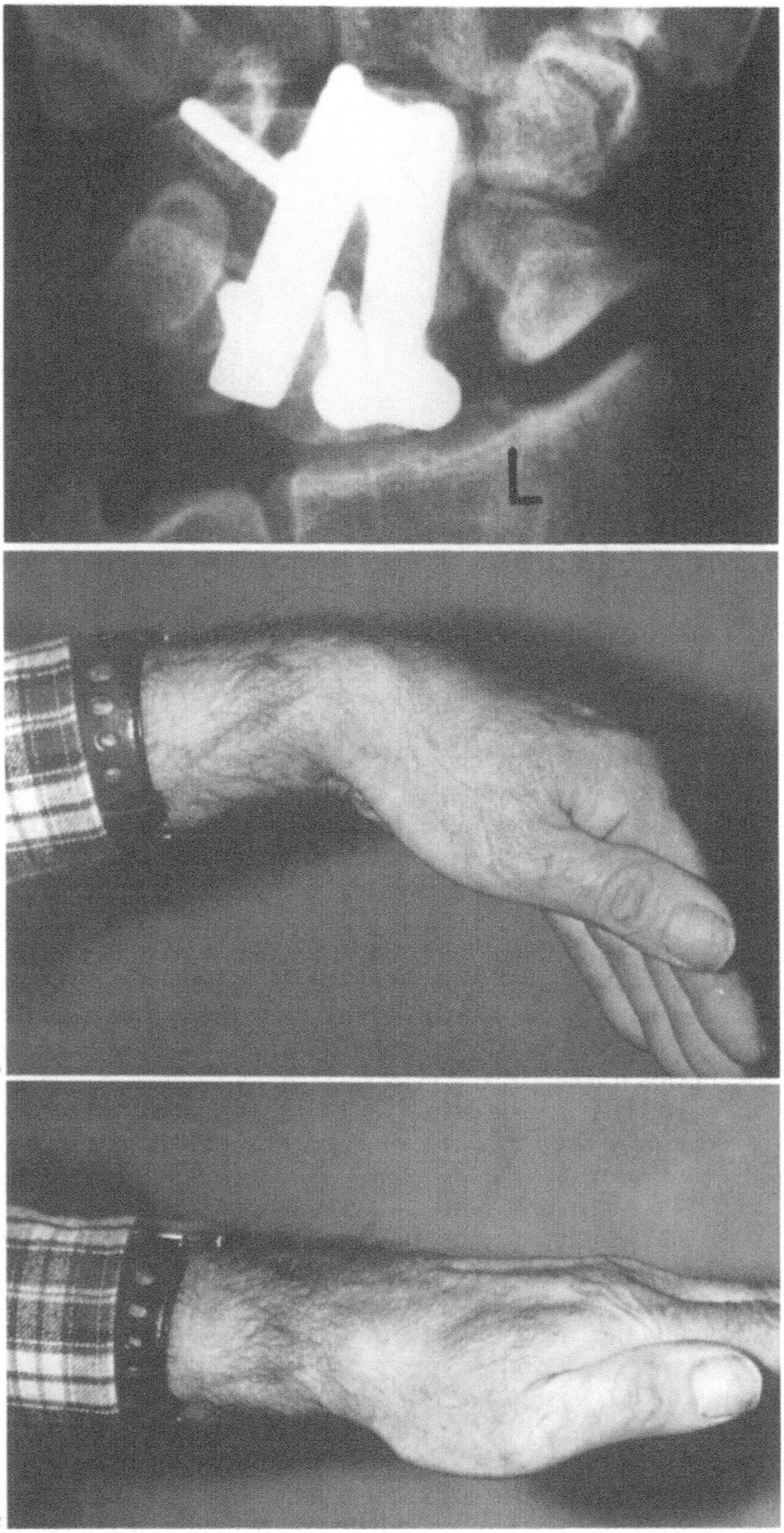

a
b
c

**Fig. V.40 a–c.** Lunate-capitate-hamate-triquetrum (LCHT) fusion: an alternative to capitate-lunate (CL) arthrodesis

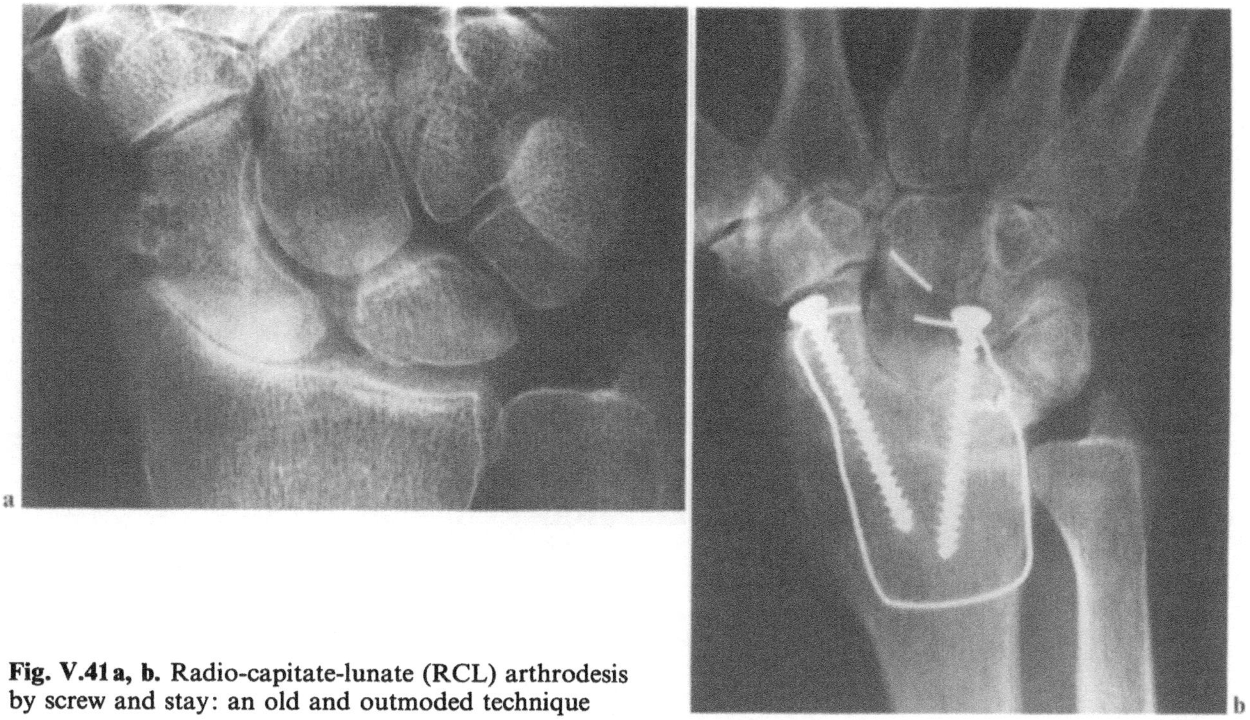

**Fig. V.41 a, b.** Radio-capitate-lunate (RCL) arthrodesis by screw and stay: an old and outmoded technique

*Old pseudarthrosis of the scaphoid, collapse and massive arthrosis.* Arthrodesis of the central column with reduction of the subluxated lunate is indicated. The scaphoid should not be interfered with; we have found the same results in patients with and without prostheses. We no longer perform resection of the proximal pole, as in the case shown in Fig. V.40.

*Note.* Styloidectomy alone is of no value; it treats a symptom and not a cause. The procedure weakens the distal V and the carpal collapse may progress. Symptomatic treatment is justified only in the absence of any possible treatment of the cause.

*Rheumatoid synovitis, ligamentous destruction and ulnar shift of the carpus.* Radio-lunate arthrodesis permits correction of the zig-zag malalignment produced by the carpal slipping. Our example (Fig. V.42), though imperfect, demonstrates the magnitude of the correction achieved (the metacarpal axis is comparable to that of the radius).

*Notes.*

1. We consider this arthrodesis to be contraindicated in post-traumatic cases (see also Fig. III.27c). A recent report by Linscheid and Dobyns (1985) supports this point of view. After five radio-lunate arthrodeses for traumatic lesions they reported two immediate failures and the appearance of a cyst in the proximal pole of the scaphoid in a third, an index of the abnormal constraints created. The authors' remarks support our working hypothesis, namely, that the intact ligaments disturb the free play of the other bones of the proximal

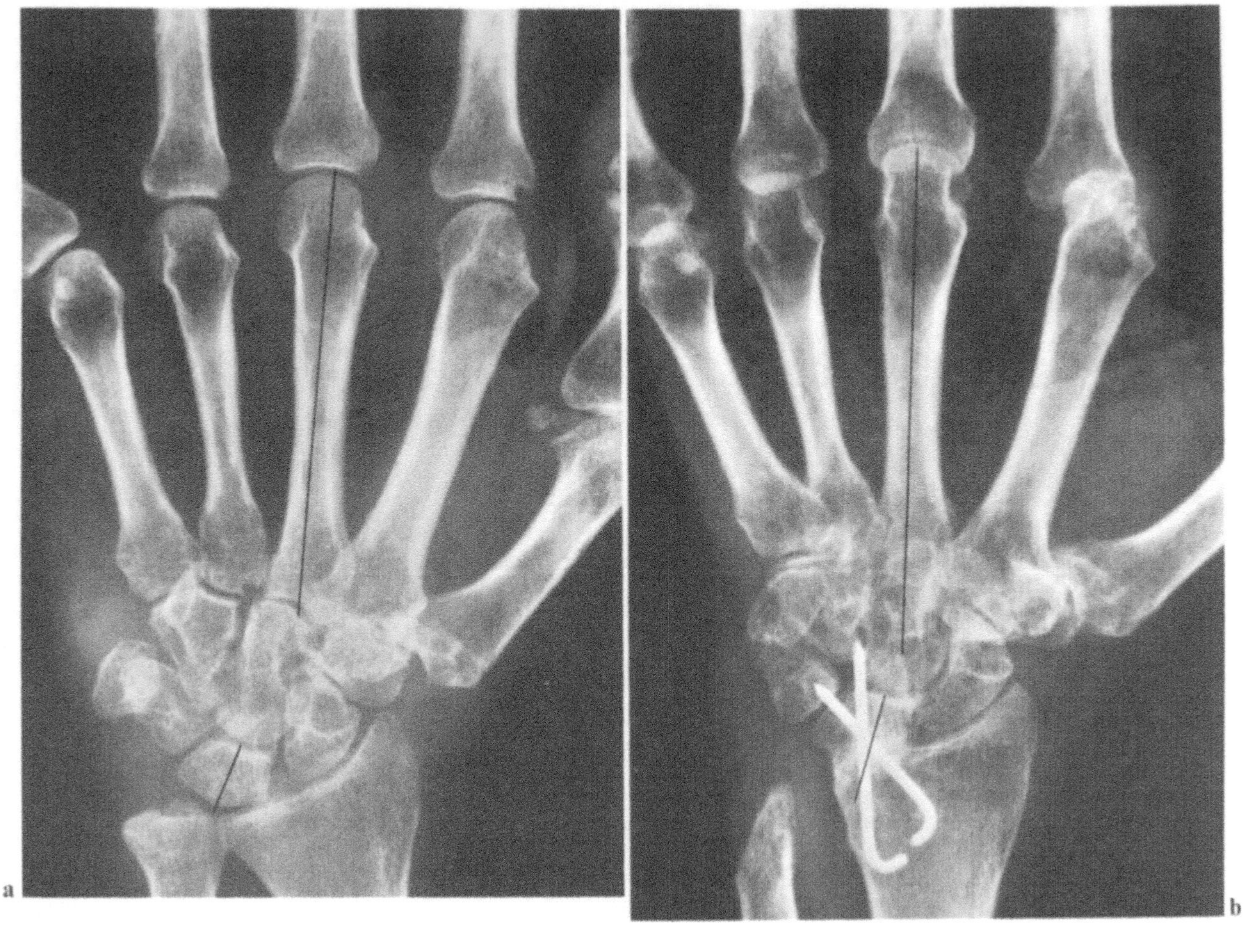

Fig. V.42. Radio-lunate (RL) arthrodesis, indicated in rheumatoid arthritis to correct and stabilize slip and to partially eliminate the zig-zag deformity

carpal row. The lunate also offers little support or stability for the capitate because of the opposing convex surfaces in the frontal plane.

2. No indication exists for scapho-lunate arthrodesis (see Fig. III.24).

*Dorso-ulnar Approach*

This approach (Fig. V.43) allows access to the triquetro-lunate and triquetro-hamate articulations. It involves opening the fifth and sixth compartments and defining the ulnar styloid and the ulnar border of the triquetro-hamate joint. From this articular margin access is gained into the articulation while preserving the dorsal capsular reinforcement of the triangular fibrocartilage. Once again, the treatment plan depends on the lesions found.

*Triquetro-lunate ligamentous lesions.* Arthrodesis is the most reliable solution (Figs. V.29 and V.44a), provided the scaphoid is correctly stabilized; otherwise, lunate-capitate (LC) fusion is preferable. The mechanics of the proximal row are not greatly disturbed, as evidenced by the relatively common congenital tri-

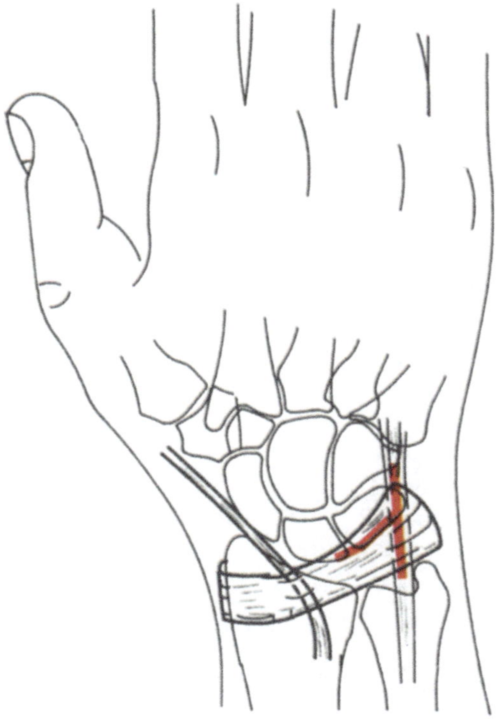

**Fig. V.43.** Dorso-ulnar approach to carpus: entry is via sixth compartment; creation of a flap of retinaculum and opening of fifth compartment is followed by opening of ulnar-carpal joint by incision along the proximal margin of triquetrum

quetro-lunate fusion. In the case in Fig. V.44b, in which the malformation was unilateral, function of the wrists was symmetrical.

The arthrodesis is easily performed with a cortico-cancellous graft and a Kirschner wire. The insertion of a screw is difficult and it may produce rotation of the triquetrum, disturbing the configuration of the mid-carpal articulation. In cases of bone tumour or infection, it is the extent of the tumour (or of the infection) that determines the size of the graft and the bones to be arthrodesed. Figure V.45 is an interesting example of this. It demonstrates the perfect integration of the graft with the passage of time and, above all, the residual mobility possible in favourable cases (Figs. V.45 and V.46).

*Triquetro-hamate lesions.* Ligamentoplasty is a good solution; the constraints are relatively minor, and the risks of secondary inadequacy of the plasty are low. This was our choice for V.F., aged 27 years, p. 77. Arthrodesis, though more difficult to perform, constitutes an excellent alternative and is imperative in the presence of arthrosis.

#### Piso-triquetral Arthrosis

This can be treated by resection of the pisiform or by piso-triquetral arthrodesis. We prefer resection, which gives rise to no detectable inconvenience.

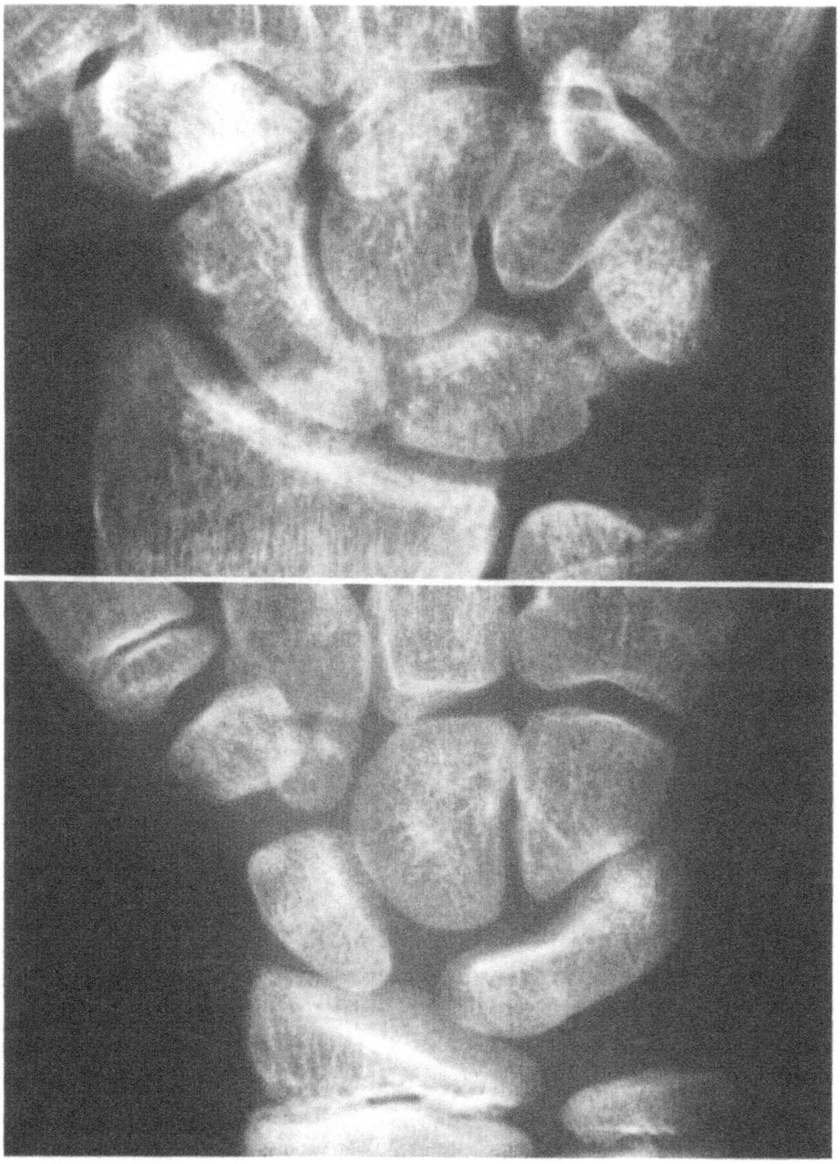

a

b

**Fig. V.44. a** Example of triquetro-lunate (TL) arthrodesis for instability. **b** Example of congenital TL fusion. The opposite side is normal; function is equal on both sides

## Skin Incisions

Regardless of the incision or approach selected, the same points of reference and the same technical problems occur. The important skin landmarks are: the radial styloid, the ulnar styloid, the radio-ulnar articulation and the second metacarpal.

The incision may be straight or zig-zag, with a step at the level of the articulation. A straight incision is advantageous with regard to blood-supply, but it must be long enough – at least 8–10 cm – to avoid any damage to the skin or nerves from retraction or ischaemia. It is centred on the snuffbox, the first web space, or the third or fifth metacarpal, as required.

The zig-zag incision gives a better view of the operative field, and if necessary the angles may be prolonged transversely. It

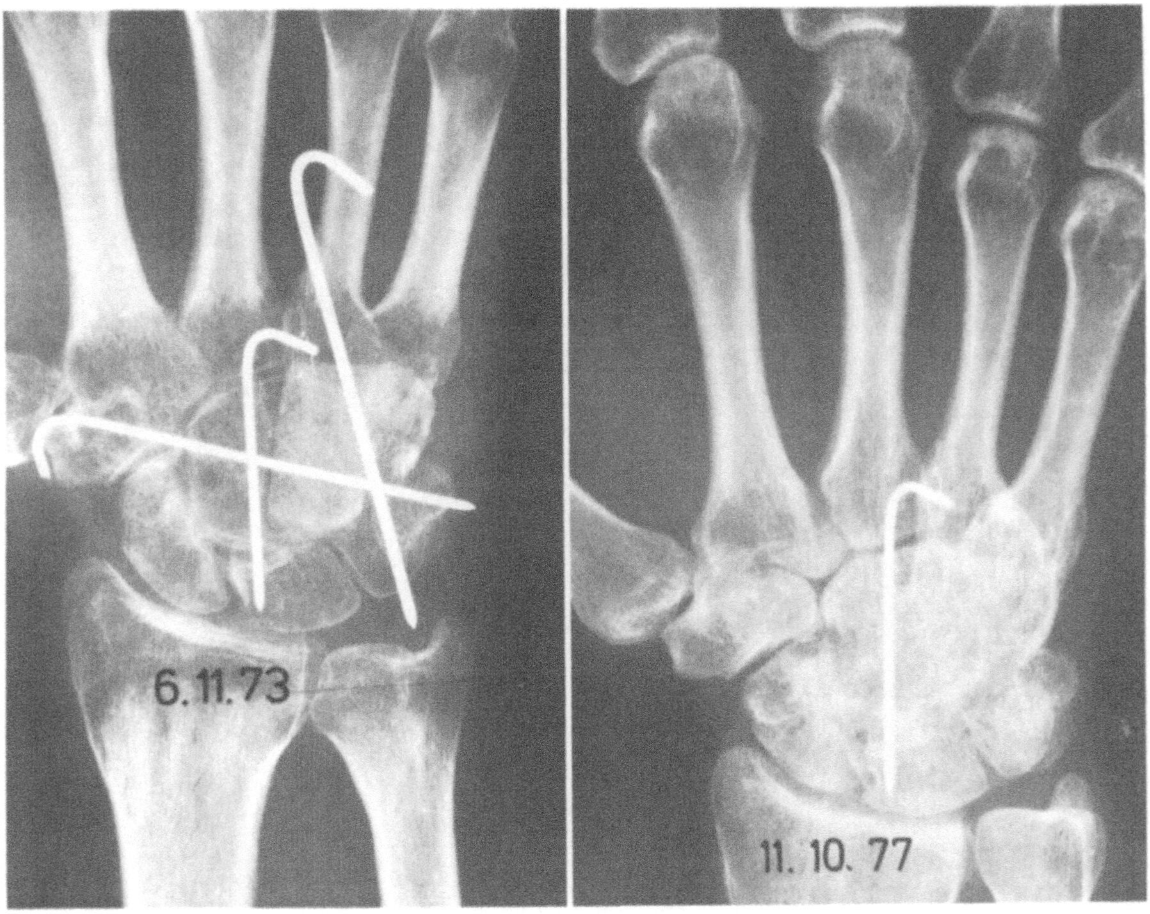

a b

**Fig. V.45. a** W.P., 28 years. This aneurysmal bone cyst of hamate was treated by resection and arthrodesis including capitate, hamate, triquetrum, lunate and fourth and fifth metacarpals. The large cortico-cancellous block is stabilized simply by the Kirschner wires. **b** Integration of cortico-cancellous graft in carpus

is definitely less favourable to the soft tissues, and skin necrosis is possible if the surgical dissection is not gentle.

The subcutaneous tissue must be incised down to the fascia. This implies that the course of the main cutaneous nerve trunks should be reviewed before each operation. The skin and subcutaneous tissue are elevated together so as not to damage the nerve branches and to reduce lymphatic damage (oedema) to a minimum.

In the radial approach, it is important to recognize the extensor pollicis longus and brevis and the branches of the radial nerve; the position, calibre and course of which are very variable.

## Conclusions

Though no hard and fast rules exist, it is possible to propose some therapeutic options based on the mechanics of the carpus, the anatomy, and clinical and surgical experience. We do not condone either the mutilating and irrevocable surgical procedure of bone resection or the more or less "useless" procedure of Silastic replacement; the first on mechanical grounds, the second because it is "dangerous" for physiological reasons: the Silastic crumbles and irritates, and the micro-particles liberated by fric-

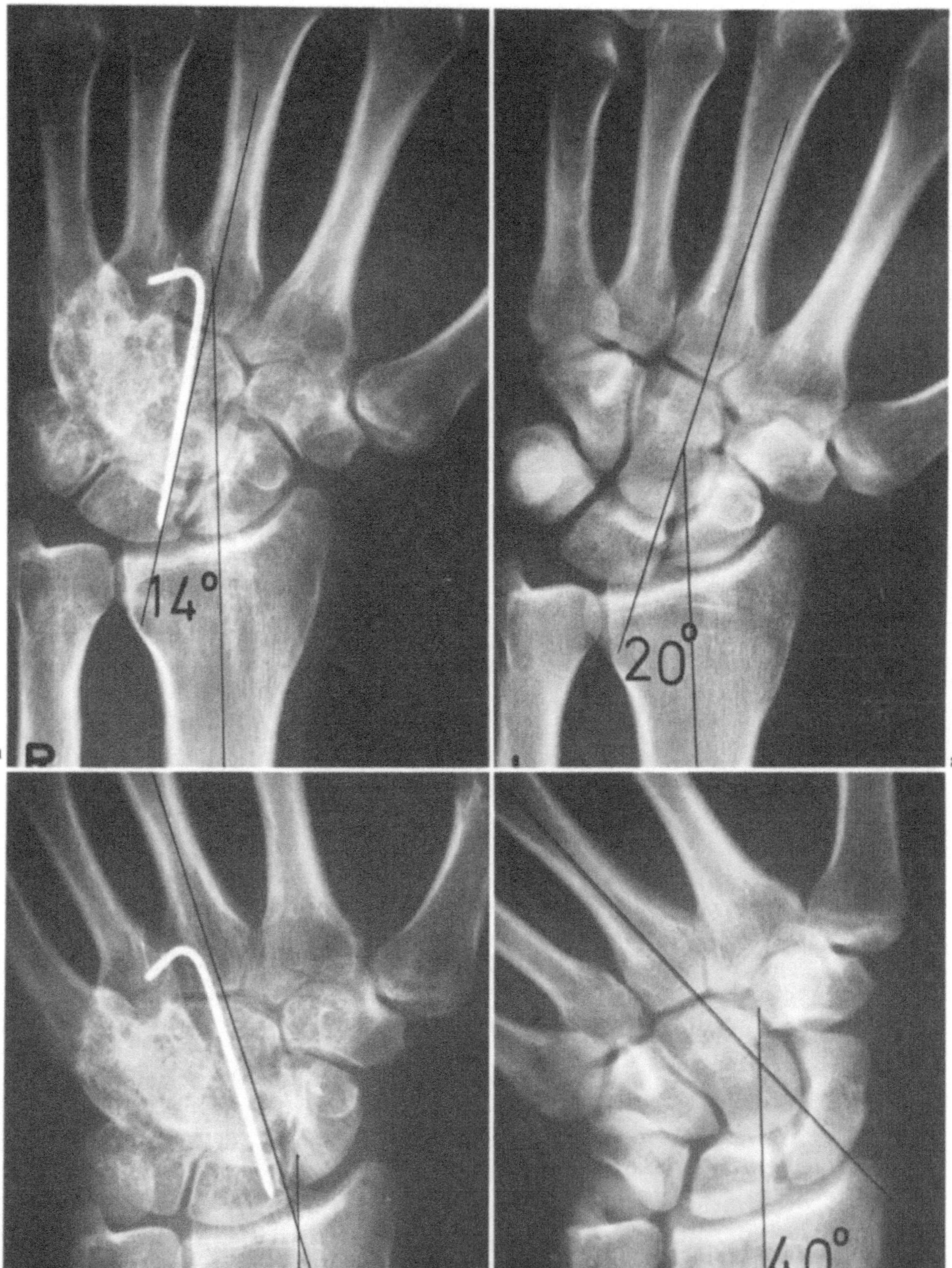


a¹ a²

b¹ b²

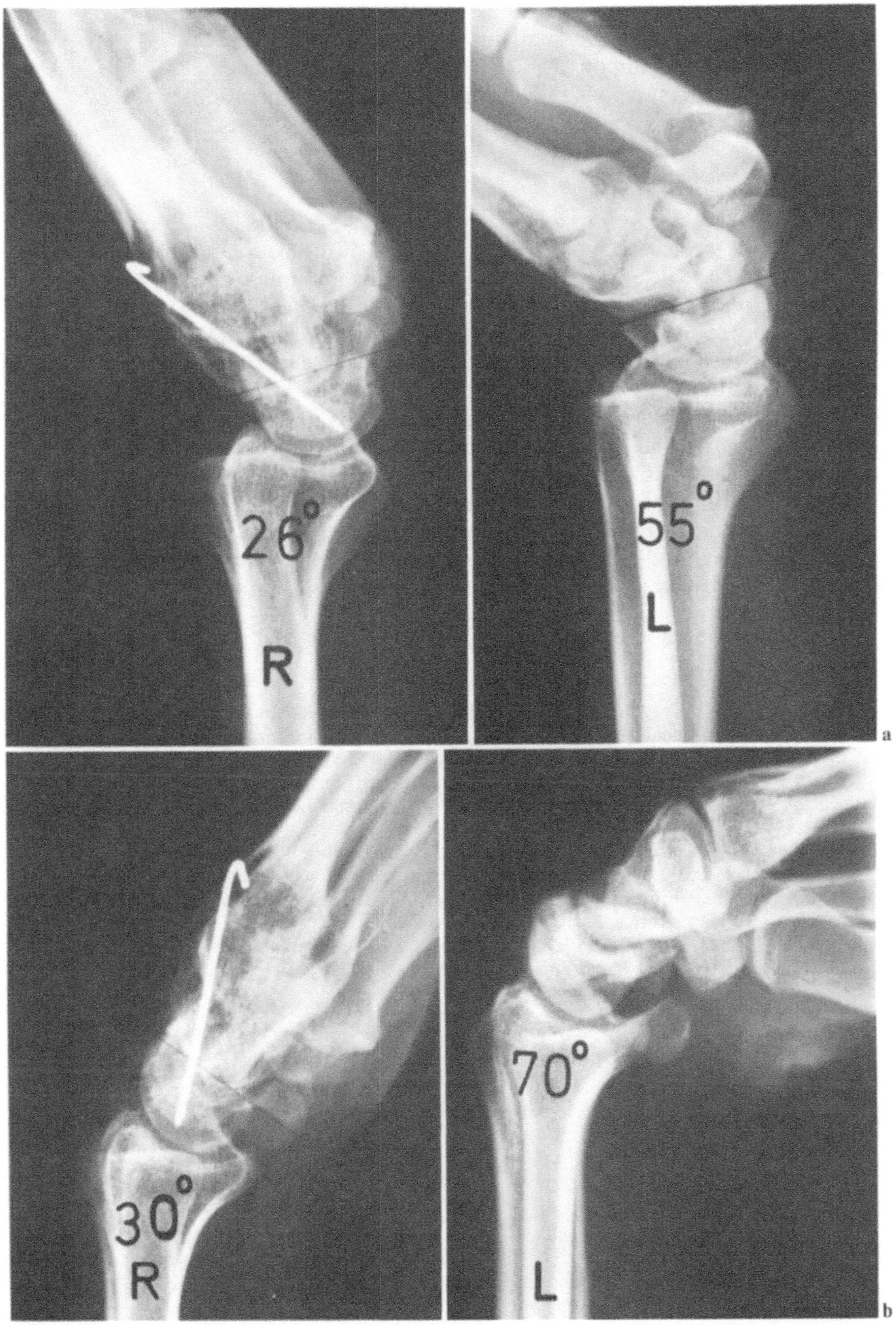


◁ **Fig. V.46 a, b.** Case shown in Fig. V.45, but 1 year after arthrodesis: AP films demonstrate wrist movement in frontal plane of operated side ($a^1$, $b^1$) compared with normal side ($a^2$, $b^2$). X-rays have been presented as mirror images to facilitate comparison. Mobility has been reduced by half

**Fig. V.47 a, b.** The same wrists are shown, but in lateral films. The range of flexion-extension is also reduced by half tion may pose a future hazard that is difficult to control. It is also important to warn the patient of the long convalescence ahead: it is not uncommon to take 1 year or more to become pain-free. The patient who is fully informed before the operation will be less likely to remind the doctor that surgery is not a panacea.

## Complications

Infections are treated classically by removal of all necrotic and infected tissue, the insertion of gentamycin beads and immobilization by external fixator (Figs. V.56 and V.57). Five weeks later one can proceed to a new partial or complete arthrodesis, either by using the external fixator or by performing a stable osteosynthesis.

Pseudarthrosis should be treated aggressively by a new graft, possibly extending the fusion to the adjacent bones, e.g. in the case of pseudarthrosis after lunate-capitate arthrodesis, one may consider including the triquetrum and hamate. The stability of the fibrous union means that a new mortice can be created under good conditions, and a stout cortico-cancellous graft inserted as for a Matti-Russe. Union is facilitated by 8 weeks' immobilization.

## References

Graner O, Lopes EI, Carvalho BC, Atlas S (1966) Arthrodesis of the carpal bones in the treatment of Kienböck's disease, painful ununited fractures of the navicular and lunate bones with avascular necrosis, and old fracture-dislocation of carpal bones. J Bone Joint Surg [Am] 48:767–774

Linscheid RL, Dobyns JH (1985) Radiolunate arthrodesis. J Hand Surg 10A:821–829

Pfeiffer KM (1982) Perilunäre, transskaphoidale, transkapitale Luxationsfrakturen (Naviculo-capitate fracture syndrome). In: Buck-Gramcko D, Nigst H (eds) Frakturen, Luxationen und Dissoziationen der Karpalknochen. Hippokrates, Stuttgart, pp 163–167

Watson HK, Ryu J, Dibella A (1985) An approach to Kienböck's disease: triscaphe arthrodesis. J Hand Surg 10A:179–187

## G. Arthrodeses of the Wrist

Even though total arthrodesis of the wrist is not commonly performed, it retains an important place in the modern surgical repertoire. It offers stability and pain relief for a good grip strength. Although a salvage procedure, it is sometimes inevitable, and must be perfectly mastered.

### Indications

1. Congenital disorders or Erb's palsy and possibly spastic hemiplegia[1]
2. Rheumatoid diseases (rheumatoid arthritis, systemic lupus erythematosus)
3. Idiopathic polyarthroses
4. Post-traumatic arthroses (in manual labourers)
5. Tumours
6. Infections (specific or otherwise)
7. Failure of partial arthrodeses
8. Loosening of prostheses[2]

### Operative Principles

The ideal position of the wrist must be defined for each patient. A dorsal approach is used to avoid nerve damage. As far as possible, the distal radio-ulnar joint should be preserved. Alignment of the axes of the second metacarpal and the radius (with slight ulnar deviation) is important. The tension band principle is utilized, the flexors being more powerful than the extensors. Rehabilitation should begin as soon as the wound has healed.

### Operative Technique

1. A straight incision, centred over the second web space, is made, and prolonged to the distal third of the radius (Fig. V.48). Care must be taken not to damage the cutaneous branch of the radial nerve at the level of the second metacarpal head if the incision has to be extended for arthrodesis with a plate as advocated by the AO (Müller et al. 1977; Fig. V.49).

---

1 In cases of spastic hemiplegia, arthrodesis should not be resorted to until after having exhausted all the possibilities of tendon transfer or elongation (Braun 1982).

2 We shall not discuss wrist prostheses, an extremely delicate subject. The number of prostheses is on the increase, but the results remain unpredictable, even in the best hands, and the life of the prosthesis is limited. Though their insertion is, and remains, a palliative procedure, it nevertheless manages to salvage several years of precious mobility. Those who undertake it must be able to undertake the responsibility of performing arthrodesis of the wrist under extremely difficult conditions, sometimes as a semiemergency if the dislocated prosthesis threatens the vitality of the skin.

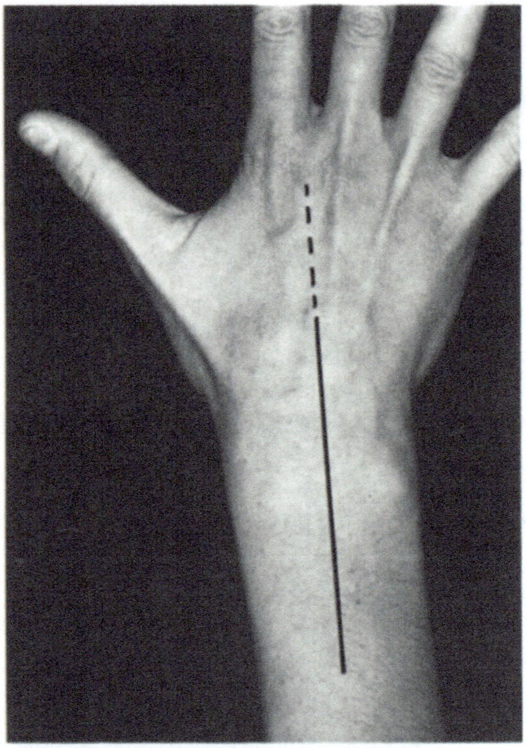

a

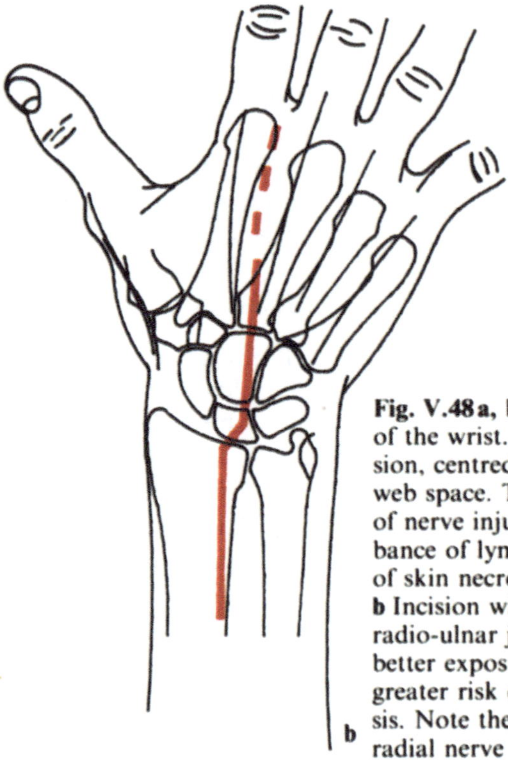

b

**Fig. V.48a, b.** Arthrodesis of the wrist. **a** Straight incision, centred on the second web space. There is no risk of nerve injury or disturbance of lymph flow; risk of skin necrosis is minimal. **b** Incision with step at radio-ulnar joint produces better exposure, but with a greater risk of skin necrosis. Note the branch of the radial nerve crossing the head of the second metacarpal

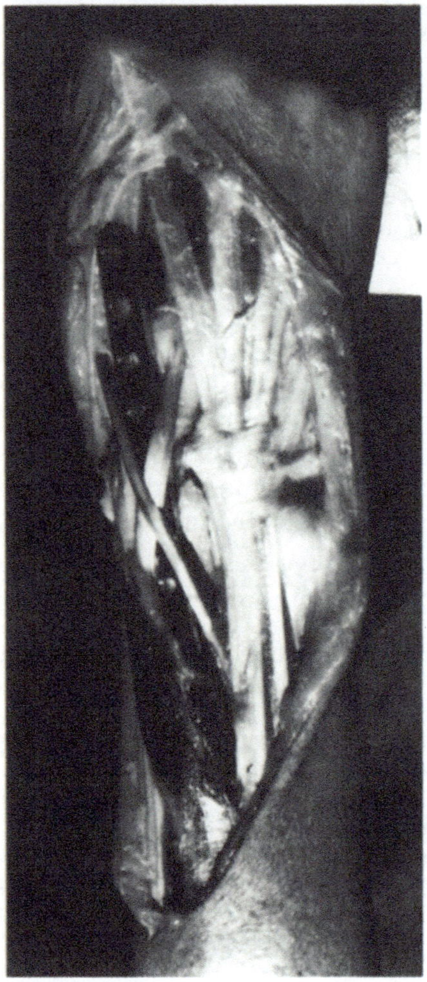

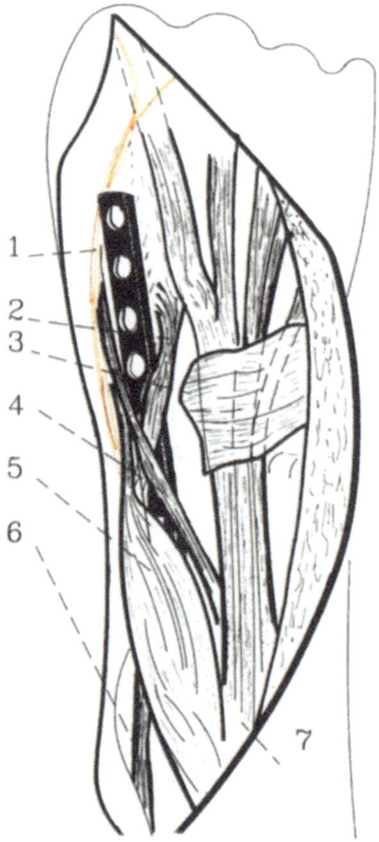


**Fig. V.49.** Arthrodesis with AO plate (3.5 mm screws). The radial wrist extensors are not resected, they shield the plate from the extensor pollicis brevis. The fourth compartment remains intact (in post-traumatic cases). The plate slides under the mass of muscles of the first compartment; watch for the branch of the radial nerve crossing the second metacarpal head

*1* cutaneous branch of radial nerve
*2* ECRB
*3* extensor retinaculum
*4* EPL
*5* EPB, APL
*6* ECRB and radial nerve
*7* EDC

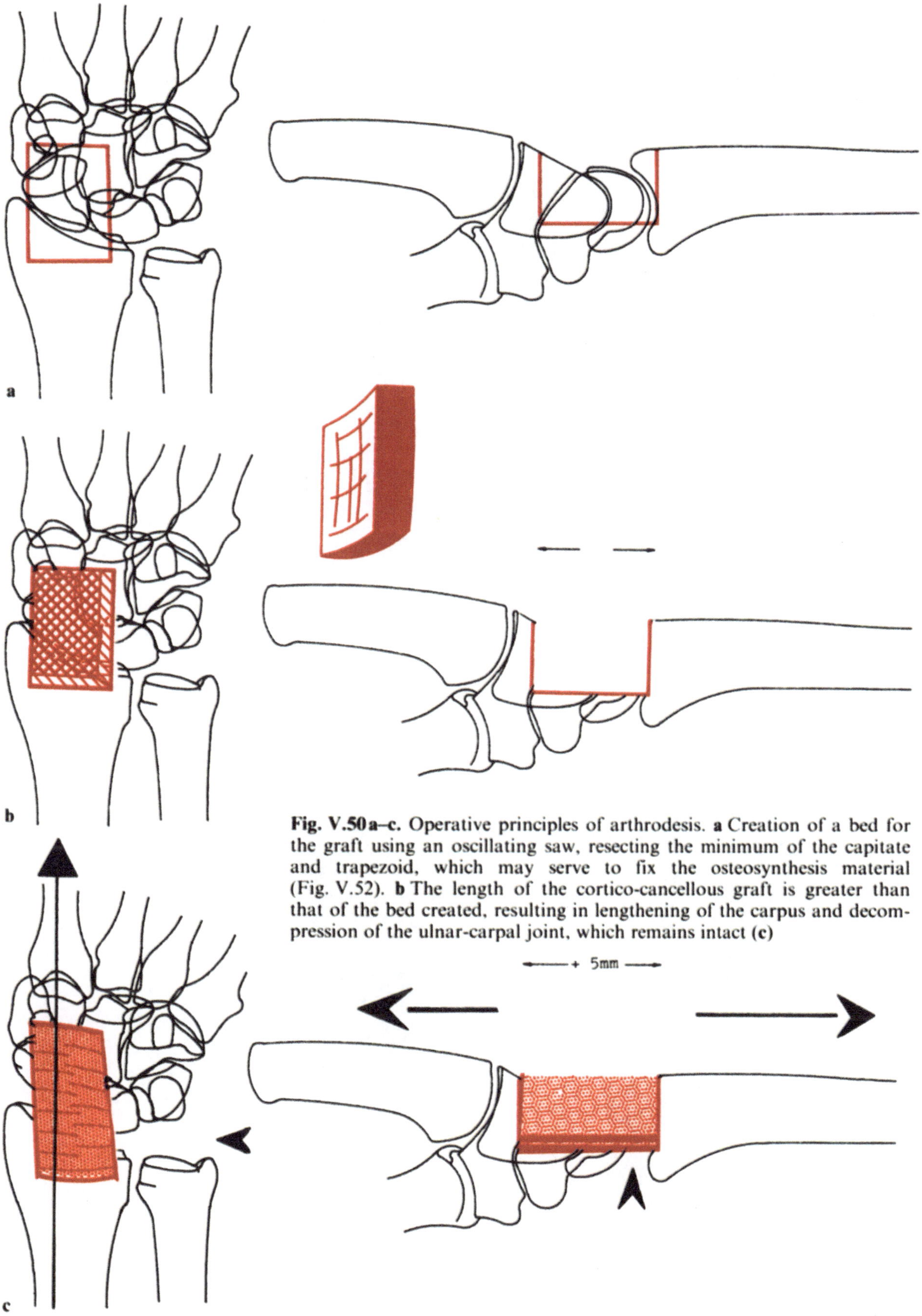


**Fig. V.50 a–c.** Operative principles of arthrodesis. **a** Creation of a bed for the graft using an oscillating saw, resecting the minimum of the capitate and trapezoid, which may serve to fix the osteosynthesis material (Fig. V.52). **b** The length of the cortico-cancellous graft is greater than that of the bed created, resulting in lengthening of the carpus and decompression of the ulnar-carpal joint, which remains intact **(c)**

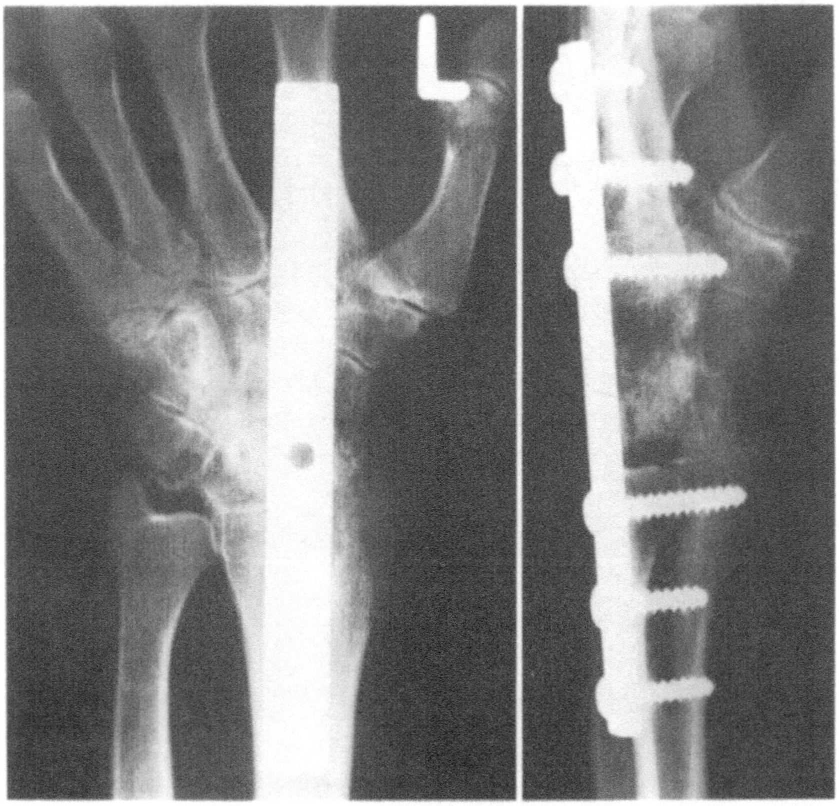


**Fig. V.51.** H.J., 58 years, polyarthrosis; example of stabilization with AO plate for 4.5 mm screws

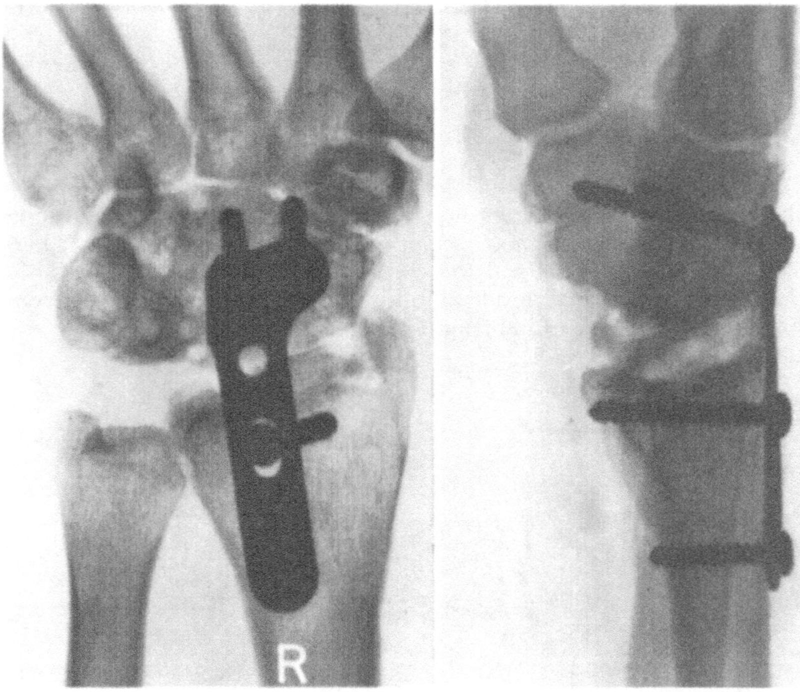


**Fig. V.52.** D.M., a 17-year-old mason; radio-carpal arthrodesis for arthrosis and weakness after failed Matti-Russe procedure. Decompression of ulnar-carpal joint was performed, and a T-plate (with ulnar flange cut off) fixed in capitate and trapezoid; the graft is clearly visible, it lengthens the carpus and decompresses the ulnar-triquetral articulation

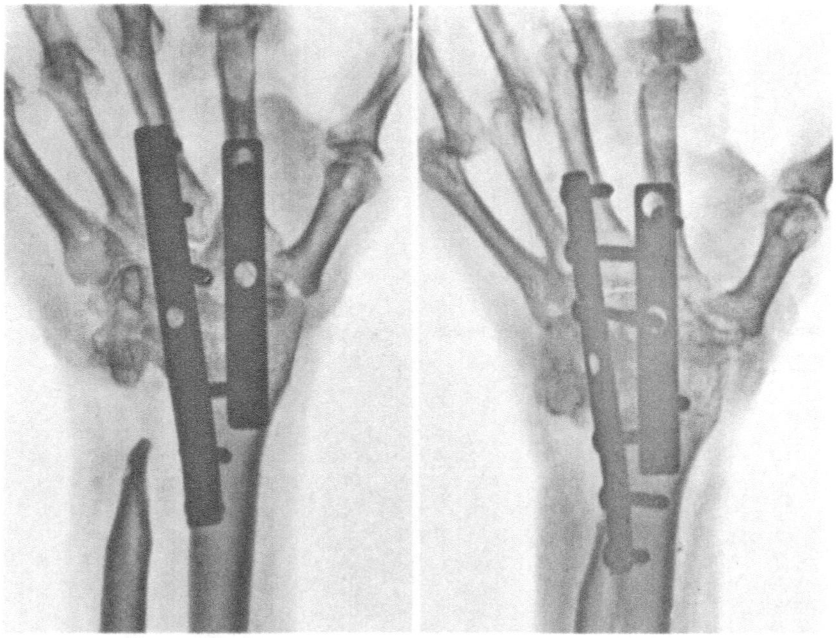

**Fig. V.53a, b.** N.B., 35 years, rheumatoid arthritis. Because of the demineralization, two third-tubular AO plates for 3.5 mm cortical screws were used. Instability and destruction of the radio-ulnar joint justified resection

2. The wrist joint is opened along the extensor carpi radialis brevis tendon.
3. Access to the radial epiphysis is gained via the third compartment, freeing the extensor pollicis longus (see also Figs. V.3–V.7). The extensor retinaculum is reflected en bloc to the ulnar side after Lister's tubercle has been shaved off; the common extensors are not exposed. On the radial side, the tendons of the two radial wrist extensors are isolated. They must be kept intact for two reasons: they originate at the distal humerus and contribute to elbow flexion, and they protect the extensor pollicis longus from the osteosynthesis material.
4. The thumb abductor group is identified, elevated and mobilized, so that the plate can be slid between the radius and this muscle bundle.
5. A bed is made for the graft with an oscillating bone saw (Fig. V.50a).
6. The graft is cut a little longer than the bed that has been dug, in order to decompress the radio-ulnar articulation (Fig. V.50b). A lengthening of 5 mm is enough.
7. The graft is inserted (Fig. V.50c), and the most suitable osteosynthesis material is chosen considering the size and muscularity of the patient, the degree of bone mineralization and any anatomical lesions. A large patient with well-mineralized bone and well-developed muscles will easily take a 4.5 mm plate (Fig. V.51). There should be no hesitation in fixing the implant to the capitate and trapezoid if the lesions permit, but the carpo-metacarpal joint should be preserved (Fig. V.52).

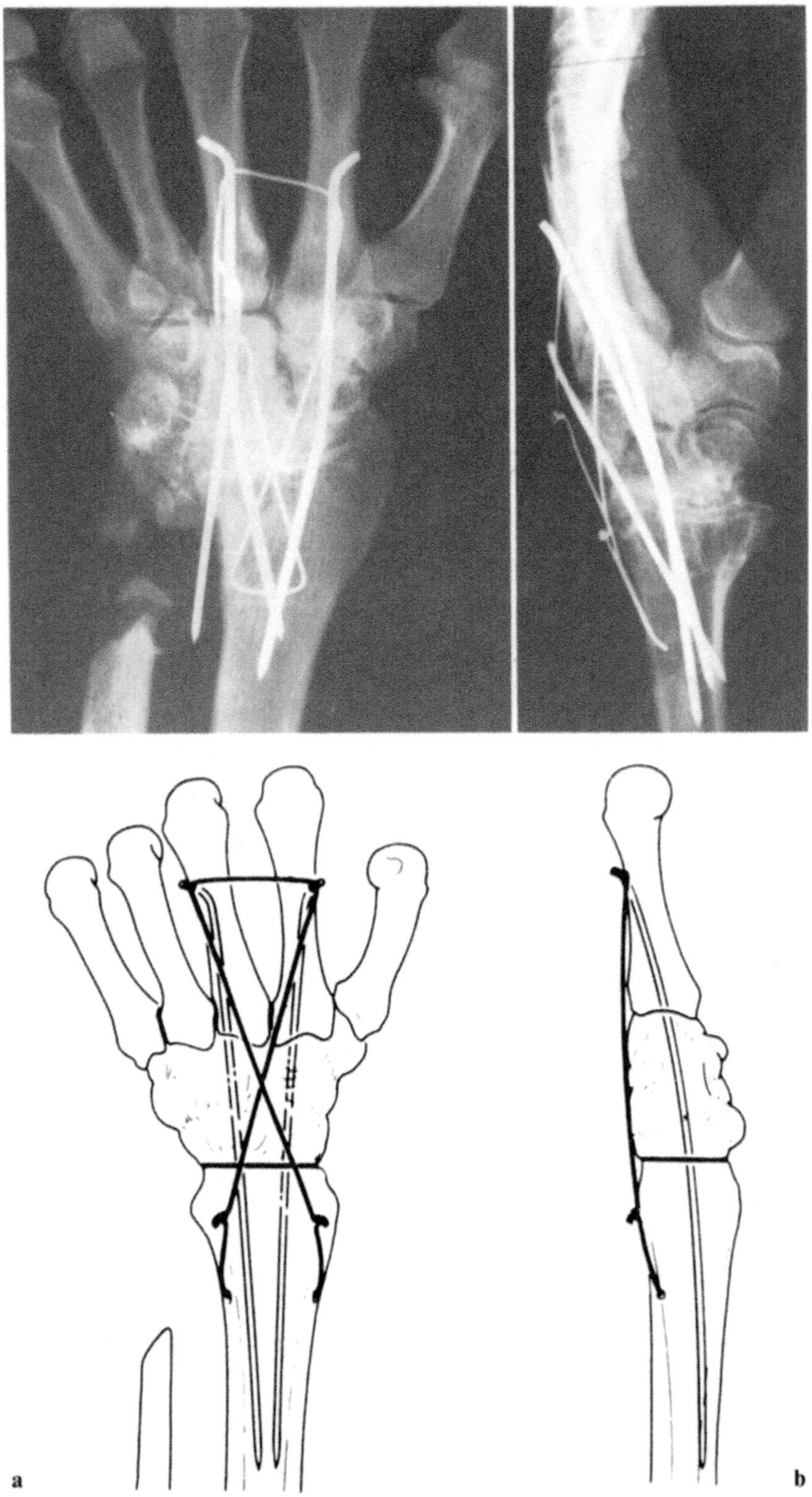

a b

**Fig. V.54a, b.** K.J., 73 years, post-traumatic arthrosis of carpus: status after Darrach's operation. **a** Fixation using tension band principle: diameter of pins 1.6 mm, diameter of wire 0.8 mm. **b** Note that the proximal anchorage of the wire is made in the cortex. If the quality of the cortex does not permit satisfactory fixation, the wire can be passed under the pins

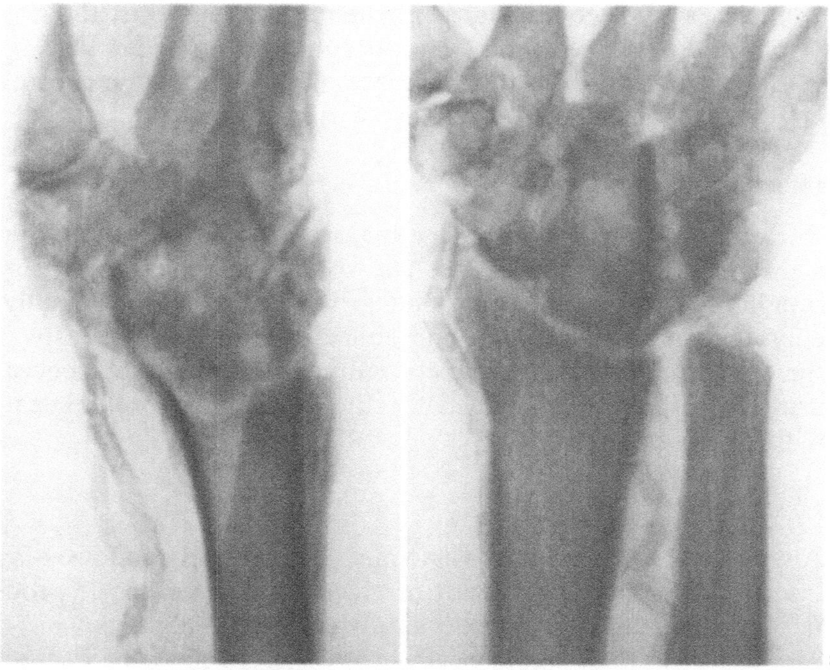

a

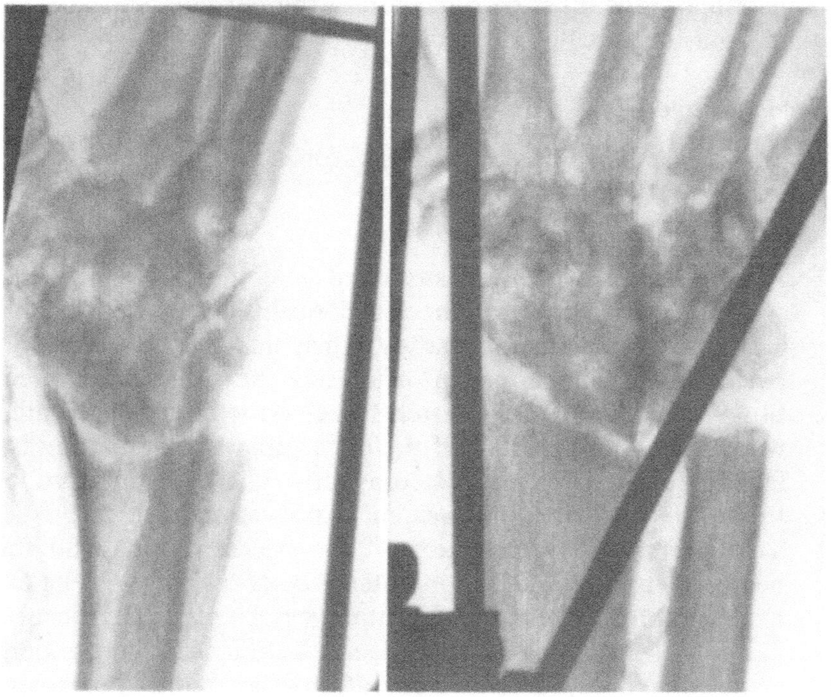

b

**Fig. V.55 a, b.** K.M., a 70-year-old diabetic: metastatic staphylococcal infection of unknown origin. **a** Debridement, stabilization by Jakob external fixator fixed in the radius and second, third and fifth metacarpal heads, as the infection involved their bases. **b** Cure with spontaneous fusion: as there is no graft, there has been shortening; the infected ulnar head has also been resected

In cases of osteoporosis, as in rheumatoid arthritis, the grip of the screws is dubious; various solutions are available, e.g. the use of two third-tubular plates (Fig. V.53), or anchoring by Kirschner wires and cerclage wiring (Fig. V.54).

### Infections of the Carpus

Regardless of the organism, the majority of cases call for total arthrodesis of the wrist, since the spread of infection is very rapid and easy, owing to the joint's ramifications. Occasionally, debridement and long-term immobilization may suffice, as was the case in a 70-year-old diabetic suffering from staphylococcal arthritis (Fig. V.55), but, usually, the problem has to be dealt with in two stages.

#### *First Stage*

All infected or necrotic tissue must be debrided followed by insertion of gentamycin beads or an analogous antibiotic product. Immobilization is by external fixator, for 3–5 weeks.

*Note.* Anchorage must be done *before* the debridement and *remote* from the focus of infection.

#### *Second Stage*

Arthrodesis is performed, using an *autogenous* graft.

### Examples

1. A 20-year-old workman sustained a complex, compound, comminuted fracture of the distal radius in a car accident. The primary treatment was by Rush nail for the ulna and plaster immobilization. Unfortunately the subsequent infection was not recognized. After 8 weeks, the patient presented with (Fig. V.56) necrosis of the distal ulna and spreading infection along the shaft, osteomyelitis of the distal third of the radius (with a "moth-eaten" appearance) and arthritis. Treatment was by: resection of the necrosed ulna and the necrosed, infected radius; maintenance of length with the external fixator; insertion of gentamycin beads; skin closure, palmar plaster splint and systemic antibiotics. The patient went home 3 days after the operation, and returned to hospital 4 weeks after debridement for removal of the gentamycin beads and reinforced autogenous (pelvic) bone graft, fixed with a 3.5 AO plate. He was discharged on the 10th day, the wounds healing uneventfully. Figure V.56d shows the range of pronation and supination and the quality of the skin cover. However, the patient has not been able to resume normal work because of the residual instability of the ulna, which we have been unable to control, despite a ligamentoplasty. This example explains our lack of enthusiasm for the Sauvé-Kapandji operation.

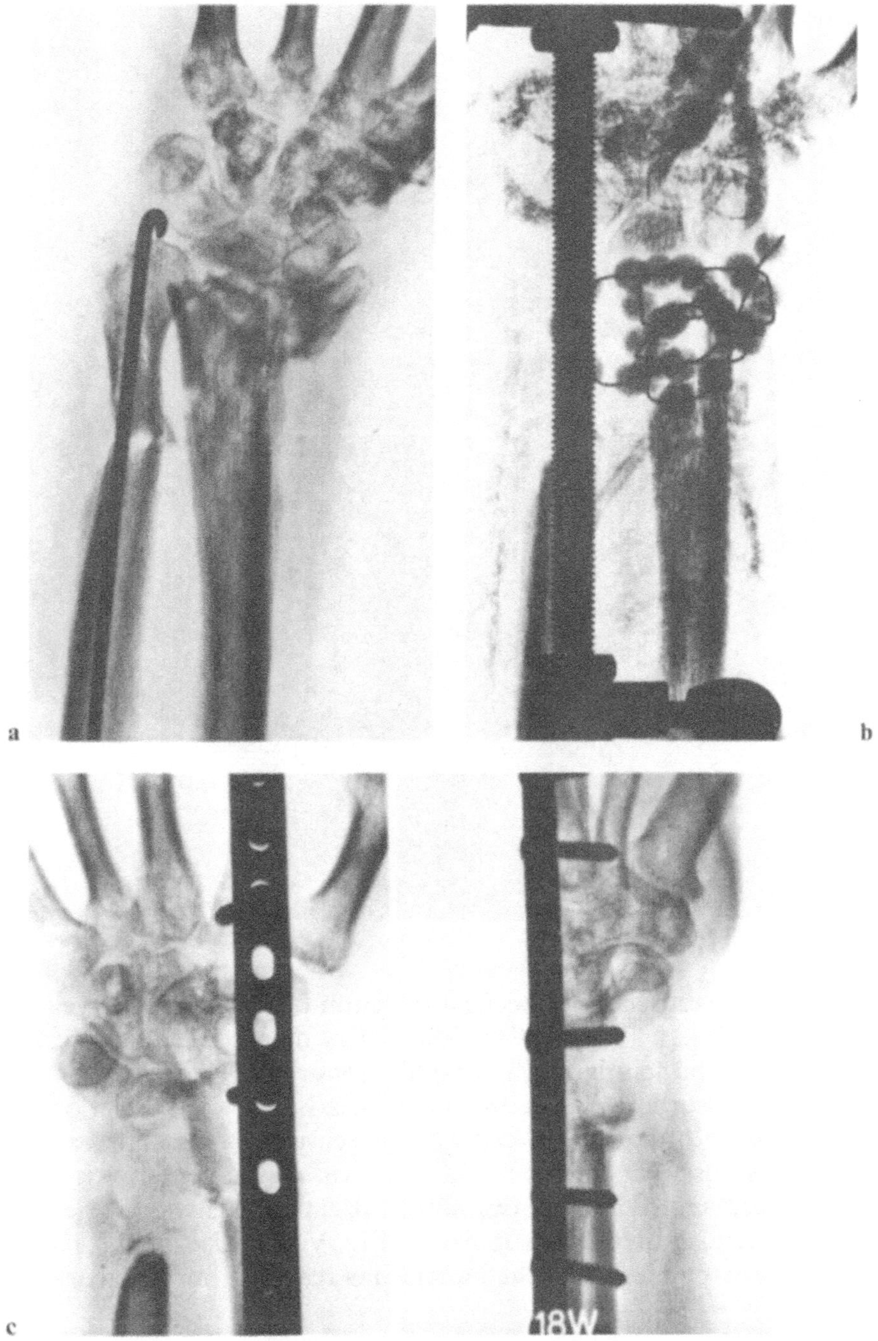


**Fig. V.56 a–c.** S.A., a 20-year-old mechanic, typical example of treatment of carpal infections. **a** Deformation of radial epiphysis, infection of distal radius (" moth-eaten" appearance, with patchy erosion and sclerosis), infection and necrosis of distal third of ulna. **b** Debridement and resection of all necrotic tissue, insertion of gentamycin beads. **c** Radiograph 18 weeks after cortico-cancellous bone graft combined with rigid fixation

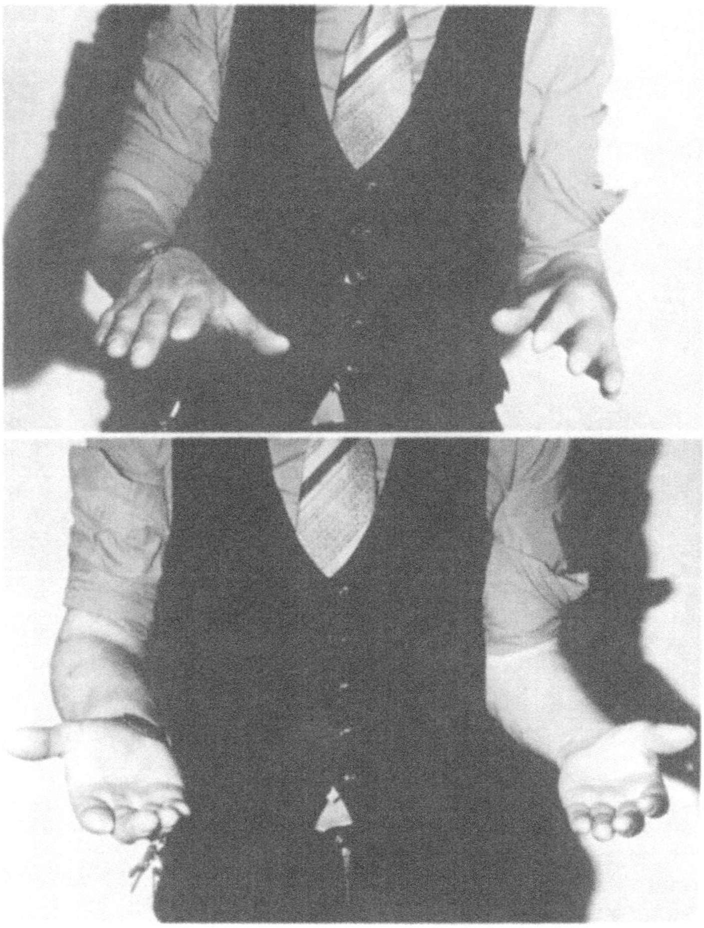

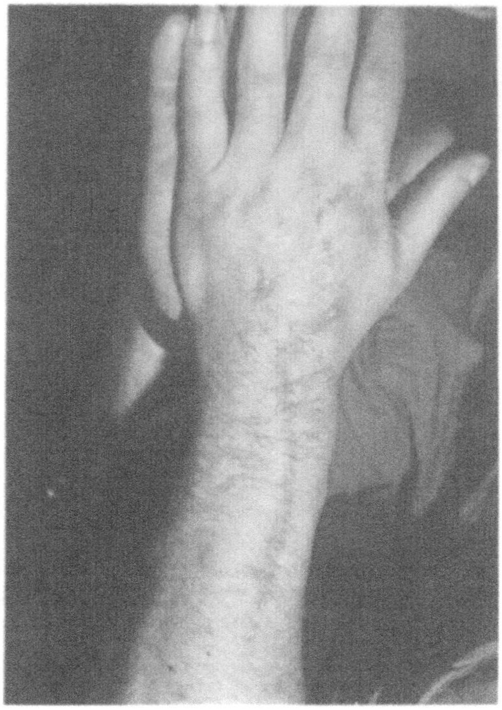

**Fig. V.56d.** Function and skin coverage at 1 year, but disabling instability of distal ulna

2. Metastatic staphylococcal infection occurred in a 60-year-old workman (Fig. V.57a). There was marked demineralization and the scintigram was highly abnormal. Here, again, it was necessary to resect the ulnar head, but this resection was made obliquely, in order to preserve the ligaments as much as possible. After 4 weeks, removal of the gentamycin beads and arthrodesis by two third-tubular plates was carried out, because of the osteoporosis (Fig. V.58). Use of the hand is now painless, and the patient has resumed normal work.

**Remarks**

The osteosynthesis does not necessarily have to include the second metacarpal, for it is then not uncommon to observe troublesome residual pain at the second carpo-metacarpal joint. The 4.5 mm screws and plate are not used routinely, only in large powerful men. The size of the plate and the diameter of the screws make their use tricky, with a risk of metacarpal fracture. The 3.5 mm screws and plate are normally used.

Compression must be done with care or the radio-ulnar joint can be damaged; this requires a graft that is sufficiently resistant and correctly shaped. Otherwise the compression should be dis-

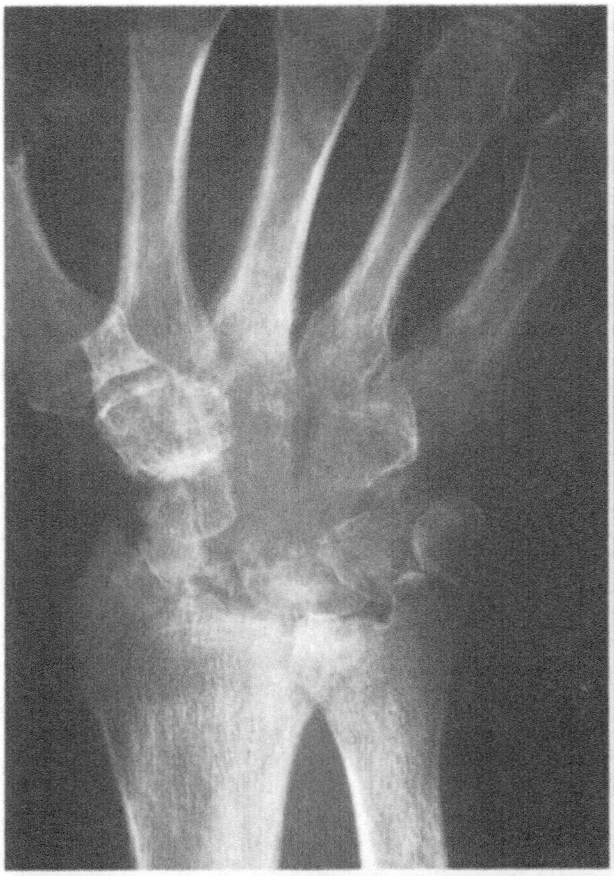
a

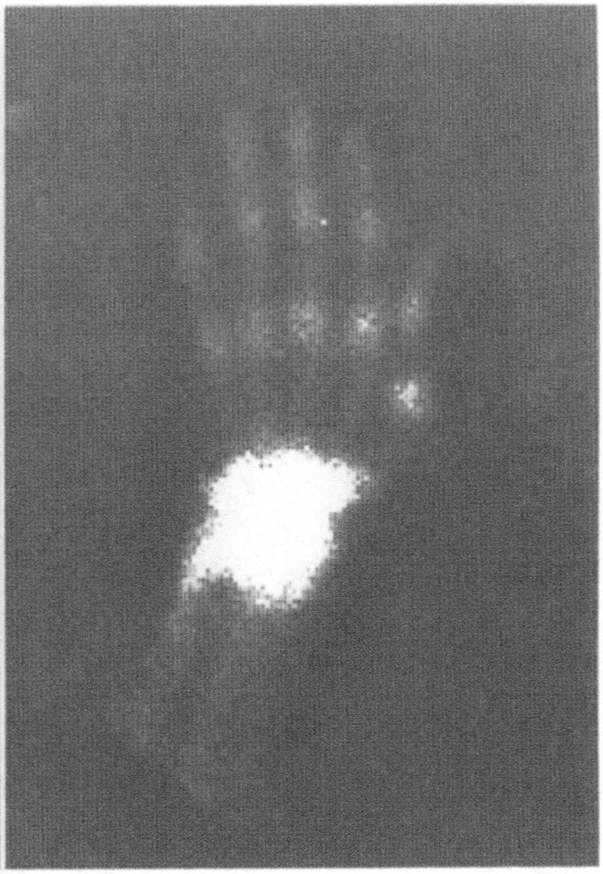
b

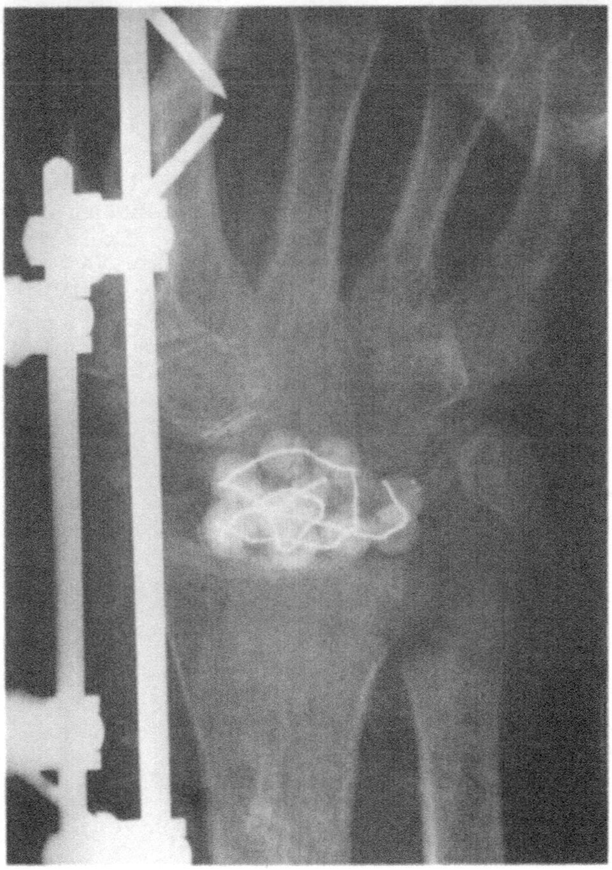
c

**Fig. V.57a–c.** F.A., 60 years, infection of carpus after contused wound and tendon suture. **a** Obvious osteolysis; **b** corresponding scintigram; **c** first stage of treatment: debridement, gentamycin beads and stabilization by Jakob external fixator; **d** cure after reinforced graft using two third-tubular AO plates

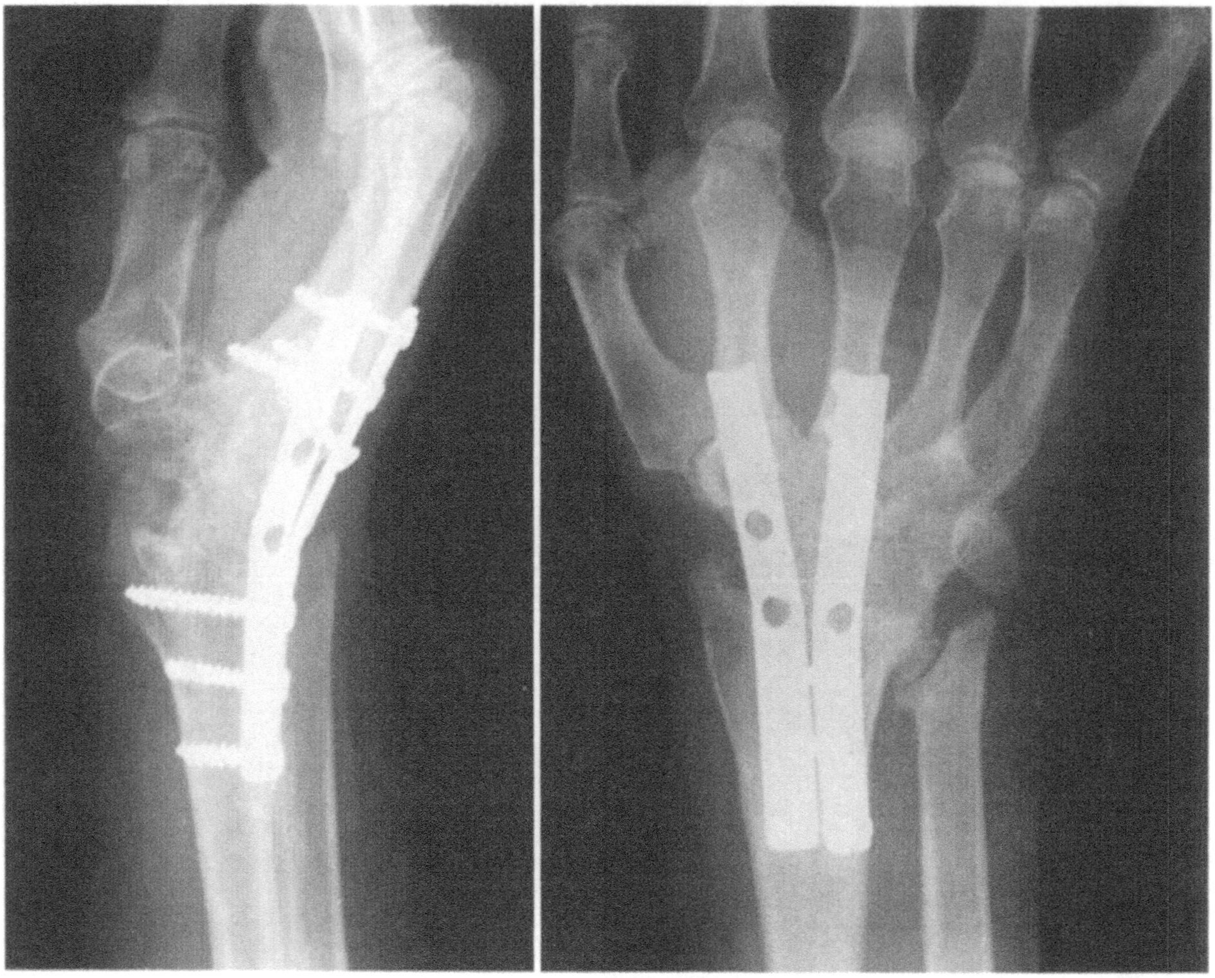

Fig. V.58. Cure after arthrodesis by two third-tubular plates

pensed with. The external fixator should be reserved for infections. It has no particular advantages, since the area is exposed anyway, and the cumbersome apparatus requires scrupulous daily care. Though our examples include numerous resections of the distal ulna, this is no longer done except for rheumatoid cases with the articulation destroyed by the disease, or in cases of infection when resection forms part of the debridement of infected tissue. The technique of Mannerfelt (1972), though useful and practical in the rheumatoid patient, does not appeal to us in the post-traumatic case. It does not permit preservation of the distal radio-ulnar joint or a refined choice of the most satisfactory position of fixation.

## References


Braun RM (1982) Rehabilitation. In: Green DP (ed) Operative hand surgery, vol 1. Churchill Livingstone, New York, pp 195–211

Mannerfelt L (1972) Nouvelle technique d'arthrodèse du poignet pour le traitement des arthrites rhumatoïdes. Rev Chir Orthop 58:471–480

Müller ME, Allgöwer M, Schneider R, Willenegger H (1977) Manual der Osteosynthese AO-Technik. Springer, Berlin Heidelberg New York, pp 387

## H. Fractures of the Radius

The treatment of fresh fractures must be distinguished from that of malunion. The aim of treatment is simple: to restore the anatomy and maintain the reduction. Though reduction is relatively easy, it is difficult to maintain (see p. 145 and the classification by mode of treatment, Table IV.15, p. 138). We shall analyse in sequence the problems of:

1. The unstable monoblock fracture (epiphysis intact = metaphyseal fracture)
2. The marginal fracture (or split epiphysis = epiphyseal fracture)
3. The comminuted fracture (or multifragmented epiphysis)

### Unstable Monoblock Fracture

In the chapter on distal radius fractures we determined that only a minority of fractures can be treated by simple plaster splintage. The main problem is the instability of the epiphyseal segment because of the gap, either absolute (crumpling) or relative (shattering), created by reduction. This "fracture gap" explains the difficulty in maintaining the reduction. Bony cohesion is not re-established, despite the osteosynthesis, and the metal bridges the "gap" (bridge plate). The functionally conditioned forces have to be taken on by the metallic implant alone, without any aid from the bone. Therefore it is illusory to try to use the tension band principle. Furthermore, the palmar cortex of the epiphyseal block is extremely thin (Fig. V.59), and does not guarantee safe support. As a result, all dorsal fixation, whether by external fixator or by plate, amounts to suspending the epiphyseal segment from the radial diaphysis. The cancellous segment does not provide a reliable grip for the OS material, so ancillary stabilization is desirable in every case. How long depends on the magnitude of the gap, the quality of the bone itself and whether a cancellous graft was used.

The palmar plate plays a double role: it provides fixation and support. However, it is considerably more risky because of the surgical exposure (compared with those encountered in the application of the external fixator) and therefore used only in patients who cannot tolerate an external device.

In conclusion, the treatment of choice for an unstable monoblock fracture remains the external fixator. Osteosynthesis is used only in exceptional cases preferably with a cortico-cancellous bone graft to ensure a stable osteosynthesis. In young patients, as the quality of the bone guarantees fixation, osteosynthesis is also a practical alternative.

*Treatment*

This must be directed towards restoring the anatomy of the radio-carpal and distal radio-ulnar joints. The stages are as follows (Fig. V.59):

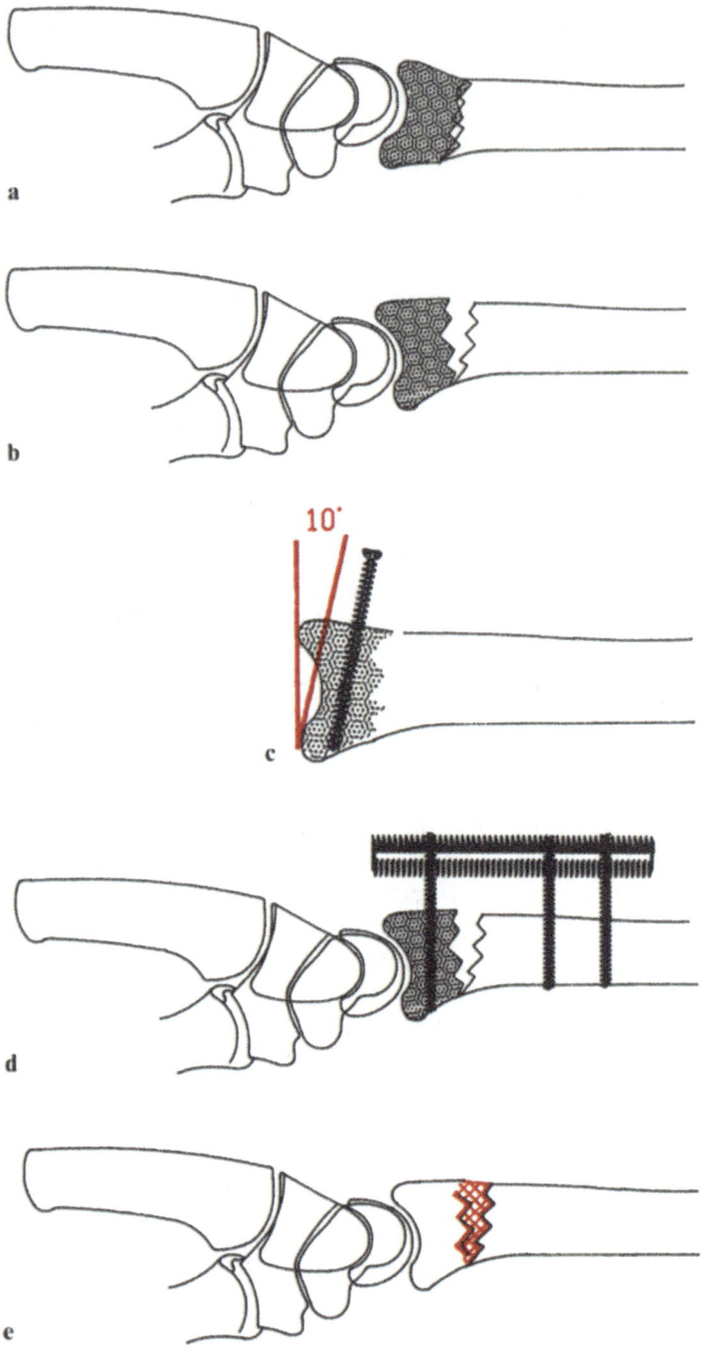


**Fig. V.59 a–e.** Principle of treatment of monoblock fracture

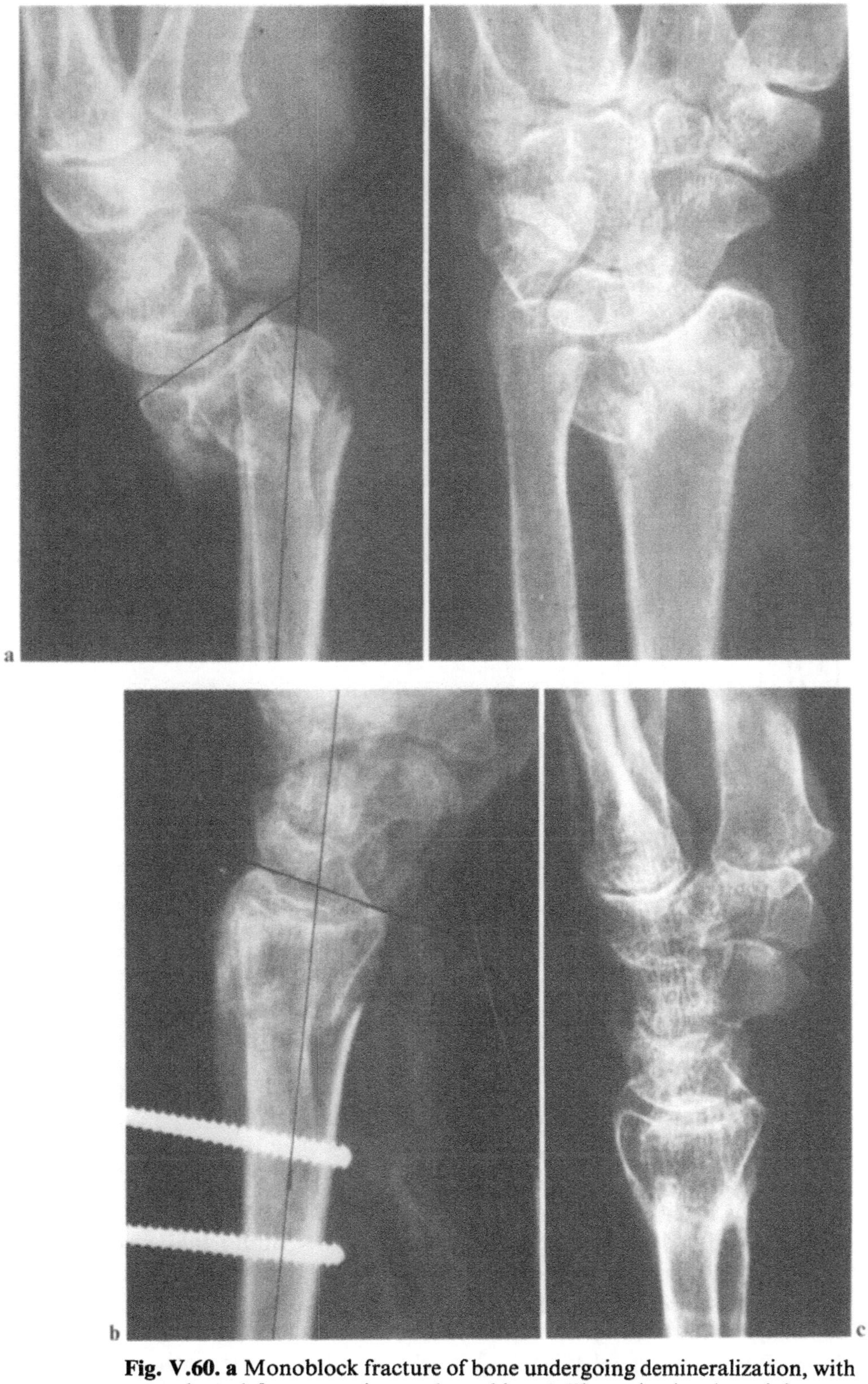

Fig. V.60. **a** Monoblock fracture of bone undergoing demineralization, with metaphyseal fragmentation and crushing. **b** The reduction is satisfactory, but the final result (**c**) is not, because of secondary tilt and shortening (see also Fig. IV.13)

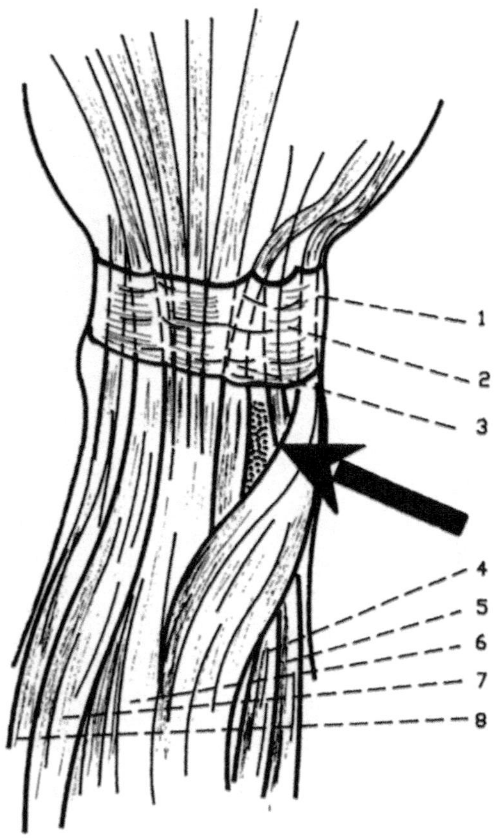


**Fig. V.61.** Site of insertion of cancellous grafts.
*1* extensor pollicis brevis and abductor pollicis longus
*2* extensor retinaculum
*3* extensor pollicis longus
*4* extensor carpi radialis brevis
*5* extensor carpi radialis longus
*6* extensor digitorum communis
*7* extensor digiti minimi
*8* extensor carpi ulnaris

1. In the initial position, the epiphyseal segment is supported on (or embedded in) the diaphysis. After manual reduction, the epiphyseal segment is maintained in position by continuous traction through Chinese fingertips or temporary wiring.
2. Fixator screws are inserted. With Weber's fixator (1985), the axis of the distal screws in the epiphyseal fragment must make a dorsal angle of 10°–15° in relation to the articulation in the sagittal plane, since all the screws must be parallel to each other once the assembly is complete.
3. The assembly is completed; the axis of the articulation is defined by the position of the screws as outlined in 2.
4. The residual gap is a problem: spontaneous filling takes at least 8 weeks, and removal of the fixator before then incurs the risk of secondary tilting (see Figs. IV.13 and V.60).

*Note.* For an external fixator, 8 weeks is a long time with increases in the risk of infection. A cancellous graft from the outset is a solution to this problem. It promotes union, limits the period during which the fixator must be used, increases stability and, thereby, diminishes the risk of secondary displacement. Moreover, it is simple to insert (Fig. V.61).

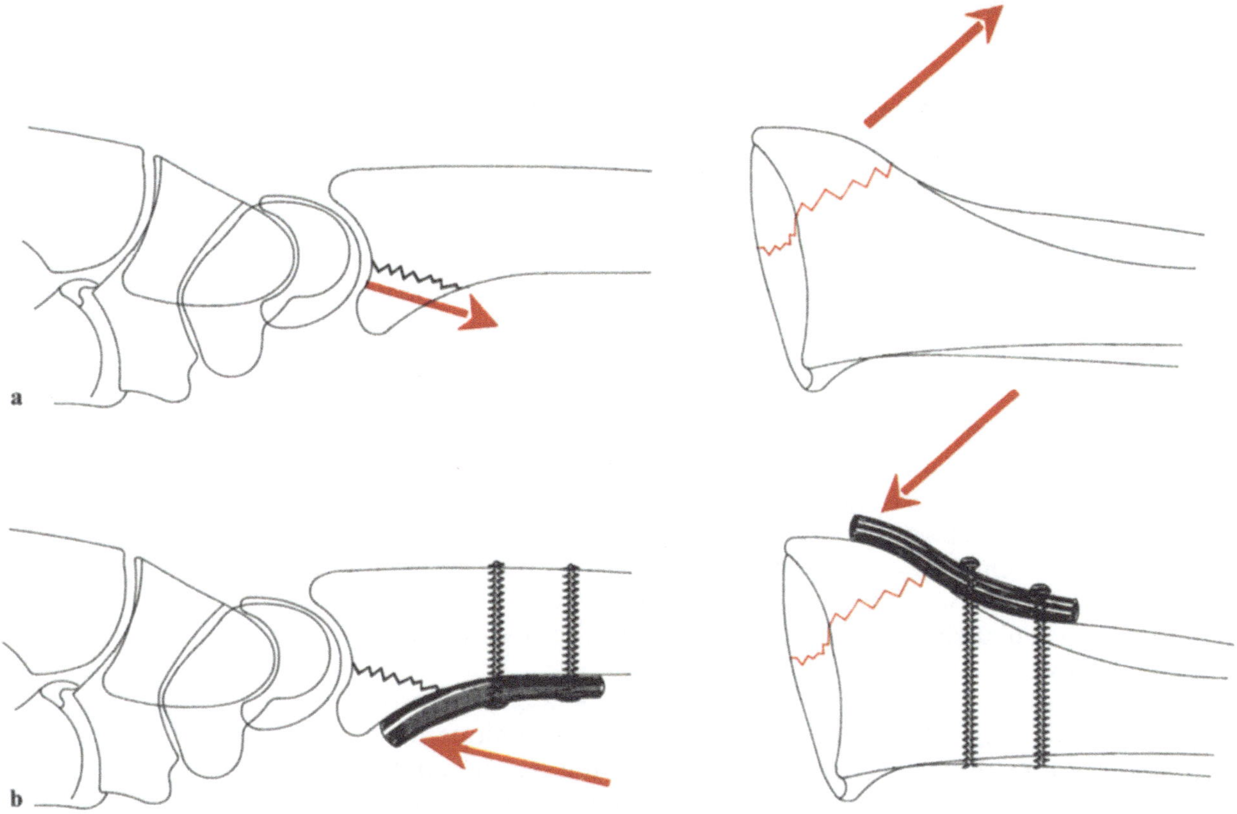


**Fig. V.62a, b.** Principle of treatment of marginal fracture (split block). **a** The marginal fragment tends to displace and produce joint incongruence. **b** A buttress-plate prevents fragment migration and, if need be, allows moderate compression

*Remarks*

Kirschner wires alone cannot be as effective as the external fixator. Their anchorage is not comparable to that of the screws of a rigid fixator or even of the threaded wires of Jakob's fixator. Moreover, this anchorage is impaired by poor mineralization, and does not stand the test of time.

In the choice of fixator, each has advantages and disadvantages. The external fixators of Jakob or Hoffmann do not call for a precise pre-operative plan, as their components can be assembled freely in any plane of space. However, the threaded wires are relatively slender, the price paid for this, occasionally essential, liberty (Fig. V.66). Weber's external fixator, though apparently simple, demands precise technique and detailed preoperative planning based on exact analysis of the X-ray films. A single error, and the operation has to be repeated. On the other hand, the assembly provides great stability, the fixation of the screws being unsurpassed. Simple bending of the rods, as proposed by Weber himself (Weber and Magerl 1985), is not practicable for the radius. My experience is that fine correction is not possible, and it risks tearing out the screws. In summary, the ideal external fixator does not exist. The surgeon who cannot or will not indulge in the luxury of owning a vast range of equipment must opt for the system with the greatest flexibility of use.

**Marginal Fracture (Split Epiphyseal Block)** (Fig. V.62)

These fractures impair joint congruence, so the goal of treatment must be retention of a perfect reduction. Whatever the site of the displaced fragment, the buttress-plate is the method of choice. It has an anti-glide effect, and, if correctly shaped, exerts a certain degree of interfragmentary compression. It is unnecessary to open the joint to ensure articular congruence; this is guaranteed by the interfragmentary compression and by perfect reduction of the extra-articular portion of the fracture. By a principle of elementary geometry, as soon as the margins on the extra-articular aspect are congruent, the same is true on the intra-articular side, especially since this fracture has no comminuted zone.

Problems may arise if the buttress-plate is used inappropriately (Fig. V.63). However, the buttress-plate technique may even prove effective in neglected marginal comminuted fractures, as shown by the example in Fig. V.64, which is 5 weeks old. If this case had been treated primarily, it would have been necessary to combine a buttress-plate with a cancellous graft to restore an adequate volume, capable of resisting pressure. In normal cases consolidation is rapid, and the osteosynthesis material can be removed as early as the end of the 3rd month.

*Note.* The external fixator or Kirschner wires do not offer the same security as the buttress-plate; their insertion is tricky, and they may produce fragmentation of the epiphyseal block which would definitively impair the final outcome. We do not advise their use in marginal fractures.

**Comminuted Fracture (Multifragmented Epiphyseal Block)**

Whether comminution is severe or not, treatment must be directed towards restoring bony volume as well as articular congruence. The problems and their solutions are as follows (Fig. V.65):

1. The comminuted fragments tend to displace in all directions.
2. Muscular forces tend to pull the carpus and the radial shaft together, causing them to penetrate and disrupt the mass of fragments. However, the capsulo-ligamentous apparatus surrounding the radial epiphysis is usually intact, and holds the bone fragments as in a bag.
3. By overcoming the effect of muscle pull, penetration by the carpus and shaft into the fracture zone is prevented.
4. Cancellous bone grafting, via a dorso-radial window (Fig. V.61), increases the bulk of the bone mass, and puts the walls of the capsulo-ligamentous sac under tension (it is essential that these walls be left intact). Such a plasty makes

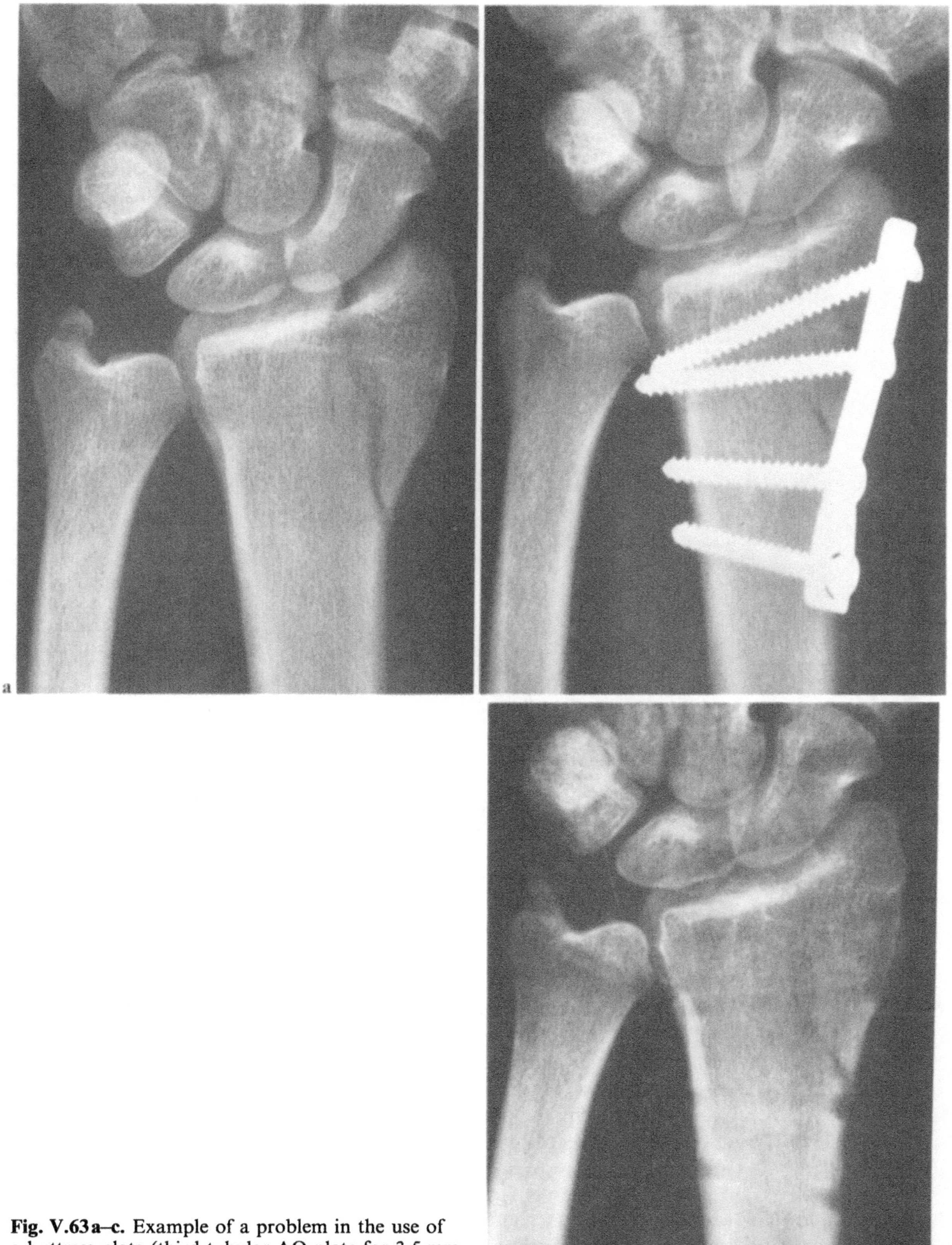

a b c

**Fig. V.63a–c.** Example of a problem in the use of a buttress-plate (third-tubular AO plate for 3.5 mm screws) for a marginal radial fracture (split epiphyseal block): one distal screw would have sufficed

a

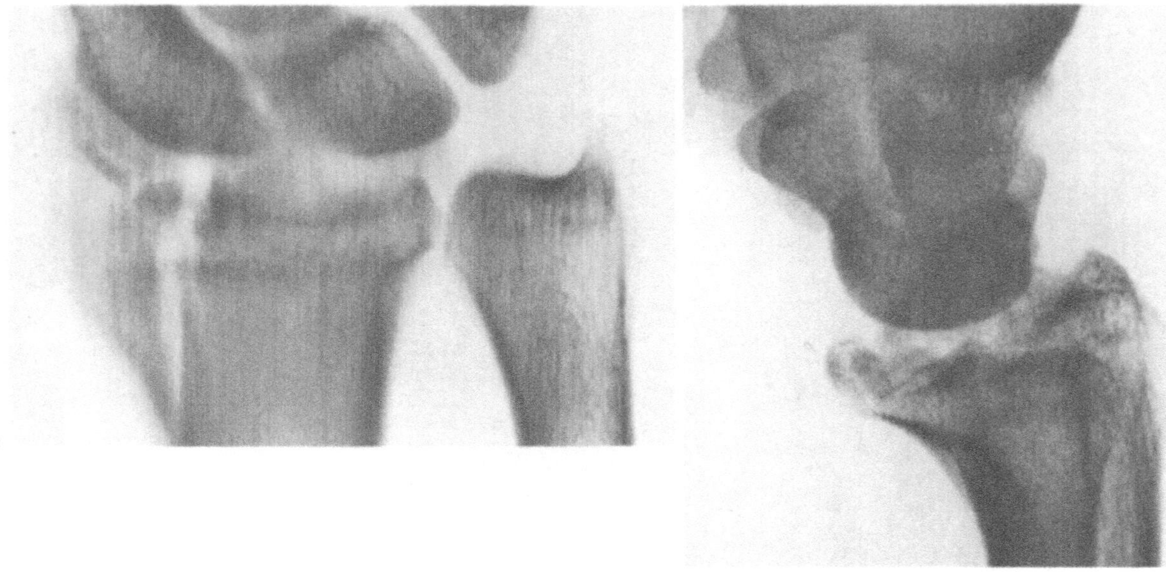

b

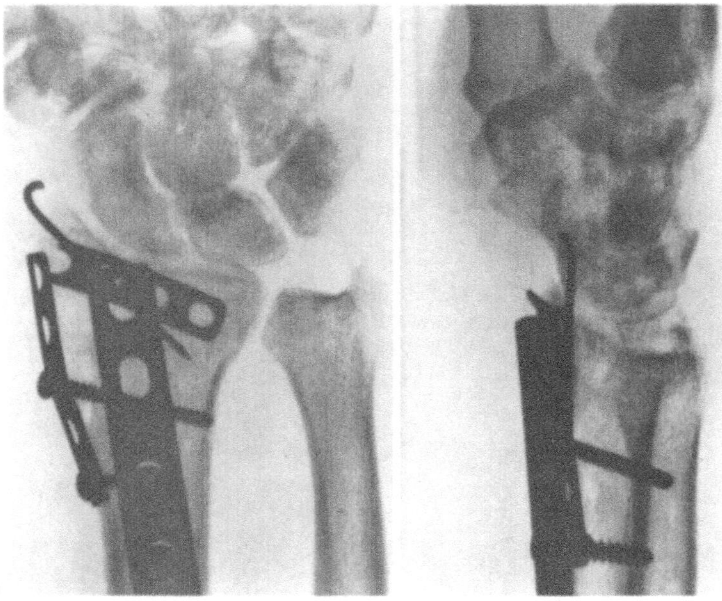

**Fig. V.64a, b.** K.L., 29 years, comminuted fracture (multi-fragmented epiphyseal block) from motorcycle accident. **a** Conservative treatment: appearance at 5 weeks. **b** Compression by palmar and radial buttress-plate. To secure reduction, it was necessary to use a thick plate for dynamic compression with 3.5 mm screws combined with a third-tubular plate. The radial buttress-plate was applied after palmar reduction and intra-operative radiological assessment of the situation

it possible to restore normal articular shape, even after some delay.

5. Reduction is maintained by the external fixator. Note that the fixator is used to neutralize the existing muscle forces; its task is not reduction itself, but the maintenance of reduction, which is obtained by manipulation and cancellous grafting.

*Two examples* illustrate our thesis:

1. The epiphyseal multifragment fracture shown in Fig. V.66, with marked separation, is composed of several fragments, two of which are relatively large. Thanks to Jakob's external fixator, these can be wired and held in as anatomic a position

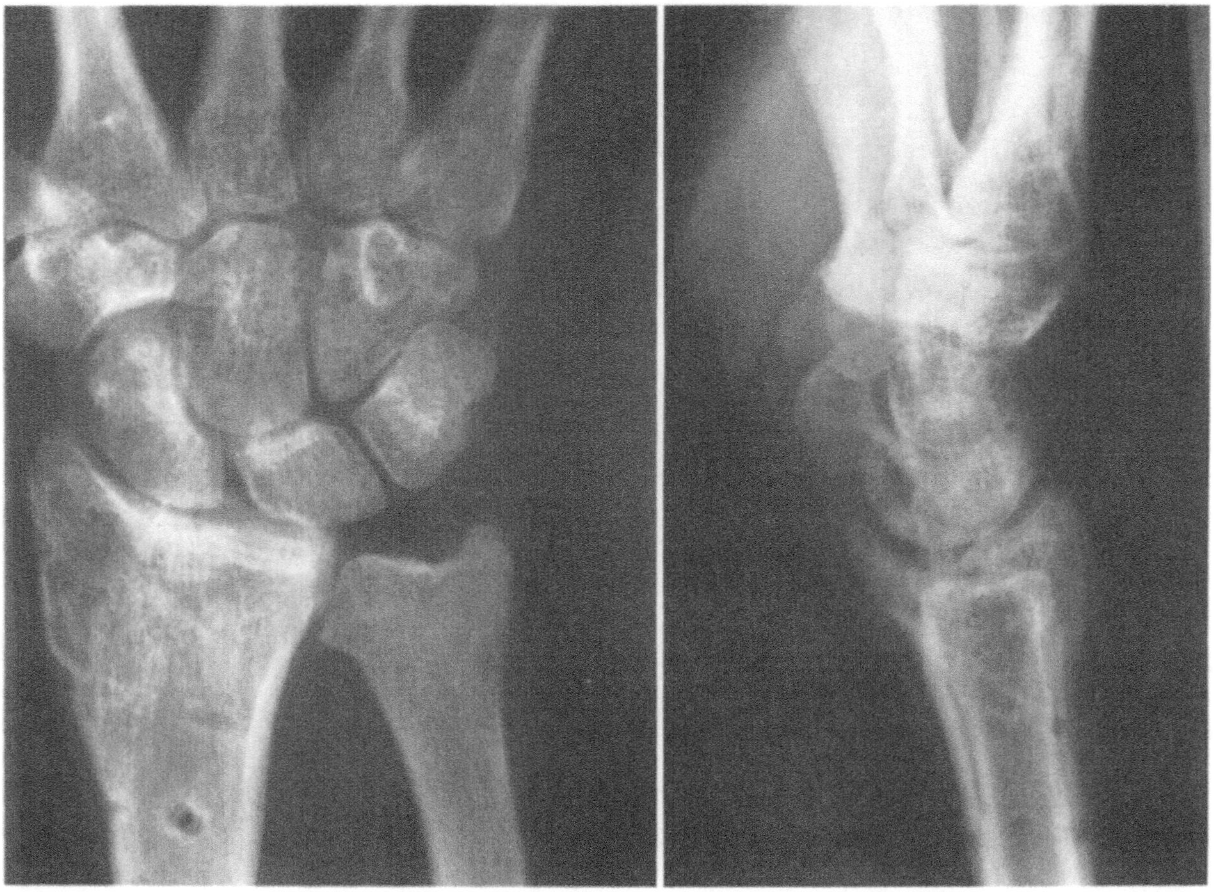

**Fig. V.64c.** Final result: articular incongruence and depression, with moderate dorsal tilt

as possible. The residual gap is filled with autogenous spongiosa. The result at 1 year, even if not perfect (dorsal tilt of 15° compared with normal, and minor joint incongruence), is evidence of the efficacy of the method.

2. The second example (Fig. V.67) perfectly illustrates the possibilities offered by bone-grafting, even when this is delayed. The patient is a 23-year-old fitter, who sustained a comminuted fracture of the distal radius that was treated by simple plaster splintage. The shattering and deformation are clearly visible in the first film (Fig. V.67a). Application of an external fixator 3 days later has stretched out the wrist, but has hardly modified the joint incongruence; in fact, the bone gaps have become more apparent (Fig. V.67b). These gaps were filled by autogenous cancellous grafts. Though the operative film (Fig. V.67c) does not make the effect of treatment obvious, the arthrogram made 6 months after the accident (Fig. V.67d) shows restoration of the joint surface. This arthrogram also reveals the existence of radio-carpal synechiae and a lesion of the triquetro-lunate ligament (Fig. V.67e). Though the radio-carpal joint has been perfectly restored, this is not the case for the distal radio-ulnar joint. This is deformed (Fig. V.67f), and exhibits a dorsal pinching that certainly accounts for the pain experienced by the

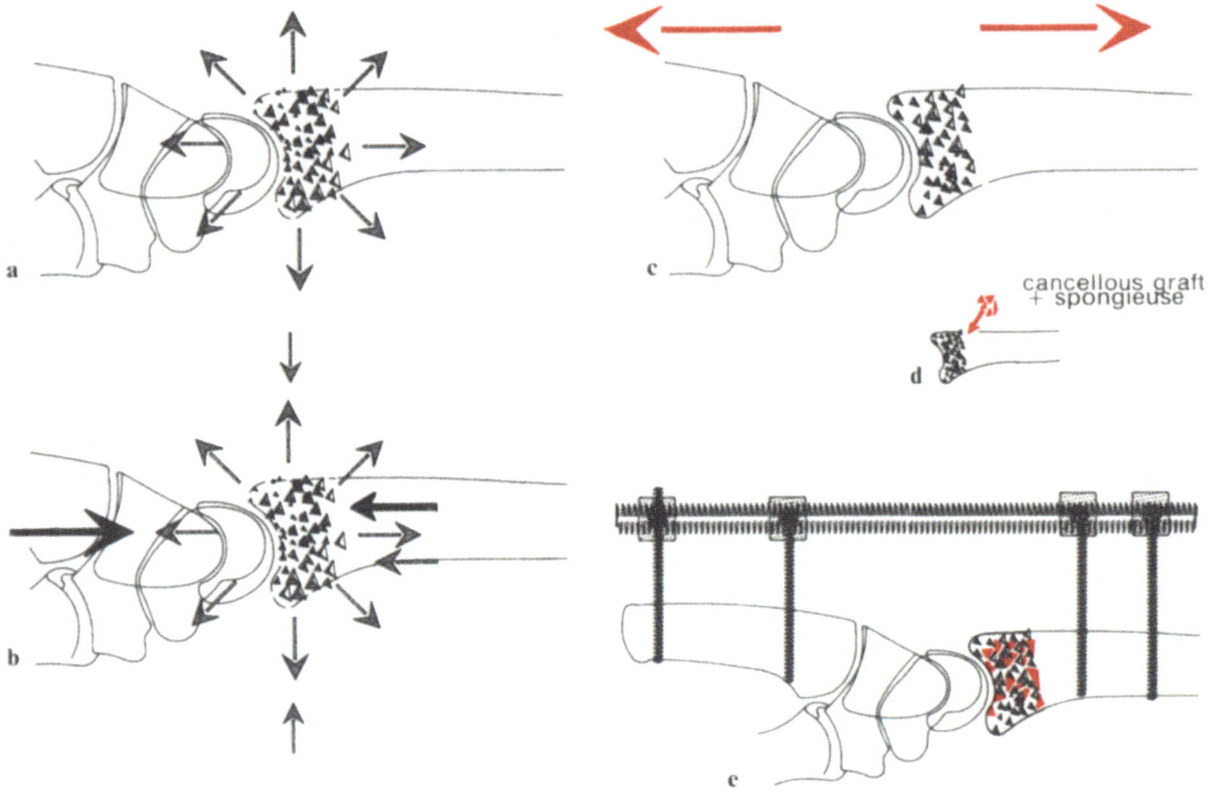


Fig. V.65 a–e. Principle of treatment of epiphyseal comminuted fractures. **a** Pathophysiology: the fragments tend to disperse in all directions. **b** The capsulo-ligamentous system surrounding the radial epiphysis contains the fragments; muscle pull produces penetration of the carpus and radial diaphysis into the fracture zone. This gives the final position. **c** Neutralization of muscle pull prevents deformity. **d** Cancellous bone plasty permits remodelling of the deformed epiphysis. **e** The external fixator, by neutralizing the muscle pull, guarantees maintenance of reduction and articular remodelling

patient – pain not relieved by shortening of the ulna. Only resection-arthroplasty of the ulna guarantees pain relief in this situation (see Fig. V.74).

*Summary*. The external fixator is the method of choice for retention of monoblock and comminuted fractures. Depending on the degree of comminution, it is inserted into either the second metacarpal or the main fragments of the fractured epiphyseal mass. There are considerable advantages of the cancellous bone grafting: shortening of the period of immobilization, better stabilization and correction of the joint deformity. Stable osteosynthesis is imperative for marginal fractures. The use of the external fixator and the buttress-plate are not mutually exclusive, the former can help in the correct positioning of the osteosynthesis material.

**Instability of the Carpus and Fracture of the Distal Radius**

Scapho-lunate dissociation associated with fracture of the distal radius must be treated according to the principles already outlined: reduction and stabilization of the radial fracture, followed by suture of the ruptured ligaments by the palmar and/or dorsal route. If a buttress-plate is ineffective and, for practical reasons, the external fixator cannot be applied until the end of the procedure, temporary stabilization can be secured by Kirschner wires.

## I. Malunion of the Radius

Malunion, i.e. consolidation of the bone fragments in faulty alignment, causes three problems (Fig. V.68):
- relative lengthening of the ulna with respect to the radius,
- articular tilt of the distal radius,
- distal radio-ulnar joint incongruence.

An additional problem, instability of the carpus or arthrosis of the distal radio-ulnar joint, may also complicate the treatment plan.

The surgical ideal, simultaneous correction of all the deformities, is not always practical, since total correction is a major procedure, carrying some risk of sympathetic dystrophy. Therefore, the proposed correction must be appropriate to the symptoms, the functional handicap, the patient's personality and the degree of mineralization of the bone. The operative risks must also be weighed against the supposed benefits.

The surgical possibilities are numerous. The lists below summarize them for each of the two bones of the forearm. It is also possible to combine these methods.

*Ulna:*

1. Lengthening osteotomy (see the discussion of Kienböck's disease)
2. Shortening osteotomy
3. Distal radio-ulnar arthrodesis (Sauvé-Kapandji; Kapandji 1985)
4. Oblique resection arthroplasty (with or without shortening)
5. Darrach's resection

*Radius:*

1. Lengthening osteotomy
2. Opening or closing wedge osteotomy (dorsal or palmar route)
3. Shortening osteotomy (see the discussion of osteomalacia of the lunate)

With all of these options, a careful choice must be made, considering the advantages and disadvantages of the various approaches and of the condition to be treated.

### Intervention Involving the Ulna

Access to the subcutaneous distal third is easy, despite the passage of the extensor carpi ulnaris along the ulnar border of the bone. The absence of large cutaneous nerve trunks limits the risks of sympathetic dystrophy or a painful scar. However, one must take care not to damage the dorsal branch of the ulnar nerve, which crosses the ulnar styloid to innervate the ulnar aspect of the dorsum of the hand.

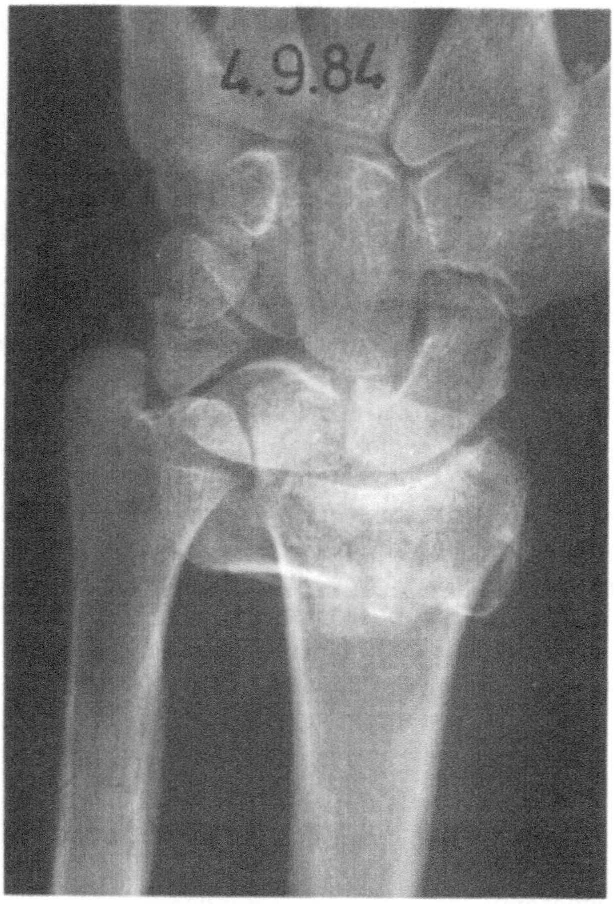


a

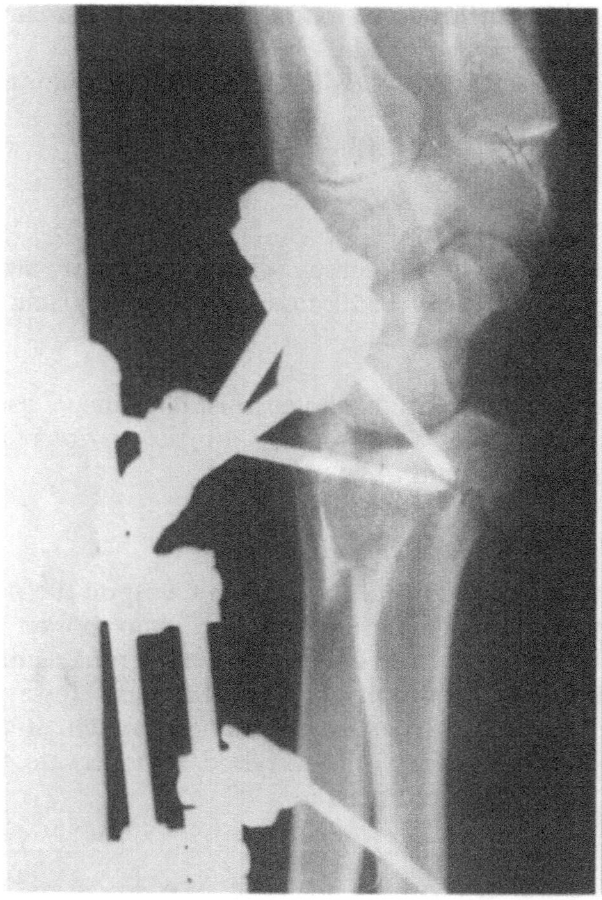

b

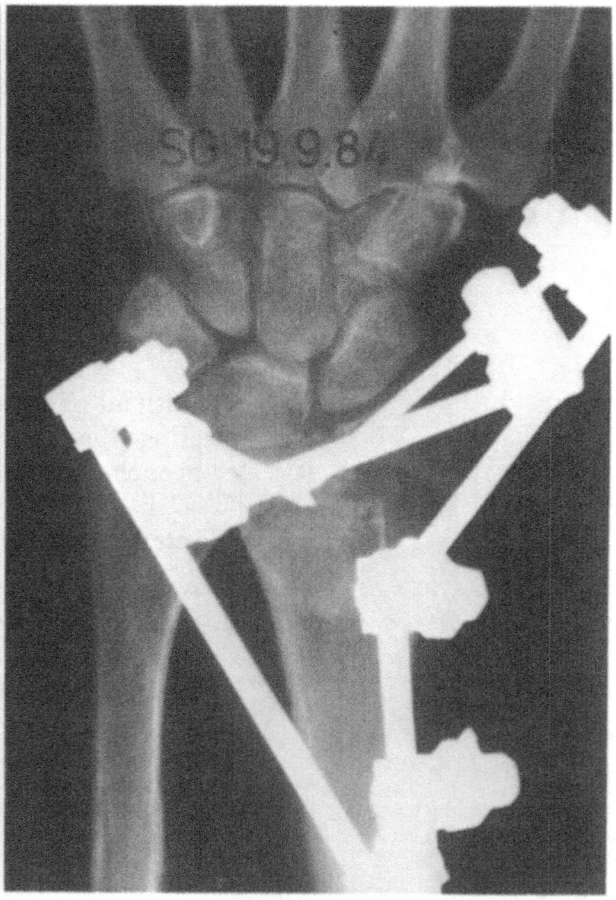

**Fig. V.66.** **a** Comminuted fracture composed of large fragments. **b** Jakob's fixator allows pinning and orientation of the main fragments, while cancellous bone grafting guarantees rapid union. **c** At 1 year the length and the joint axes are virtually normal

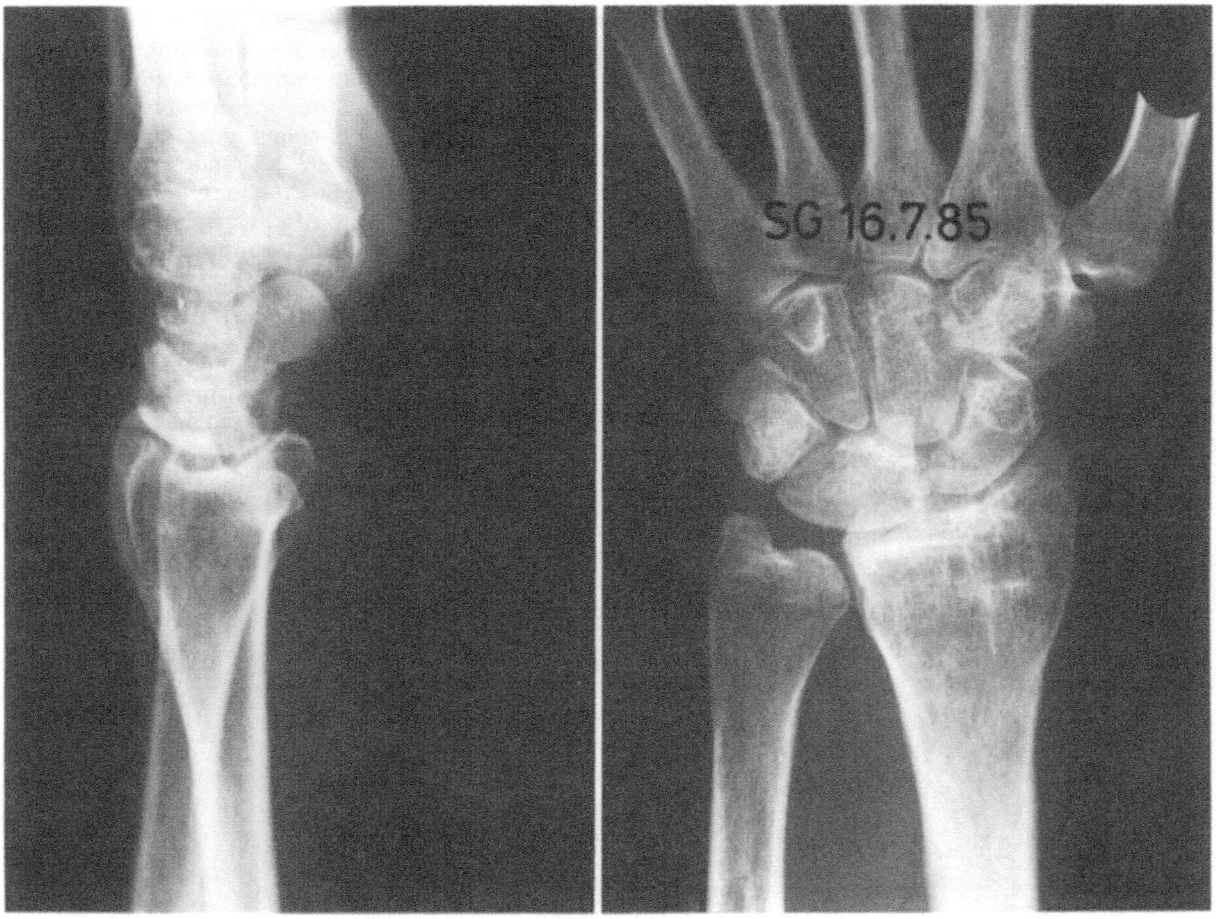


c

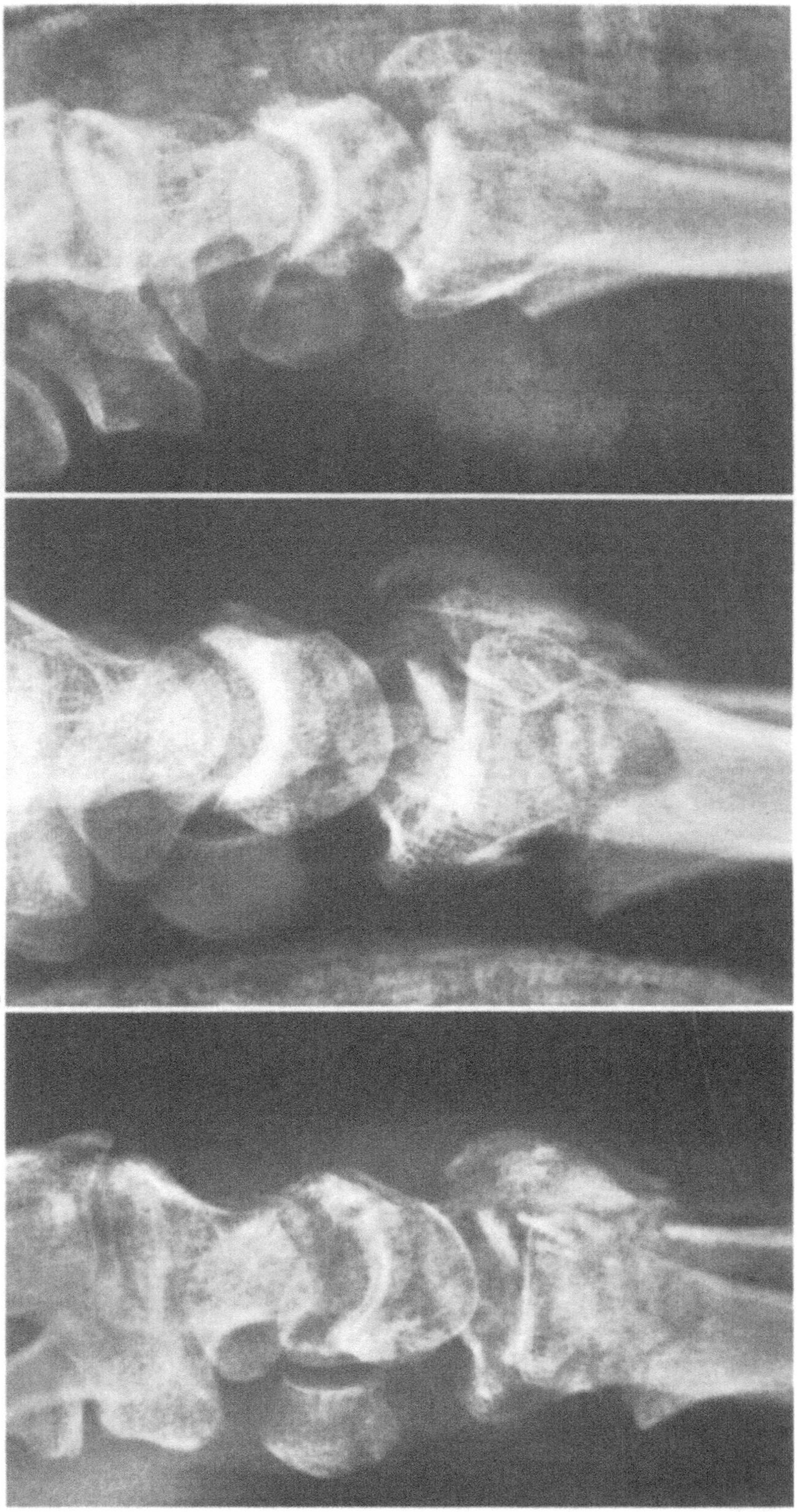

a

b

c

**Fig. V.67 a–f.** The importance of cancellous bone grafting. **a** Joint deformation 3 days after conservative treatment of a comminuted epiphyseal fracture. **b** Traction has not modified the joint deformation. **c** After cancellous grafting the gap disappears. **d, e** Arthrography brings proof of the efficacity of remodelling by cancellous plasty; note the intra-articular synechiae preventing diffusion of contrast medium into the radial compartment. **f** Limitation of method despite cancellous plasty: inadequate restoration of radio-ulnar alignment with joint incongruence, dorsal subluxation and pain

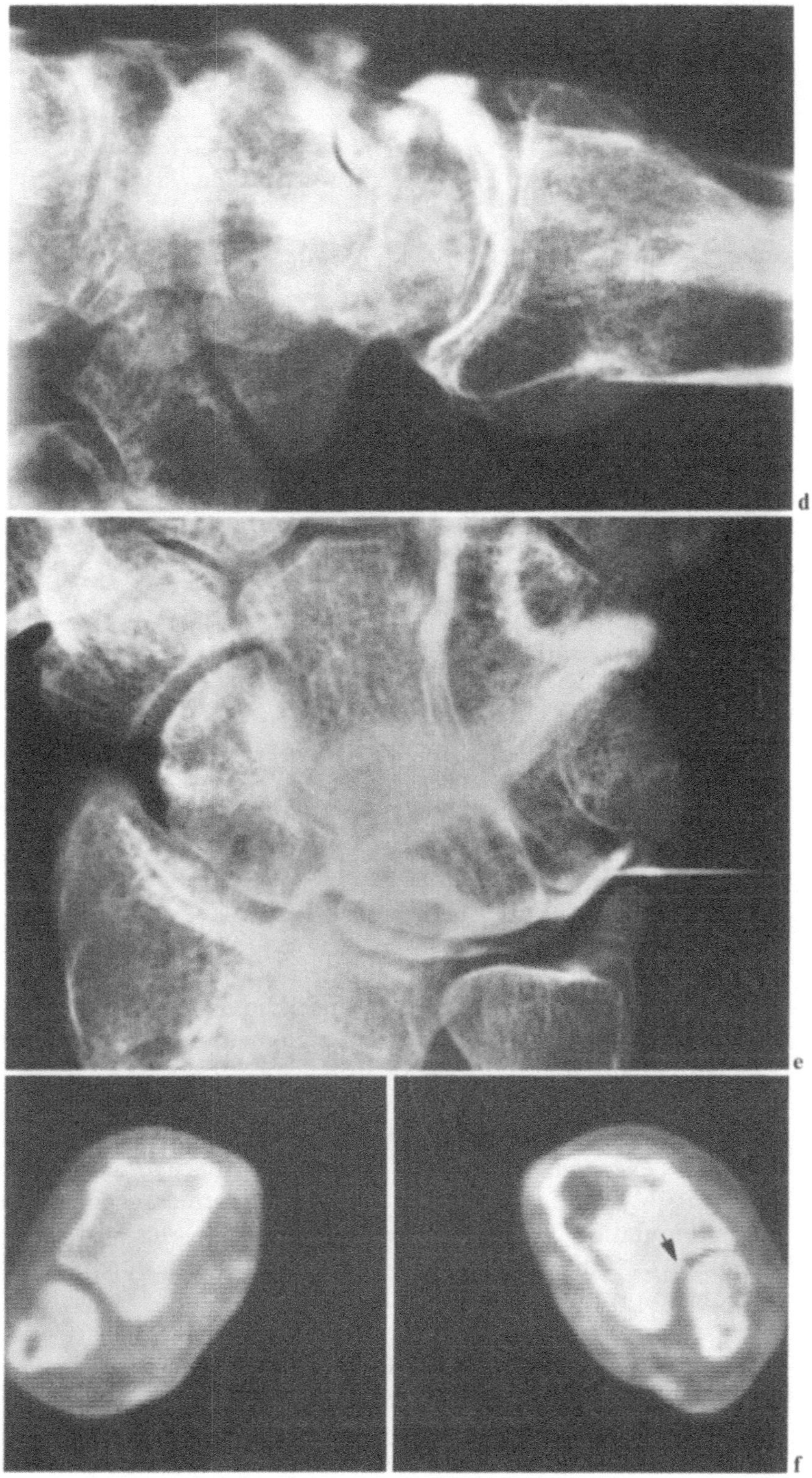

d

e

f

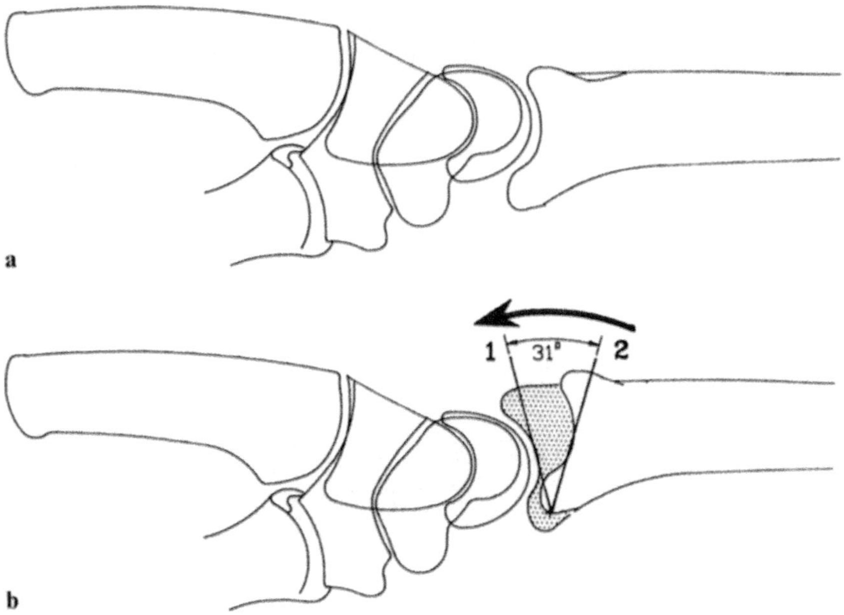


Fig. V.68a, b. Problems of malunion. **a** Loss of substance: articular tilt, carpal subluxation and shortening. **b** Global correction: lengthening and correction of tilt
*1* ideal angle
*2* actual angle
*1–2* desired correction

*Techniques of Shortening the Ulna* (Fig. V.69)

The stages involved are:
1. An incision centred on the ulna, slightly longer than the plate intended for osteosynthesis
2. Drilling of two or three distal holes, and incision of the interosseous membrane to remove any obstacle to shortening (Fig. V.69a)
3. Marking of rotation with a bone chisel or, alternatively, (Fig. V.69b, c) with two parallel Kirschner wires
4. Osteotomy at right angles to the axis of the bone (the advantage being its simplicity), or an oblique osteotomy (Fig. V.69d–g) (advantages: better interfragmentary stability, and oblique lag-screw)

*Note.* It is wise always to use a clamp to manipulate the distal fragment, even when the screws are in place; this avoids stressing and possibly tearing them out if bone mineralization is poor or manipulation vigorous. The use of an AO tension device does not appear necessary; if it is used, the incision must be prolonged proximally by a third.

*Indications.* Two examples illustrate our approach:
1. S.N. (Fig. V.70), a 40-year-old civil servant, suffered the following sequelae of a fractured radius: permanent subluxation of the distal radio-ulnar joint, pain on pronation-supination and loss of power. The radial articular surfaces are, however, correctly orientated.
   *Question:* is there distal radio-ulnar instability? If in doubt, we prefer to limit ourselves to a shortening osteotomy of around 0.8 cm.

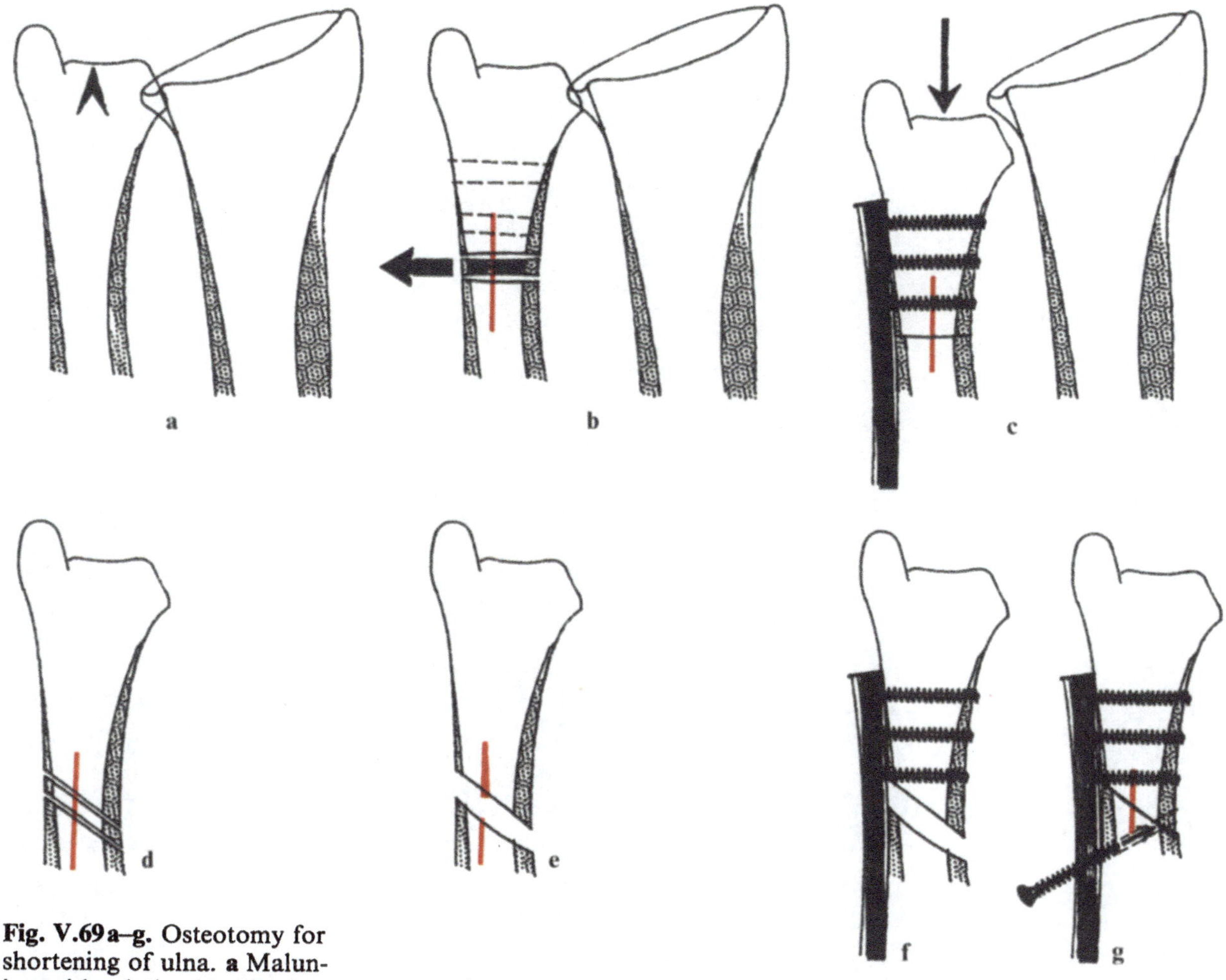


**Fig. V.69 a–g.** Osteotomy for shortening of ulna. **a** Malunion with relative lengthening of the ulna produces excessive ulnar-carpal pressure, sometimes subluxation and instability of the distal radio-ulnar joint (Fig. V.70). **b**, **c** The solution is transverse osteotomy: drilling of two or three holes distally, marking of rotation (*red line*) with chisel, section of distal interosseous membrane and resection (*arrow*) of a disc of bone whose thickness corresponds to the desired shortening (**b**). **c** Shortening with or without compression device, manipulation of distal fragment (*arrow*) using a clamp despite screws.
**d–g** An alternative solution is oblique osteotomy, performed as in **b**, but with oblique shaping of the fragment to be excised (**d**); **e** and **f** are managed as for **c**, plus the possibility of completing the assembly with an oblique lag-screw (**g**)

*Result:* reduction of the subluxation resulted in restoration of power and the disappearance of pain. The patient is once more 100% fit for work.

2. L.E., a 26-year-old post-office employee (Fig. V.71), sustained two fractures of the radius, a monoblock fracture with dorsal and radial tilt, and a fracture of the proximal third of the shaft. The result was limitation of supination and permanent pain at the ulnar styloid.
   *Question:* should all the deformities be corrected, a large-scale operation, or is it enough initially to shorten the ulna and level it? As this woman was complaining only of the ulnar head syndrome, and was rather apprehensive, we suggested making a start by readjusting the inferior radio-ulnar joint by means of a shortening osteotomy.
   *Result:* this was so favourable (with disappearance of the pain and normalization of forearm rotation) that it was not necessary to consider supplementary correction.

*Conclusion:* Readjustment of the appropriate lengths of the radius and ulna is essential. This should be the first surgical procedure to be undertaken if multiple corrections of uncertain outcome are being considered.

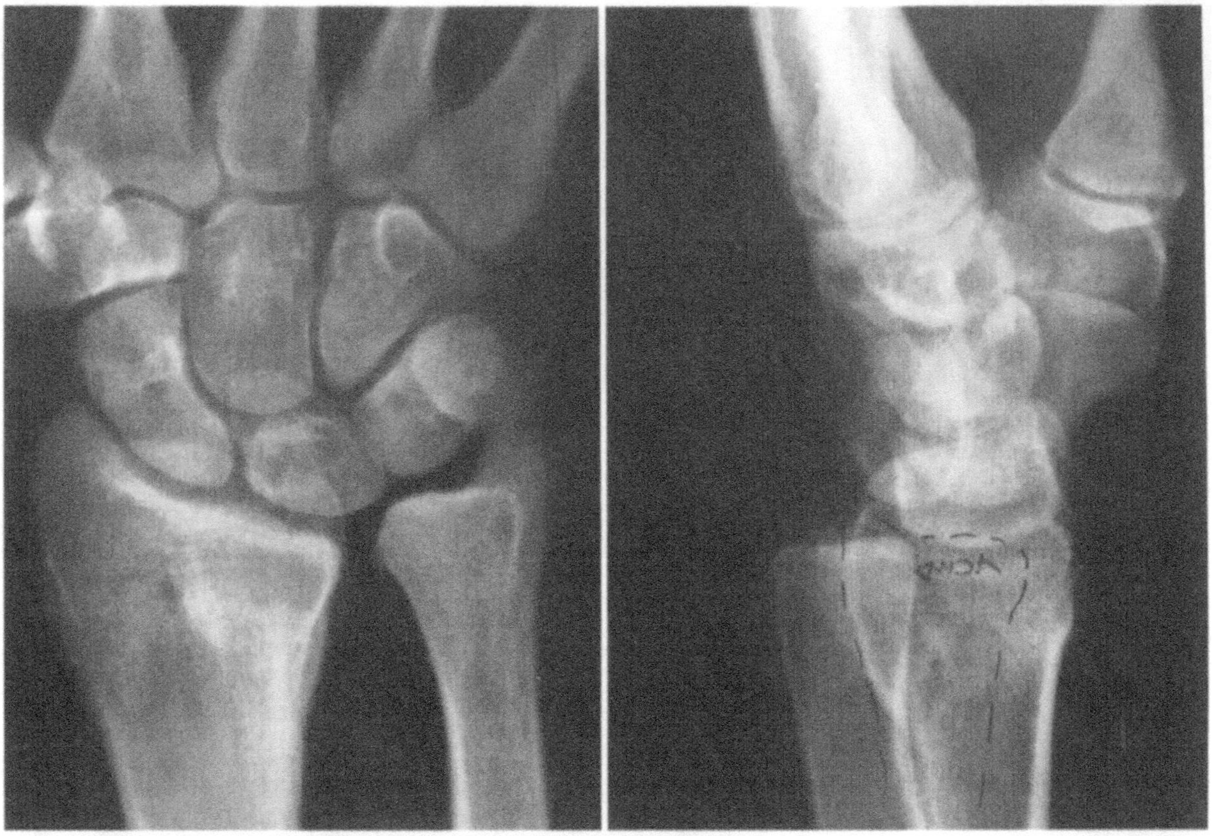

a

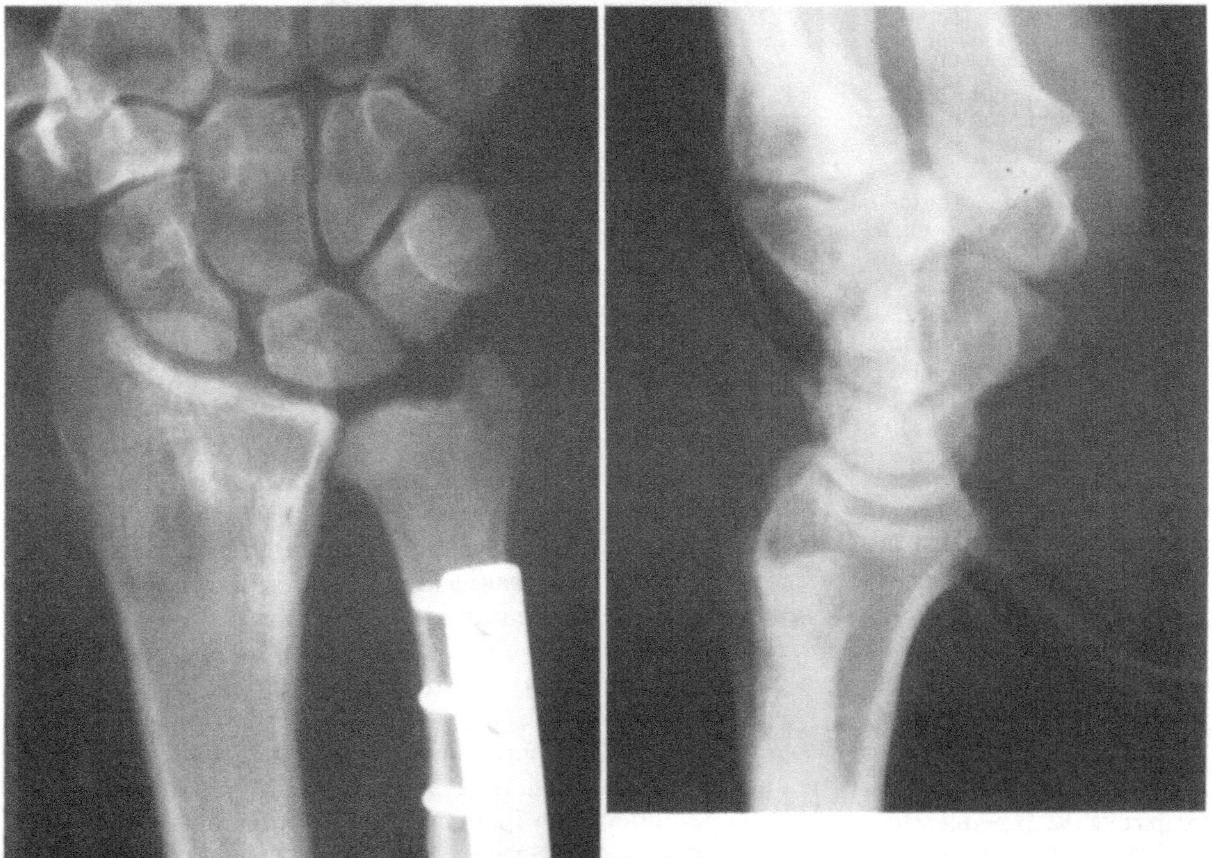

b

Fig. V.70 a, b

**Fig. V.71 a, b.** L.E., a 26-year-old post-office employee, with ulnar head syndrome after fracture of the radius at two levels. **a** Complete incongruence of distal radio-ulnar joint. **b** Appearance after simple shortening (see text). **c** Functional result

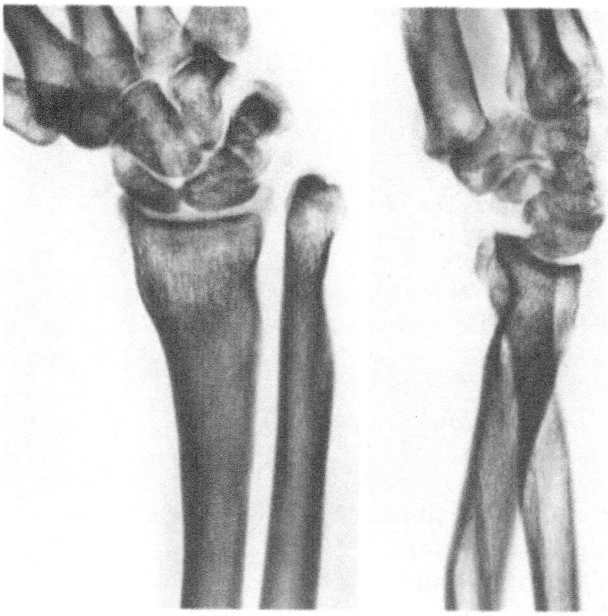

a

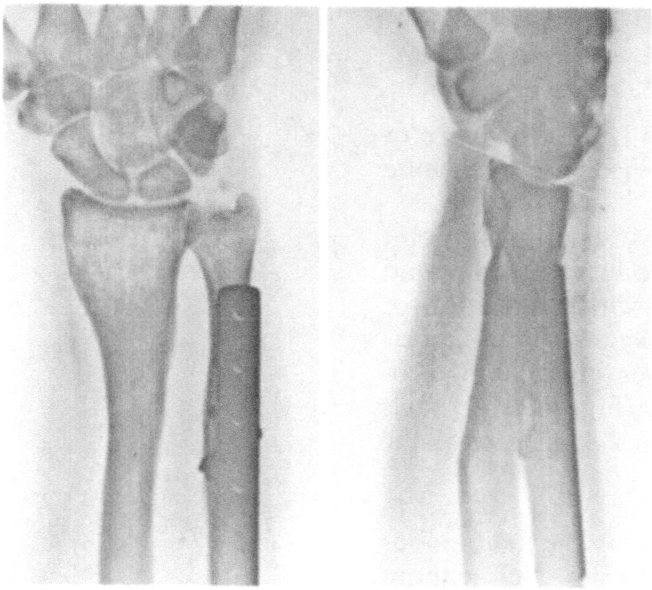

b

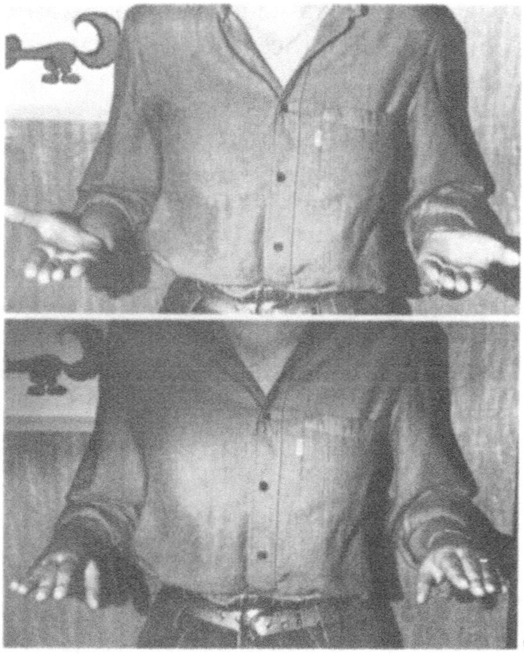

c

◁ **Fig. V.70 a, b.** S.N., a 40-year-old civil servant, with ulnar head syndrome after monoblock fracture and conservative treatment. **a** Lengthening and subluxation of ulna. **b** Clinical and structural normalization after shortening (without other procedure)

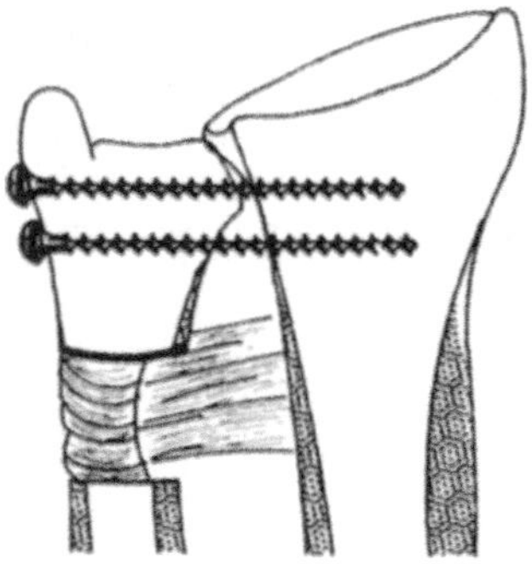

Fig. V.72. Sauvé-Kapandji principle. The ulnar head is reduced and fixed to the radius, 2 cm of the ulna is excised and the pronator quadratus is interposed. The problem is the doubtful stability of the ulnar stump

### Sauvé-Kapandji Technique (1985)

This is shown schematically in Fig. V.72. We do not use it, since stabilization of the proximal fragment of the ulna is uncertain. We have seen difficult cases of painful instability of the ulna following this procedure, and remain sceptical of the value of the method.

### Technique of Oblique Resection Arthroplasty

We have modified the technique of Bowers (1982) for cases of post-traumatic arthritis. It can also be combined with shortening of the ulna if the need arises.

Case O.B., aged 23 years, demonstrates this point (Fig. V.73a). A motorcycle accident had produced a compound fracture of the distal third of the radius, with dislocation of the ulnar head. Despite reduction and ligamentous suture, post-traumatic arthrosis developed, limiting power, and making pronation-supination painful. The radiograph (Fig. V.73b) shows some intra-osseous cysts without other signs of arthrosis; the joint incongruence is obvious.

What is to be done:

- Perform a shortening? This would not modify the joint lesions although it might adjust the joint mechanics, but without guarantee of improvement.
- Resort to Darrach's resection? This procedure often results in painful contact between the ulnar stump and the radius, a syndrome well described by Bell et al. (1985). Besides, this operation produces marked loss of power.
- Cap the head of the ulna with a Silastic prosthesis? This introduction of a foreign body requires definitive bone resection, and in the event of failure (which is common, since it is extremely difficult to stabilize the prosthetic cap) it is necessary to resort to Darrach's operation, and possibly to stabilization of the ulnar stump.

*The advantages of resection-arthroplasty* are as follows:

1. Preservation of the ulnar styloid and attachments of the proximal V

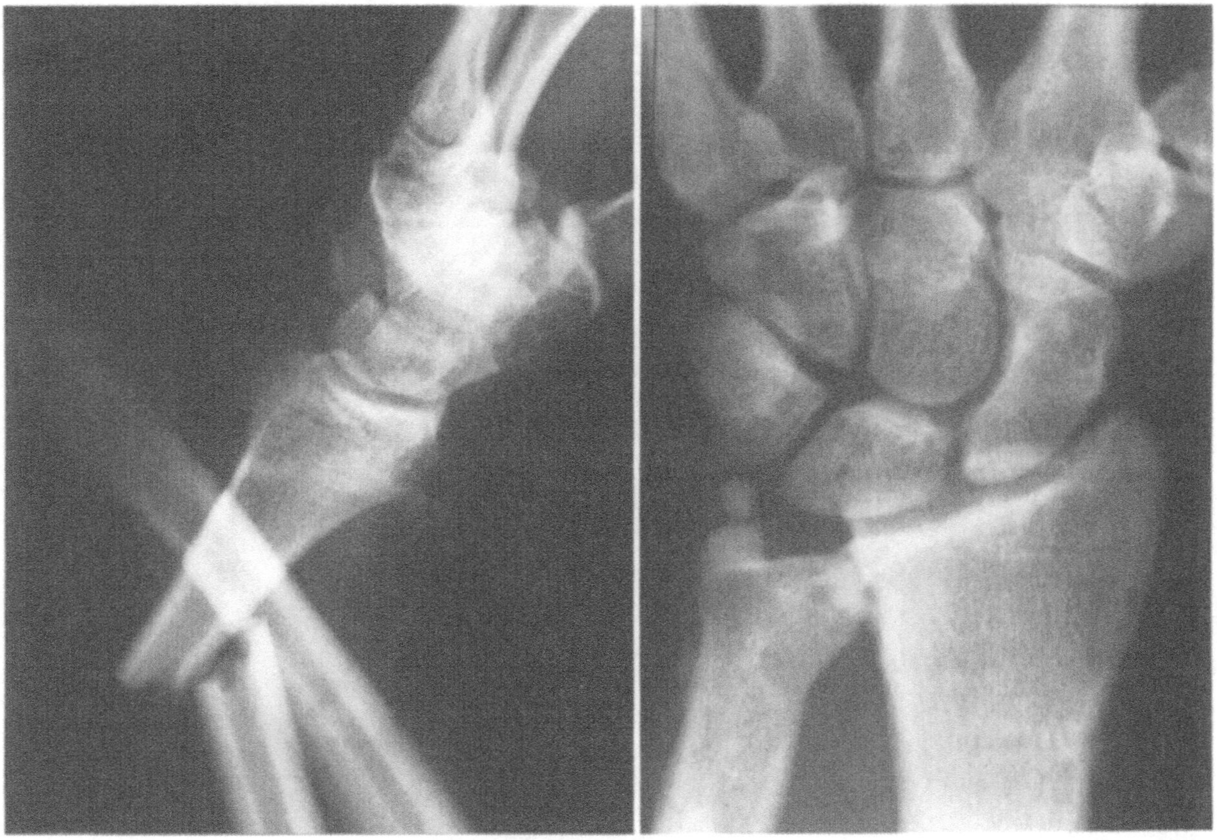

a b

**Fig. V.73.** **a** Fracture-dislocation on admission. **b** One year later there is severe pain at the distal radio-ulnar joint on pronation and supination, with subchondral cysts of the ulnar head

2. Stabilization of the ulna
3. Intra-articular interposition of a strip of retinaculum (preventing abduction of the ulna)
4. Relative simplicity of technique.

*Operative technique* (Fig. V.74). The procedure comprises:

1. A long incision (Fig. V.74a), with a flap based on a palmar ulnar hinge to avoid any nerve damage
2. Identification of the extensor retinaculum (Fig. V.74b), and developing a tongue whose base is the attachment to the triquetrum, and whose radial extent is the tubercle of Lister (Fig. V.74c)
3. Freeing of extensor carpi ulnaris (ECU) by Z-incision of the sheath (Fig. V.74d)
4. Identification of the ulna, and release of its head (Fig. V.74e) *Note:* the incision must respect the triangular fibrocartilage, particularly its dorsal ligament.
5. Plotting the line of excision of the articular portion of the ulnar head (Fig. V.74f)
6. Identification of the palmar or anterior joint capsule (Fig. V.74g). The tongue of retinaculum is fixed to the palmar capsule, and the whole is reinforced with the posterior capsule (Fig. V.74h)
7. Closure in layers, with care to close the tunnel for the ECU again

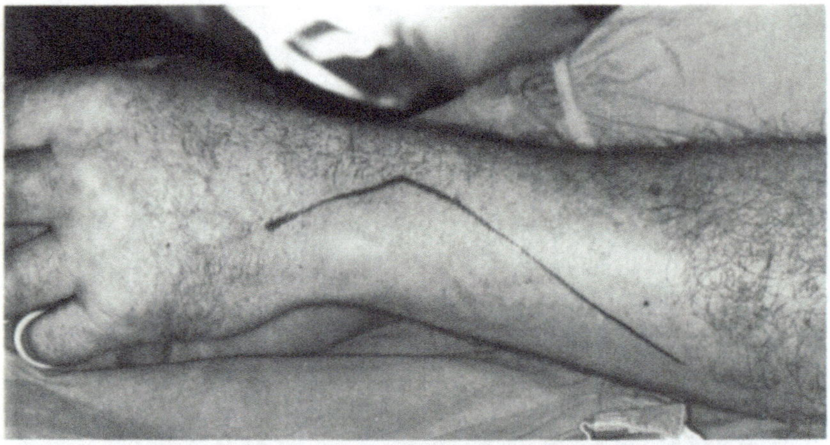

a

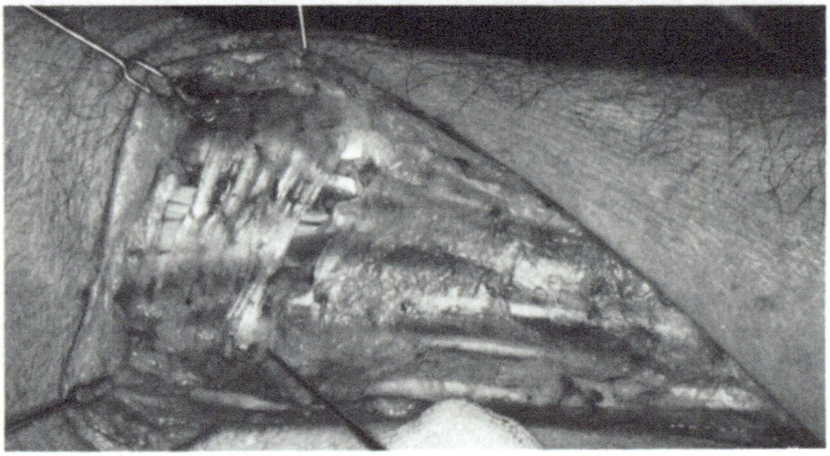

b

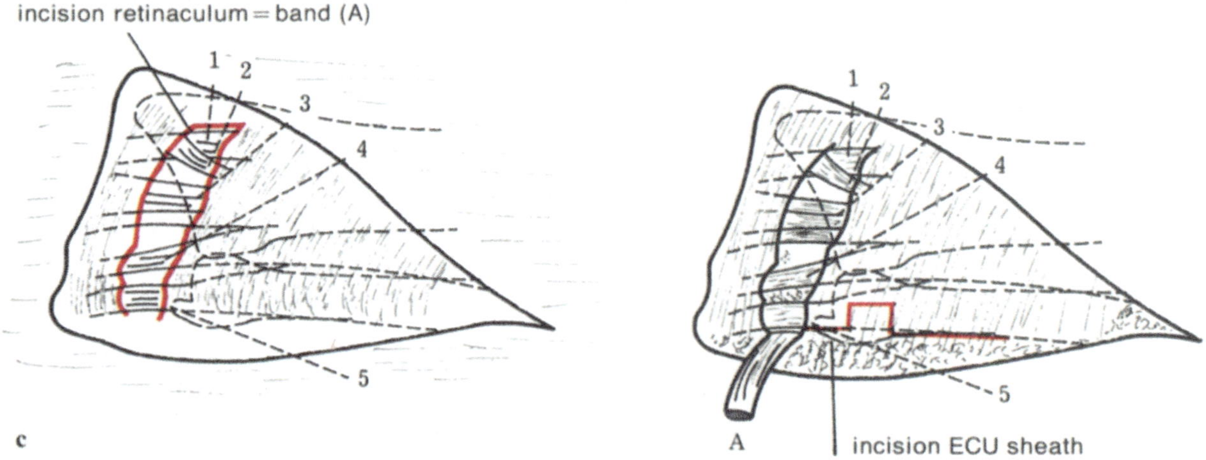


c

**Fig. V.74a–e.** Modified oblique resection-arthroplasty for previous case. **a** Incision with ulnar flap; it must allow for concomitant shortening osteotomy. **b** Identification of extensor retinaculum and dissection of strip (*A*) with ulnar hinge. **c** Elevation of this strip exposes extensor carpi radialis (ECR) brevis, extensor pollicis longus (EPL), extensor digitorum communis, extensor digiti minimi and extensor carpi ulnaris (ECU), whose sheath is opened with a Z-incision. **d** After Z-incision of sheath of ECU. **e** Retraction of the tendons exposes the capsulo-ligamentous system of the ulna; the line of incision must respect the dorsal capsular reinforcement of the triangular fibrocartilage (*6*)

*1* ECR brevis
*2* EPL
*3* extensor digitorum communis
*4* extensor digiti minimi
*5* ECU
*6* Retraction of the dorsal triangular fibrocartilage

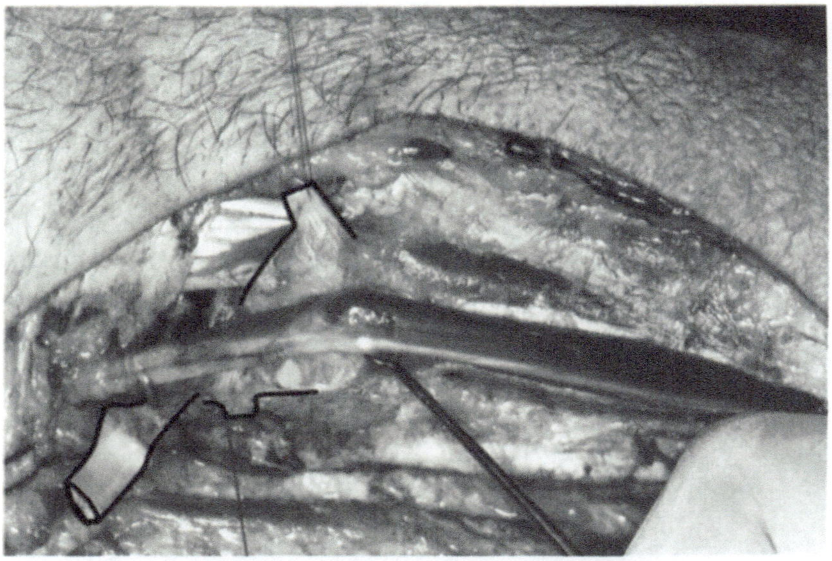

d

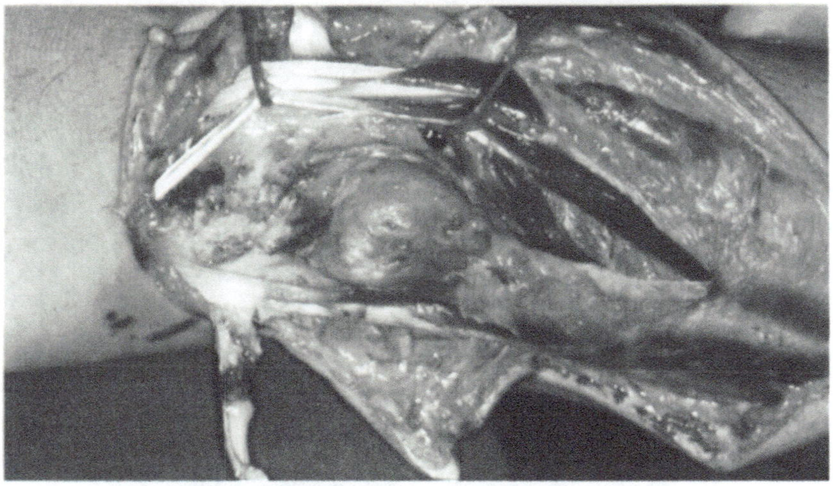

e

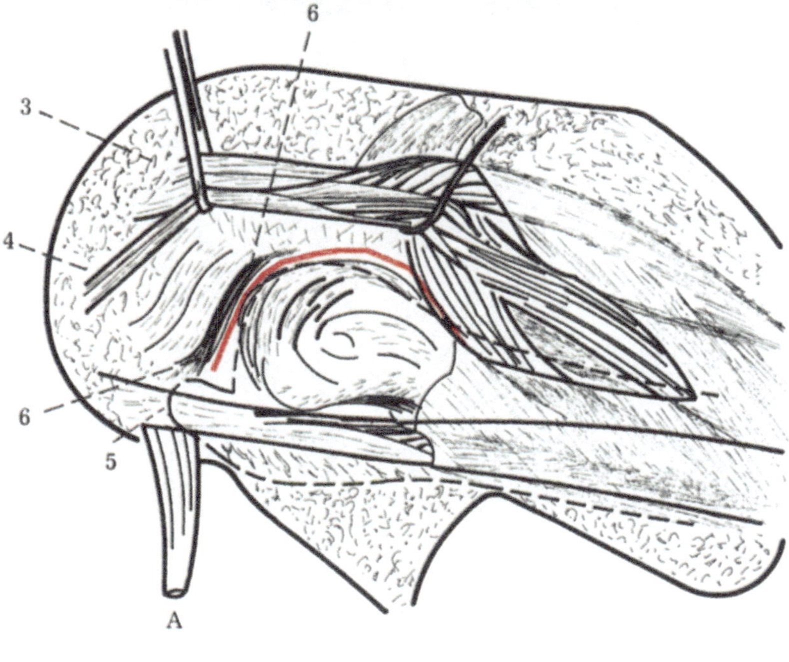

Fig. V.74f. Inspection of lesions, oblique line of resection (*red*). **g** Identification of palmar capsule. **h** Suture of strip of retinaculum to palmar capsule

*7* radius
*8* anterior articular capsule
*9* posterior articular capsule
*10* ulna
*11* reflected articular capsule

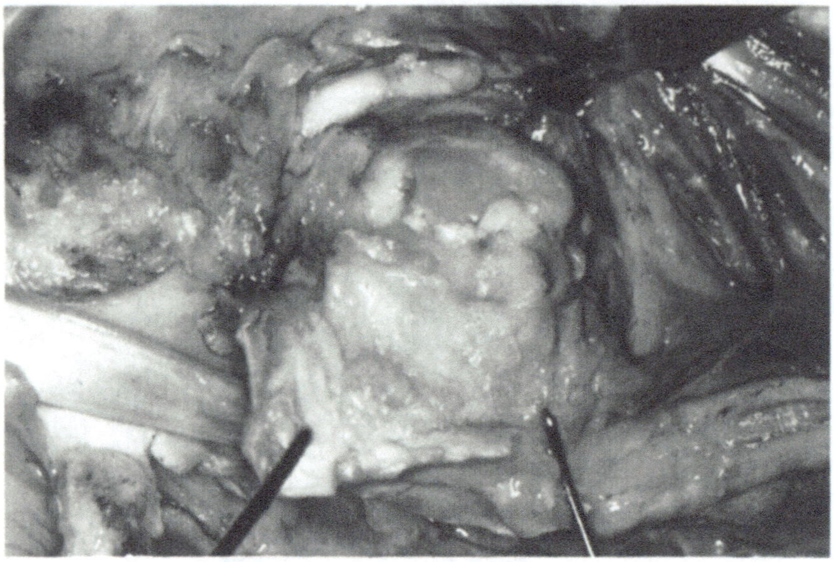

f

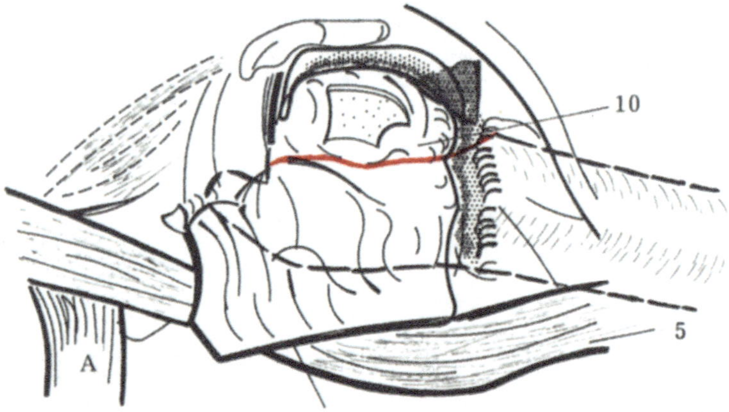


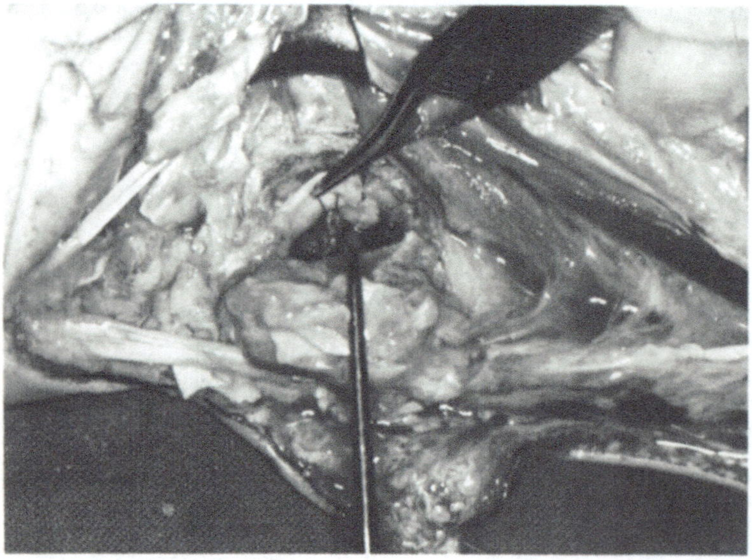

g

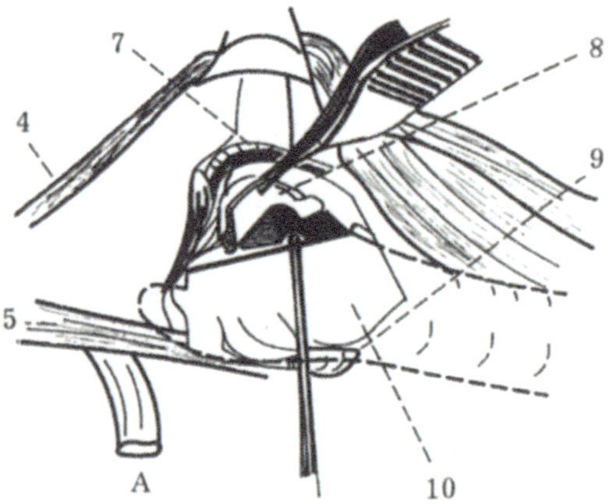


**Fig. V.74f, g**

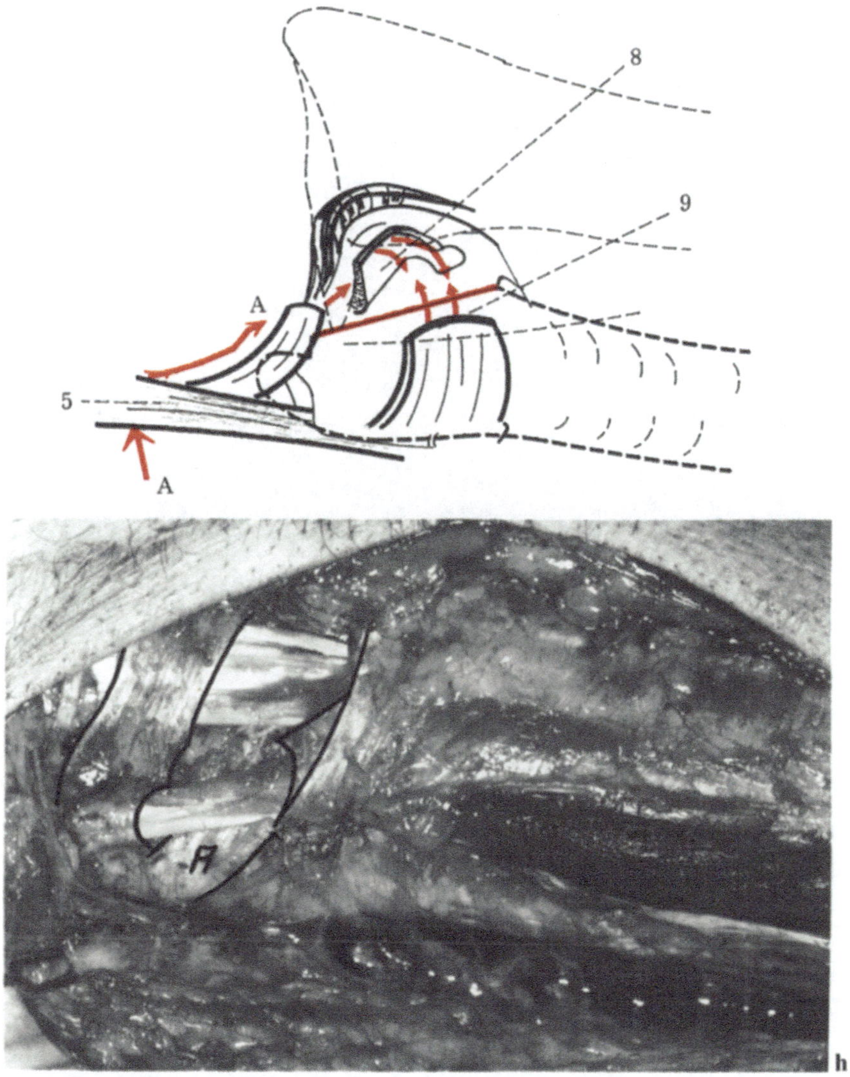


**Fig. V.74h**

*Result:* Five weeks after the operation, forearm rotation was complete and painless (Fig. V.75a). Figure V.75b shows a radiograph at 6 months. The patient was able to resume work as a forester.

**Darrach Resection**

This is no longer indicated in post-traumatic cases, but we still perform it in cases of rheumatoid arthritis, having found no satisfactory alternative.

*Note.* We reserve stabilization by the method of Linscheid (Hui and Linscheid 1982) or that of Boyes/Bunnell (Boyes 1970) for post-traumatic posterior ulnar instability.

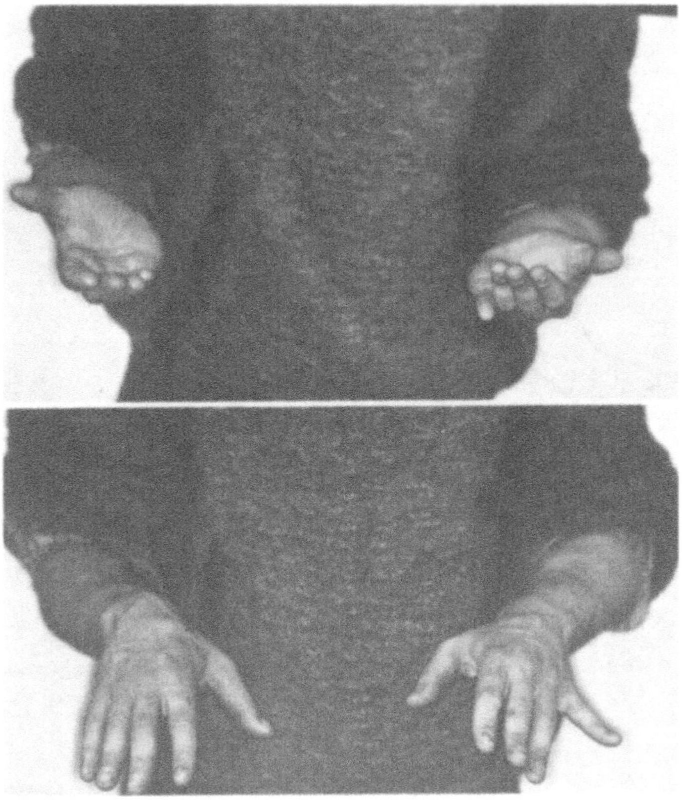

a

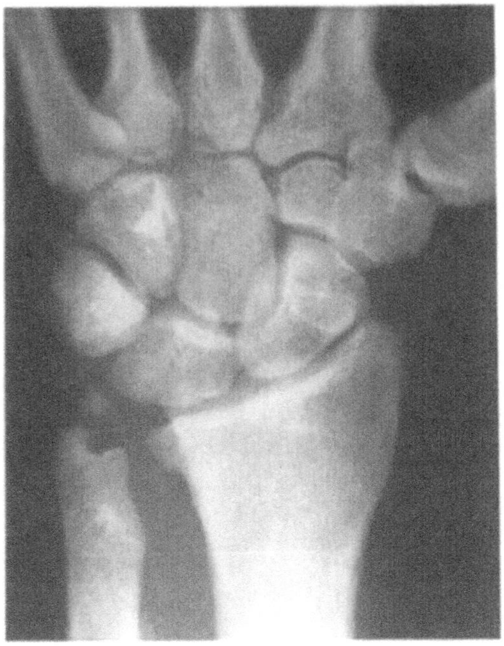

b

**Fig. V.75. a** Same case, pronation-supination at 6 weeks. **b** X-ray at 6 weeks: no sign of radial deviation of ulna

## Intervention Involving the Distal Radius

### *Dorsal Approach*

Difficulties may be posed by the extensor retinaculum and the muscle bellies of the extensor and abductor pollicis longus. The *solution* (Figs. V.3–V.7) is to free the extensor pollicis longus from the third compartment, divide Lister's tubercle, elevate the retinaculum en bloc and elevate the muscle bellies so that the plate may be slid under them. This is a more tricky approach, and requires delicate operative technique. The risk of algodystrophy is minor, and the scar is generally painless.

NB: This route is particularly indicated for correction of malunion, since it makes it possible to directly fill the gap created by the injury.

### *Palmar Approach* (Fig. V.15c)

The structures which may present difficulty are: the flexor retinaculum, the median nerve, the major tendon bundle, pronator quadratus, flexor pollicis longus and the palmar branch of the median nerve. The solutions are: to perform a generous ulnar skin incision (at least 10 cm) and a Z-incision of the flexor retinaculum (Fig. V.30a–c), to identify the flexor pollicis longus and to incise the pronator quadratus 0.5 cm from its insertion on the radius in order to facilitate reattachment. With this ap-

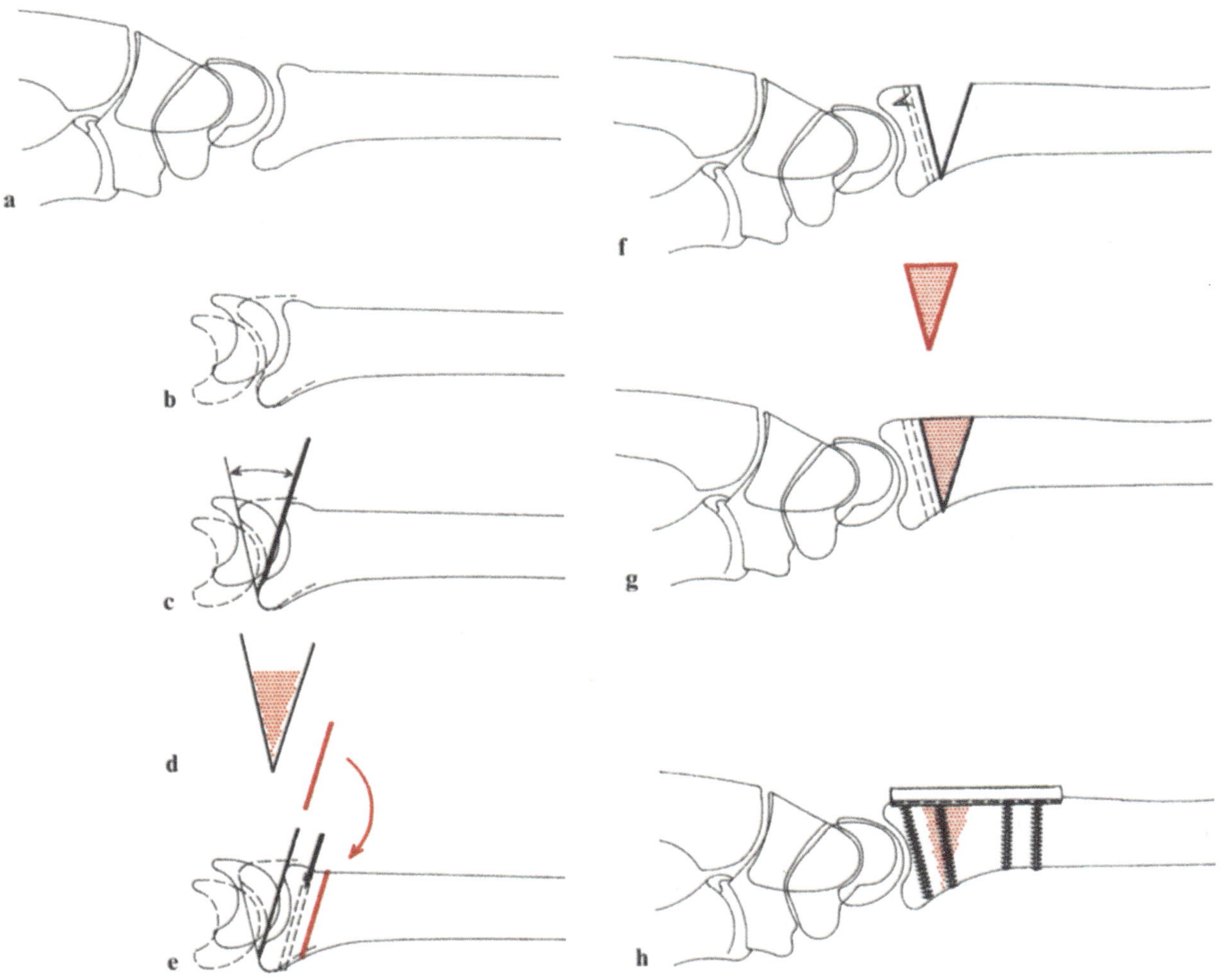


**Fig. V.76a–h.** Dorsal opening wedge osteotomy. **a** Articular deformation in sagittal plane. **b** Superimposed tracings of normal and injured sides. **c** Calculation of angular difference. **d** Shaping of graft on basis of pre-operative calculations. **e** An intra-articular Kirschner wire gives the joint inclination. **f** Correction of the axis opens a gap. **g** Graft inserted into gap. **h** Fixation by plate (or screw, fixator, cerclage wiring and stay)

proach, the operative risks are greater, i.e. irritation of the median nerve with the risk of subsequent sympathetic dystrophy. Removal of the osteosynthesis material is also more difficult.

*Note.* Using the palmar route, a dorsal opening wedge osteotomy is impossible, but a closing osteotomy is easy. Correcting the articular tilt is possible but the shortening of the radius is compounded. Correction of the relative lengthening of the ulna then becomes imperative, which adds to the duration and difficulty of the operation.

*Discussion.* Dorsally, the radius is easily accessible to the surgeon, and without excessive risks. This cannot be said of the palmar route, which produces irritation of the median nerve to a varying degree depending on the mode of dissection. In our view, it is not justified to risk sympathetic dystrophy unless there is an associated carpal tunnel syndrome, or if it is impossible to obtain the homogenous or autogenous cortico-cancellous graft that is necessary with the dorsal approach.

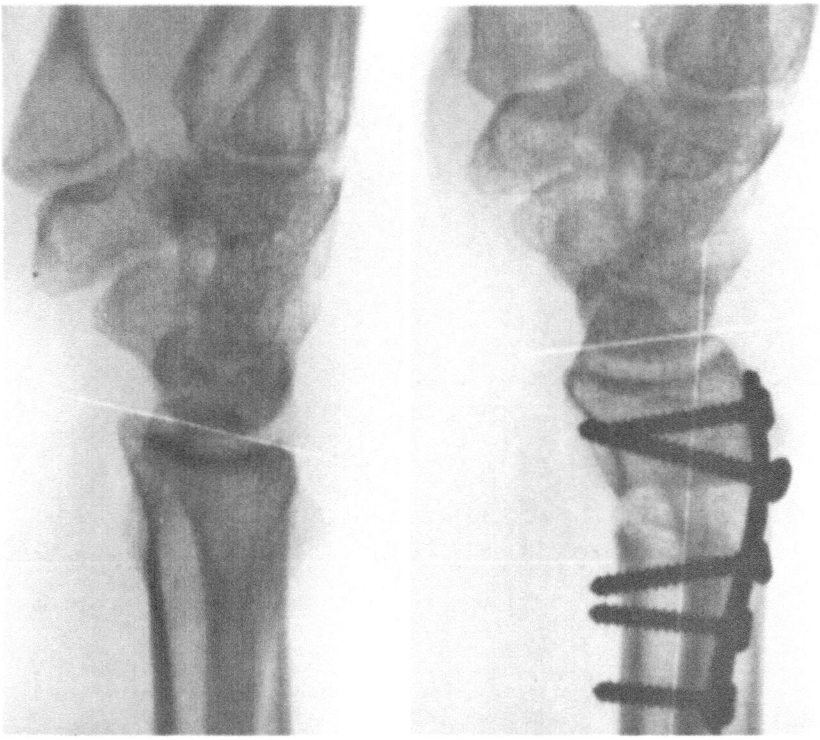

**Fig. V.77.** Lengthening and imperfect angular correction

*Dorsal Open Wedge Osteotomy*

The tilt of the epiphyseal block after distal radius fracture provokes a subluxation (not an instability) of the carpus, a shortening of the radius in relation to the ulna and a tilt of the joint axes (Figs. V.68 and V.76). The aim of correction is simple: to restore the length and the joint angles by inserting a cortico-cancellous graft. Comparative outlines of the normal and injured sides make it possible to calculate exactly the sagittal angular differences and the size of the graft necessary to correct them.

*Note.* It is impossible, in the frontal plane, to make similar preoperative calculations, as any posterior tilt modifies the apparent frontal angle. The true angle is therefore impossible to calculate. Thus, precise correction is practicable only in the sagittal plane; correction of the frontal angle is empirical. This is why we shape the bony polyhedron in such a way that its dorso-radial border is 10% longer than its dorso-ulnar border.

*Operative technique* (Fig. V.76). A cortico-cancellous graft, either homogenous or autogenous, is removed according to the preoperative calculations (Fig. V.76d). The joint slope is marked with a Kirschner wire slipped into the articulation (Fig. V.76e). Two anchorage holes are drilled, the axis of the holes being parallel to the articular plane. The osteotomy is made 2.5 cm proximal to the ulnar articular margin, at right angles to the articulation and to the previously drilled holes. The epiphyseal

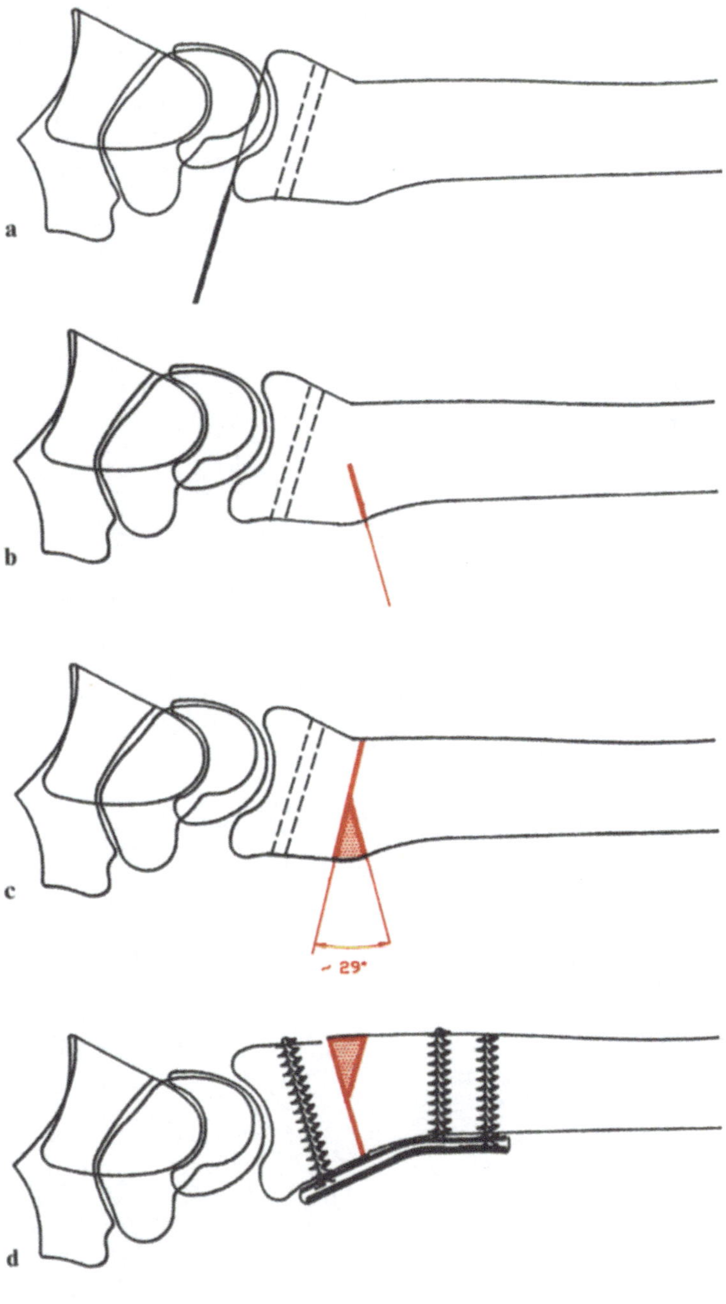


**Fig. V.78 a–d.** Palmar closing wedge osteotomy. **a** The articular slope is determined, and holes are drilled in the epiphyseal block parallel to the joint axis. **b** Axis and length of desired osteotomy (in *red*), to correspond to normal articular slope. **c** Second osteotomy, parallel to articular axis to be corrected, yields a bony wedge (*red area*). **d** The wedge is turned around, and an AO T-plate for 3.5 mm screws is applied. The desired correction is obtained. Note that preliminary shortening of the ulna is essential

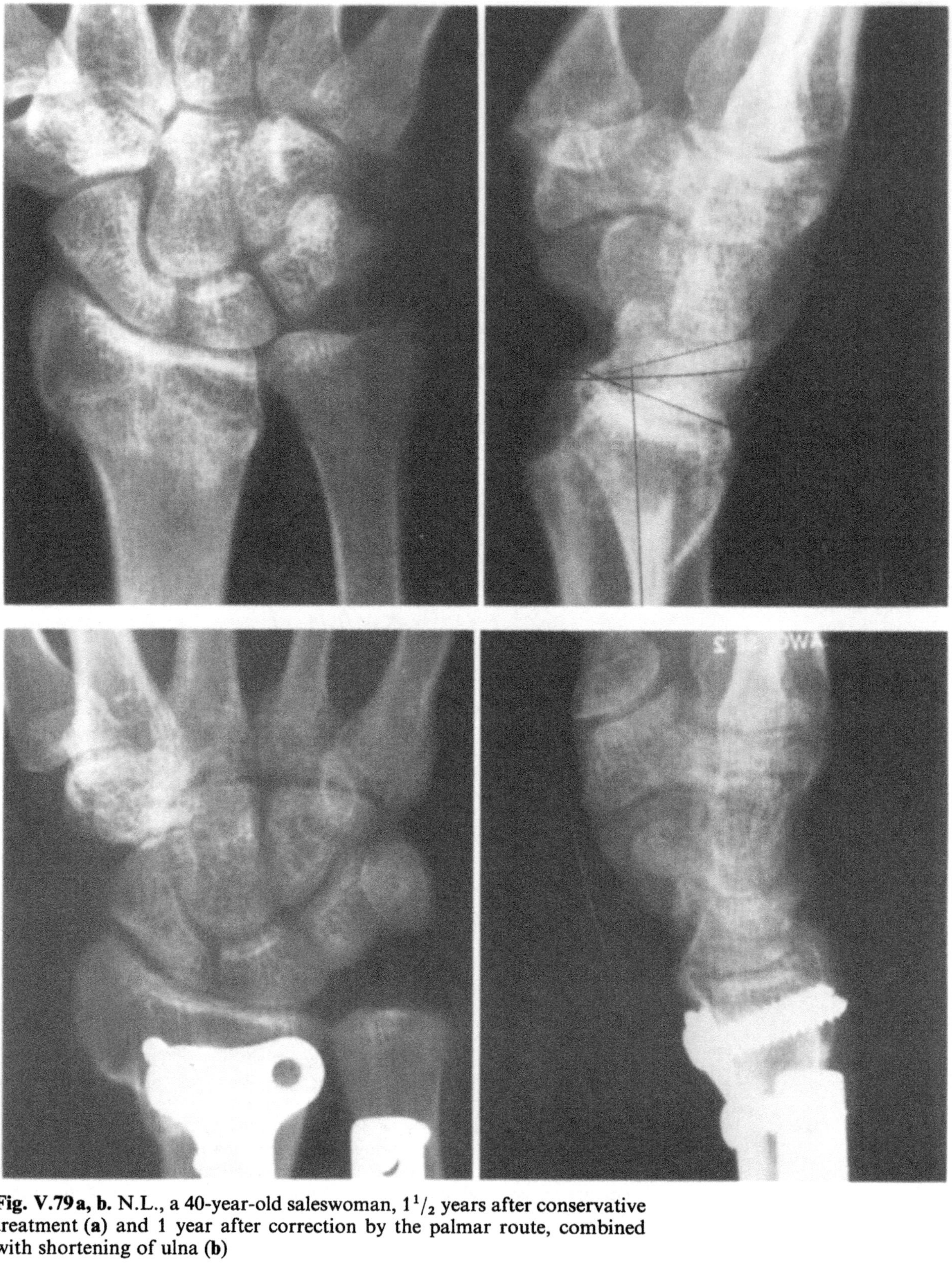

a

b

**Fig. V.79 a, b.** N.L., a 40-year-old saleswoman, $1^1/_2$ years after conservative treatment (**a**) and 1 year after correction by the palmar route, combined with shortening of ulna (**b**)

**Fig. V.80 a–c.** A 20-year-old female manual worker. **a** Deformity after conservative treatment. **b** Correction obtained. **c** Pronation-supination 2 years after correction

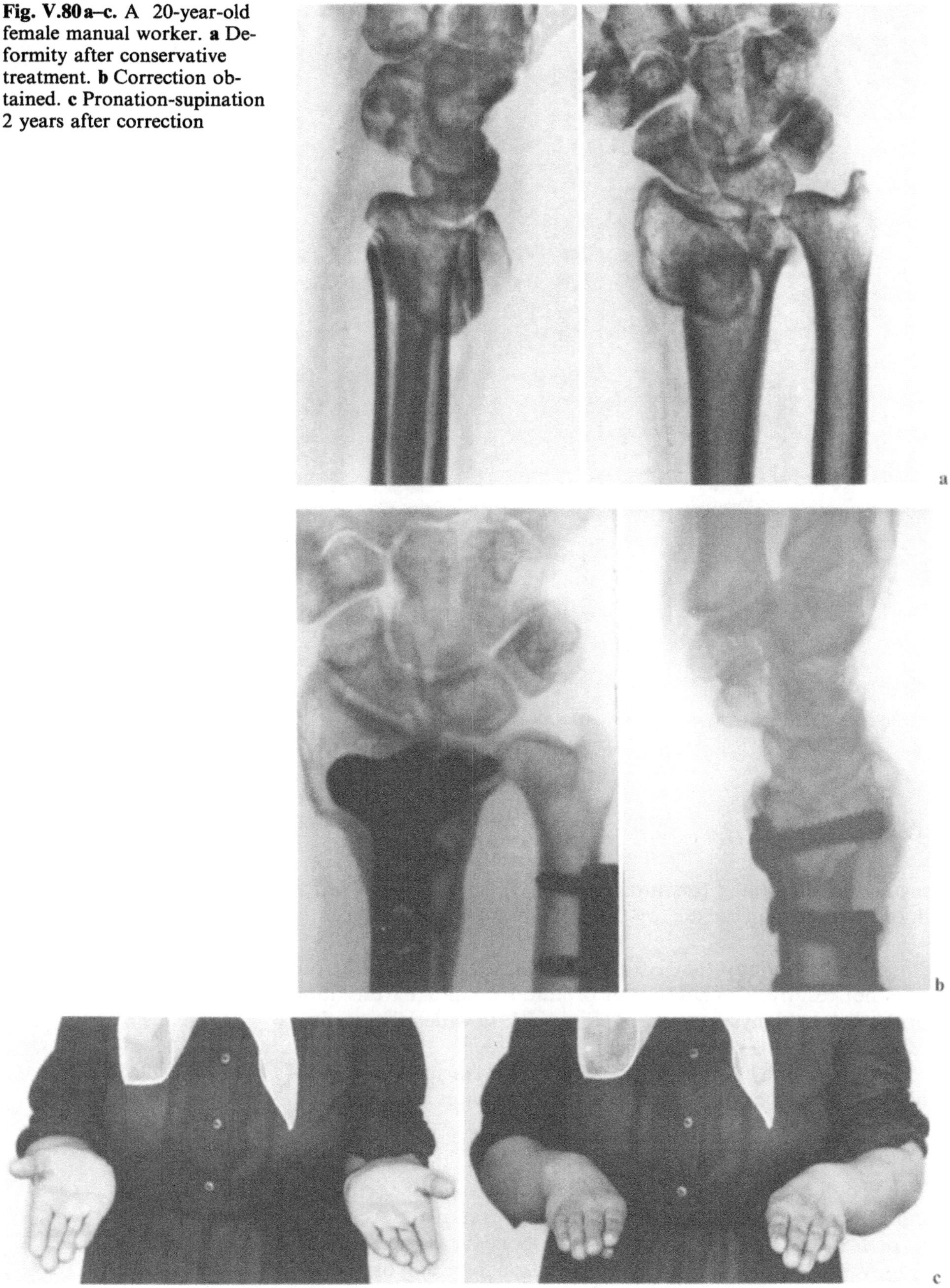

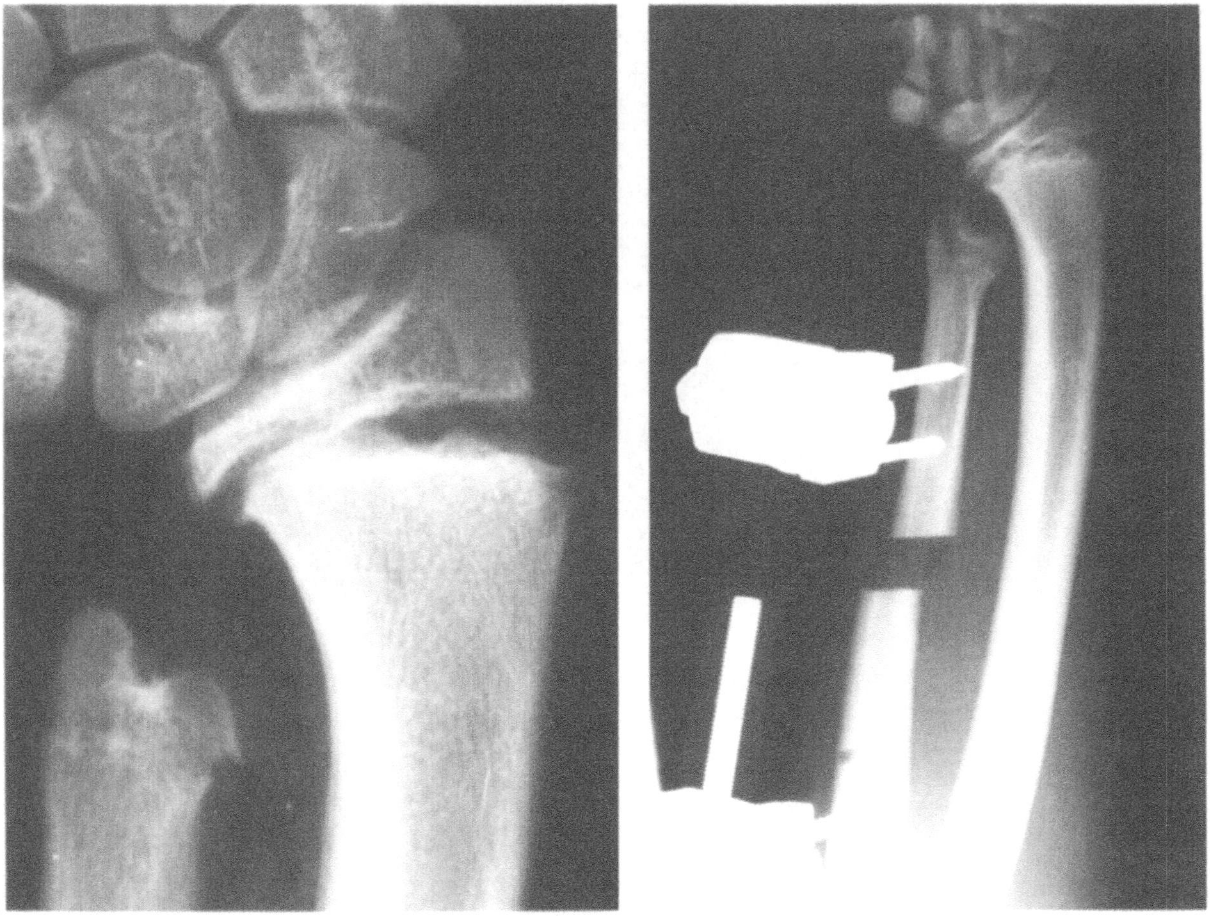

a b

segment is then tilted forward (Fig. V.76f), and the graft introduced into the gap created by the correction (Fig. V.76g).

*Note.* An osteotomy that is too proximal corrects the tilt, but does not restore the anatomy. It produces a palmar translation of the distal epiphyseal segment (Fig. V.77, in which the cortico-cancellous graft is clearly visible).

Fixation is by plate (Fig. V.76h) or by tension band technique using one or two screws or Kirschner wires.

*Palmar Closed Wedge Osteotomy* (Fig. V.78)

This procedure succeeds in obtaining the best angular correction, but is always accompanied by shortening, even if the technique is perfect and the palmar wedge of bone is turned around (Fig. V.78c). This is why we believe that a shortening osteotomy of the ulna should always be performed before considering correction of the radius.

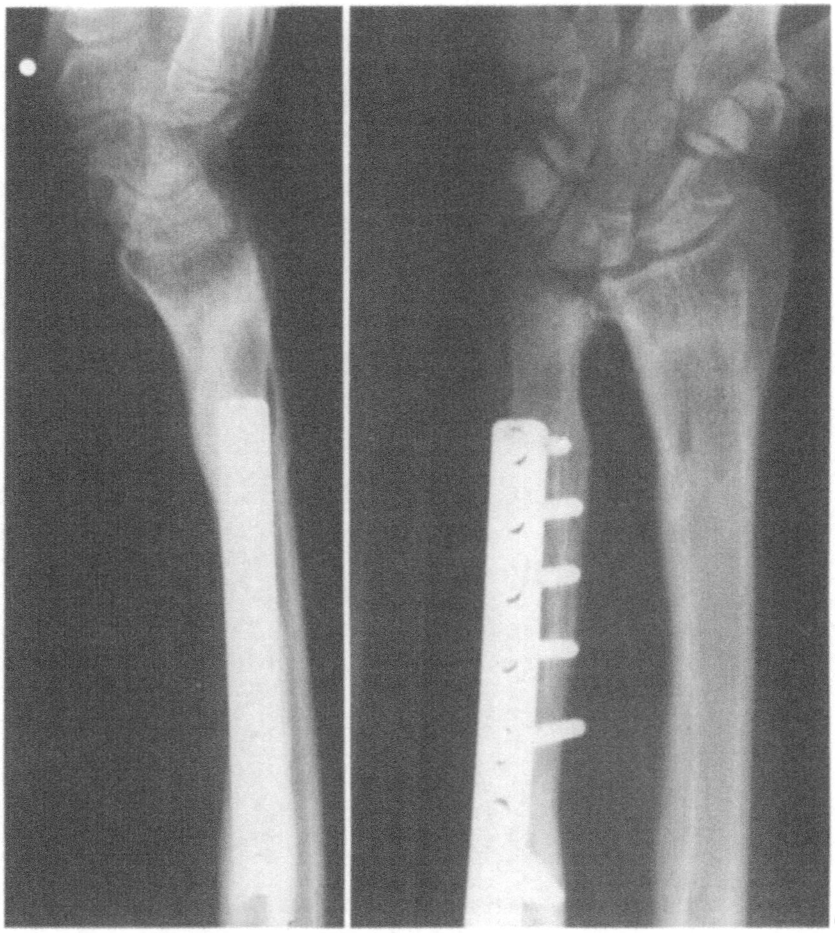

c

**Fig. V.81 a–c.** Special problems: T.M., aged 18 years, injury at age 15 years. **a** Sequel to fracture of the radius: closure of entire growth-plate of ulna. **b** Progessive lengthening by Wagner's apparatus. **c** Result 1 year after starting correction (there is also correction of the distal radius in the frontal plane) was: pronation-supination moderately restricted, extension normal, flexion diminished by half. *NB:* The treatment plan is the same if the arrest of growth involves the radius

*Operative technique.* The steps involved in the osteotomy are as follows:

1. Calculation of the desired correction is made.
2. The axis of the articulation is estimated, using a Kirschner wire (Fig. V.78 a).
3. Drilling and tapping of the distal holes is carried out parallel to the axis of the joint.
4. The plane of the first osteotomy line corresponds to the desired joint axis (i.e. to that of the normal side). Note that one must stop half-way through (Fig. V.78 b).
5. The freed bony wedge is turned around, in order to fill the gap created by the palmar tilt (Fig. V.78 d). It is important to bear in mind that this fragment is of poor quality and friable.
6. The T-plate is fixed in the previously prepared holes, making sure that the palmar bony contact is perfect.
7. Immobilization with a plaster splint is maintained until the wounds have healed.

Two examples illustrate our thesis. The first patient, a 40-year-old saleswoman with an ulnar head syndrome and troublesome limitation of pronation-supination (70-0-0), also had definite

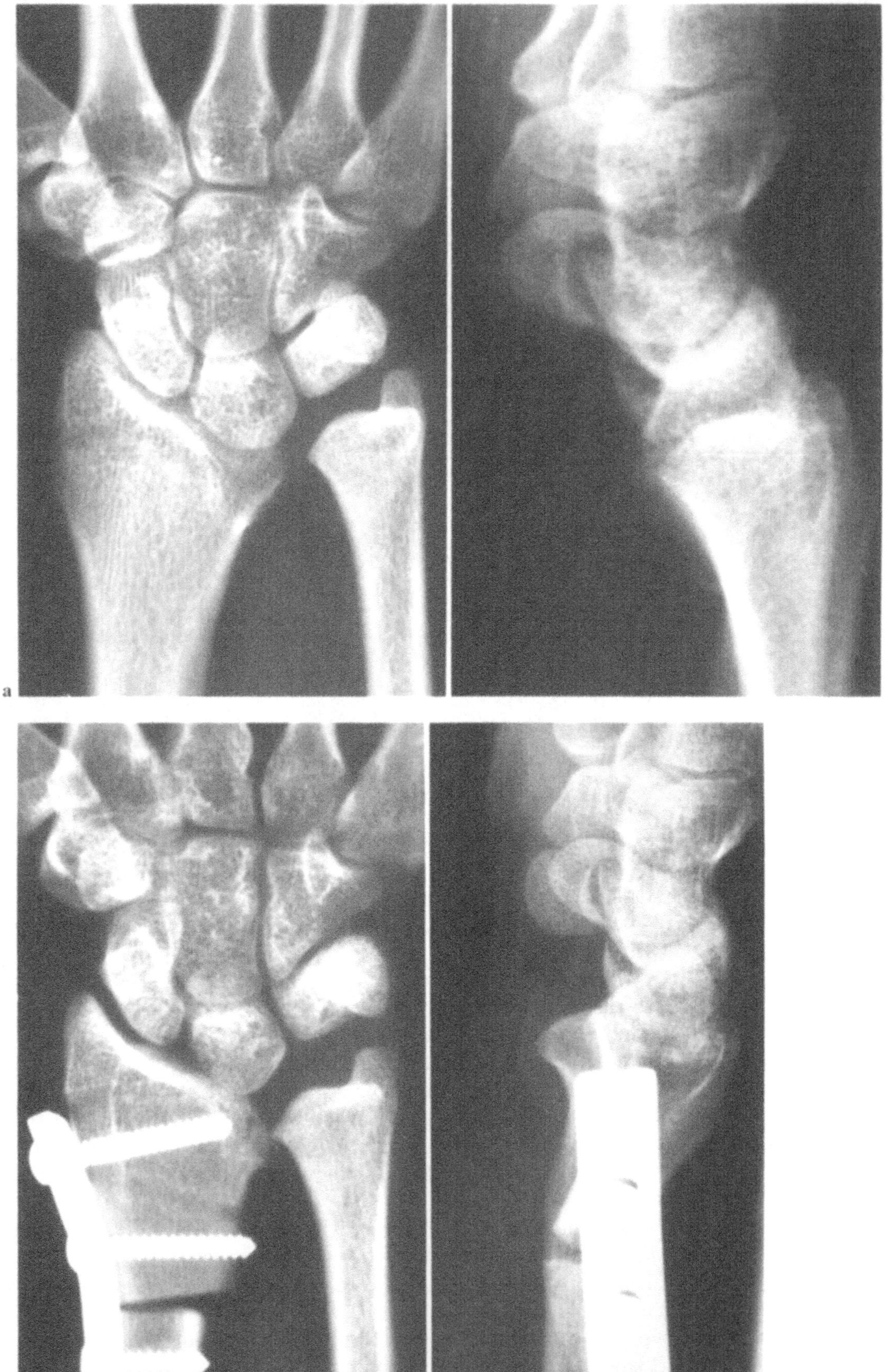
a
b

sensory disturbance in the median nerve territory, justifying correction by the palmar route (Fig. V.79a). Correction was satisfactory (Fig. V.79b), restoring pronation and supination and abolishing pain on effort. However, the joint remains sensitive to changes in the weather.

The second case, a young 20-year-old woman, is a striking example of failure of conservative therapy. She was unable to resume work due to ulnar head syndrome, carpal tunnel syndrome and restriction of pronation-supination; making operation inevitable (Fig. V.80a). Despite difficult rehabilitation, complicated by moderate sympathetic dystrophy, she resumed work 4 months later. After 2 years it is impossible to distinguish the healthy from the injured side (Fig. V.80b, c).

*Special Therapeutic Problems*

*Fracture with growth disturbance.* A patient with a fracture of the wrist at the age of 15 years (Fig. V.81) had traumatic closure of the growth plate of the distal ulna and cessation of growth, with progressive deformity of the distal radius (a similar case is shown in Fig. IV.8a, b). The patient consulted us 3 years later. What should be done?

The wrist itself was normal, so we decided to lengthen the ulna progressively with Wagner's apparatus, leaving an intact periosteal cuff. Each day the patient lengthened the bone by 1 mm until the ulna was at the level of the radius. Stabilization (without cancellous graft) was by eight-hole AO plate with 3.5 mm screws. An open-wedge osteotomy of the radius on the ulnar side, with bone graft and T-plate, restored the angles of the radio-carpal joint. The hand regained its normal appearance; minor bilateral restriction of pronation-supination persists, but is not troubling the patient.

*Conclusion.* Whether the growth arrest affects the radius or the ulna, and whatever the age of the patient, it is possible to preserve function by one or more lengthening osteotomies. Of course, it is important to advise both parents and child to disinfect the pin sites twice daily but we have encountered no particular problems regarding management of the apparatus.

## K. Madelung's Deformity

◁ **Fig. V.82a, b.** Madelung's deformity. **a** Correction of deformation of axis of distal radius by AO dynamic compression plate for 3.5 mm cortical screws. **b** No cancellous graft is needed; the method of bending and mounting the plate determines correction

This is an autosomal dominant congenital condition, more common in girls. It results from premature closure of the medio-palmar portion of the growth-plate of the distal radius. The typical clinical picture is that:

1. The forearm is abnormally short.
2. The distal radial epiphysis exhibits a double curvature, palmar and ulnar, associated with: (a) ulnar subluxation of the carpus, (b) dorsal subluxation of the distal ulna and (c) distal radio-ulnar instability.

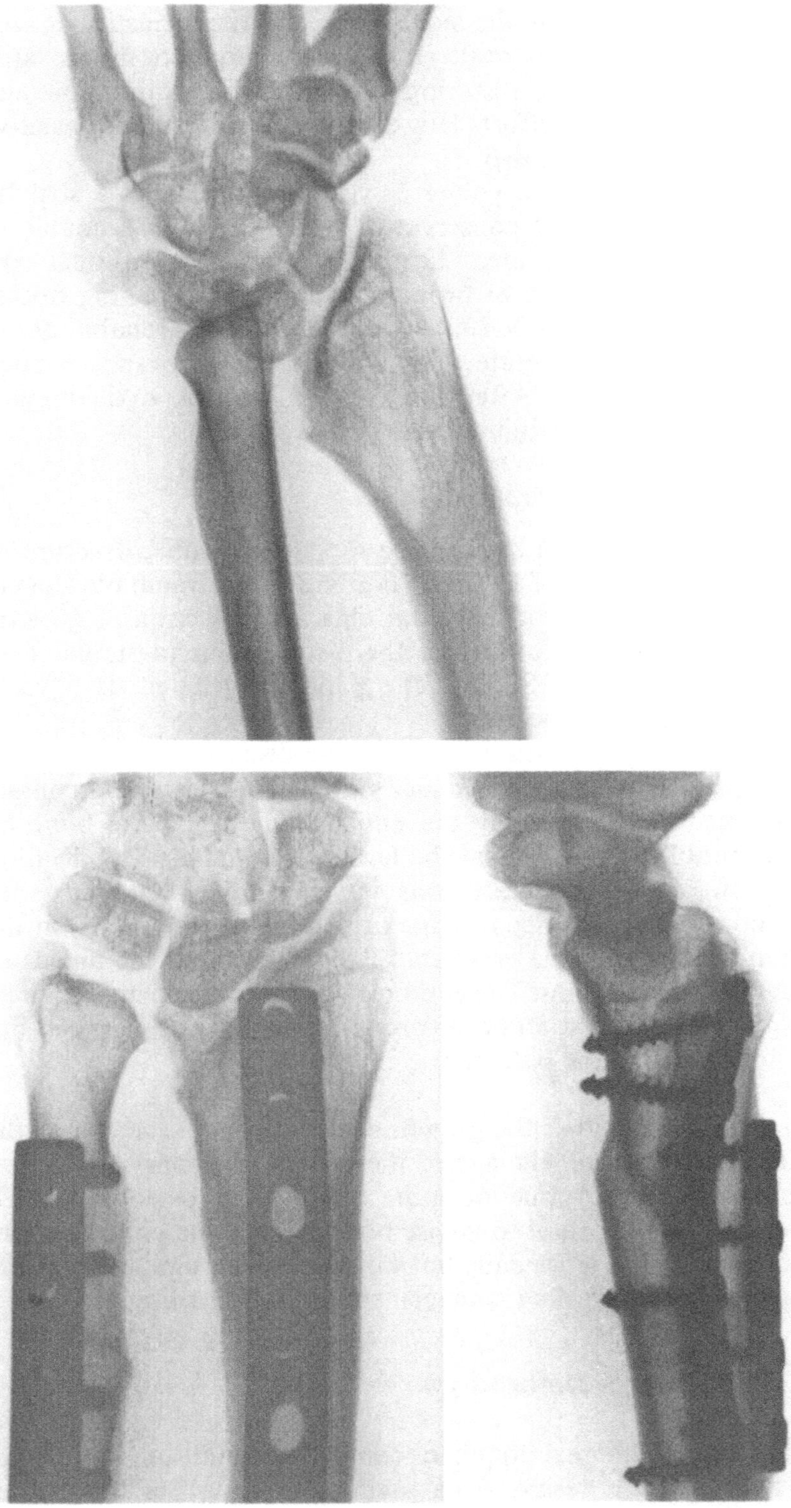

a

b

**Fig. V.83. a** In severe Madelung's deformity, combined ulnar shortening may prove indispensable. **b** The plate may be placed dorsally on the same principles, but correction of the radius is less satisfactory, since the dorsal route does not permit correction of the definite rotatory component also present in this deformity

These malformations, bilateral but not symmetrical, lead to premature wear of the joints and subluxation of the tendons. These complications then require combined arthrodesis and tendon repair. Therefore, prompt correction of the deformities as a prophylactic measure is desirable. This correction must be made on the radius, as it is the cause of the deformity. Angulation of the distal end of the radius in a dorsal and lateral direction suffices in most cases. The operative technique is as follows:

1. A dorsal or dorso-radial approach is used.
2. The radial epiphysis is freed via the third extensor compartment.
3. An AO plate for 3.5 mm screws with five holes is used.
4. The plate is bent at 30°, giving the correction desired in the frontal plane (when the plate is fixed on the lateral border of the radius).
5. Before performing the osteotomy, the plate is placed on the radial border of the epiphysis, with a dorsal angle of 30° in relation to the shaft; this angle corresponds to the desired correction in the sagittal plane; its apex is distal.
6. The plate is removed, rotation is marked out, and the osteotomy performed.
7. The plate is reapplied distally, and fixed proximally in the axis of the shaft.

*Note.* We never perform resection of the distal ulna. A cortico-cancellous graft is unnecessary in young patients, if the osteotomy is made distally enough in the metaphyseal zone (Fig. V.82).

## References


Bell MJ, Hill RJ, McMurtry RY (1985) Ulnar impingement syndrome. J Bone Joint Surg [Br] 67:126–129

Boyes JH (1970) Bunnell's surgery of the hand, 5th edn. Lippincott, Philadelphia, pp 229–302

Bowers WH (1982) Distal radio-ulnar joint. In: Green DP (ed) Operative hand surgery, vol 1. Churchill Livingstone, New York, pp 754–756

Hui FC, Linscheid R (1982) Ulnotriquetral augmentation tenodesis: A reconstructive procedure for dorsal subluxation of the distal radioulnar joint. J Hand Surg 7:230–236

Jakob RP (1982) Der kleine Fixateur externe. AO Bulletin

Kapandji A (1985) L'opération de Kapandji-Sauvé. Technique et résultats dans les indications non rhumatologiques. 21st annual meeting of the GEM, Paris

Weber BG, Magerl F (1985) Fixateur externe. Springer, Berlin Heidelberg New York Tokyo, pp 89–932

# Epilogue

This book will not have been written in vain if you approach the carpus and the radius with a new attitude of mind, convinced that the clinical and radiological approach must be standardized. Treatment will continue to develop, thanks to the elaboration of a common language as the basis for progress and research.

Let me recapitulate the most important points to be retained:

- Analysing the anatomy of the carpus based on a clinical and therapeutic perspective leads to a concept of stability with practical applications.
- The treatment of ligamentous instability of the carpus is in a state of transition and burdened by contradictions. Yet, it is possible to derive a mode of treatment through simple and methodical reasoning. With our concept of stability, the most appropriate solution should become apparent to the surgeon.
- The Matti-Russe procedure, currently the treatment of choice for non-union of the scaphoid, has its anatomical and biomechanical limitations. To overcome these, it is necessary to cope with ligamentous inadequacy. Ligamentoplasty combined with internal fixation may be an adequate procedure for meeting this need.
- Once it has been resituated in its anatomical, biological and mechanical contect, according pre-eminence to the consequences of osseous and ligamentous inadequacy, the study of distal radial fractures leads to a new system of classification, on the basis of which treatment may be logically deduced.

# Subject Index

GPSR Compliance

*The European Union's (EU) General Product Safety Regulation (GPSR) is a set of rules that requires consumer products to be safe and our obligations to ensure this.*

*If you have any concerns about our products, you can contact us on ProductSafety@springernature.com*

In case Publisher is established outside the EU, the EU authorized representative is:

Springer Nature Customer Service Center GmbH
Europaplatz 3
69115 Heidelberg, Germany

**Batch number: 10838288**

Printed by Printforce, the Netherlands